SECTION EDITORS

Janet B. Cahill, PT, CSCS

Section Manager
Inpatient Therapy
Department of Rehabilitation
Hospital for Special Surgery
New York, New York

John T. Cavanaugh, PT, MEd, ATC

Advanced Clinician
Sports Medicine Perfomance and Research Center
Department of Rehabilitation
Hospital for Special Surgery
New York, New York

Deborah Corradi-Scalise, PT, DPT, MA

Section Manager
Pediatric Rehabilitation
Department of Rehabilitation
Hospital for Special Surgery
New York, New York

Holly Rudnick, PT, Cert MDT

Advanced Clinician
Sports Medicine Performance and Research Center
Department of Rehabilitation
Hospital for Special Surgery
New York, New York

Aviva Wolff, OTR/L, CHT

Section Manager
Hand Therapy
Department of Rehabilitation
Hospital for Special Surgery
New York, New York

Handbook of
Postsurgical Rehabilitation Guidelines
for the Orthopedic Clinician

Hospital for Special Surgery
Department of Rehabilitation

EDITORS

JeMe Cioppa-Mosca, PT, MBA

Administrative Editor
Assistant Vice President
Department of Rehabilitation
Hospital for Special Surgery
New York, New York

Janet B. Cahill, PT, CSCS

Administrative Editor
Section Manager
Inpatient Therapy
Department of Rehabilitation
Hospital for Special Surgery
New York, New York

Carmen Young Tucker, PT

Administrative Editor
Director
Inpatient Division
Department of Rehabilitation
Hospital of Special Surgery
New York, New York

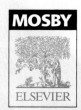

MOSBY
ELSEVIER

11830 Westline Industrial Drive
St. Louis, Missouri 63146

HANDBOOK OF POSTSURGICAL REHABILITATION   ISBN: 978-0-323-04939-9
GUIDELINES FOR THE ORTHOPEDIC CLINICIAN

Notice

Neither the Publisher nor the Authors assume any responsibility for any loss
or injury and/or damage to persons or property arising out of or related to
any use of the material contained in this book. It is the responsibility of the
treating practitioner, relying on independent expertise and knowledge of
the patient, to determine the best treatment and method of application for
the patient.

The Publisher

Library of Congress Control Number 2007938503

Acquisitions Editor: Kathryn Falk
Associate Developmental Editor: Sarah Vales
Publishing Services Manager: Melissa Lastarria
Senior Project Manager: Joy Moore
Design Direction: Teresa McBryan

Printed in the United States of America
Last digit is the print number: 9 8 7 6 5 4 3 2 1

This book is dedicated to all the past,
present, and future therapists
in the Rehabilitation Department
at Hospital for Special Surgery.
Their spirit and commitment
to clinical excellence was,
is, and will be the legacy
of this book.

Preface

Postsurgical Rehabilitation Guidelines for the Orthopedic Clinician was published as a complete textbook in June 2006. Comprehensive and dynamic, this book was written to offer a thorough understanding of how to develop an individual postsurgical plan that provides your patients with the best possible outcomes and function. Now that the foundation is set, we are pleased to present busy practitioners and students alike with this streamlined version, *Handbook of Postsurgical Rehabilitation Guidelines for the Orthopedic Clinician*. This handbook will take you from the desk to the treatment area, where you can apply what you've learned with full confidence that the information you need is right at your fingertips (or more likely, in the pocket of your lab coat).

The handbook highlights the easy-to-follow phase-guideline tables found in the original textbook, encapsulating crucial information into phases of healing and rehabilitation that incorporate Goals, Precautions, Treatment Strategies, and Criteria for Advancement. Please keep in mind that this handbook is intended as a companion to, and by no means a replacement of, the didactic, evidence-based content found in the original textbook. We strongly recommend that the concepts introduced in *Postsurgical Rehabilitation Guidelines for the Orthopedic Clinician* be thoroughly read and understood before the information outlined in the handbook is put into practice. You will also find the original text an invaluable resource for addressing questions and troubleshooting, in addition to the not-to-be-missed DVD featuring over 60 minutes and over 100 clips of video presentations demonstrating specific treatment strategies, tests, and measures.

Founded in 1863, Hospital for Special Surgery (HSS) is the world's leading specialty hospital for orthopedics and rheumatology. Ranked number one in the Northeast and with over 17,000 procedures performed per year, the Hospital affords the HSS Rehabilitation Department with the remarkable opportunity to garner first-hand, in-depth experience with essentially every musculoskeletal disease known. With a commitment to the pursuit of knowledge and the advancement of rehabilitative care that it brings, the department plays an integral role in the multidisciplinary approach to patient care and research at the Hospital. HSS is proud to provide a wide array of comprehensive services by a leading team of therapists.

The mission of the HSS Rehabilitation Department is to provide the highest quality of rehabilitative and restorative care to maximize patient function and promote education, clinical research, and community service. Furthermore, the department aims to excel in educating colleagues and future colleagues, and this handbook is a natural extension of that aim.

We are extremely pleased to offer this resource to you, our colleagues, in a format that will allow you to apply what you've learned in your day-to-day treatment plans. As with the original textbook, it is our expectation that the therapists and health care professionals that follow these guidelines have a basic foundation of the diagnosis, special tests, and/or surgical procedures that may be warranted for these orthopedic conditions. This is the transitional piece that will help you make the most of the information presented in *Postsurgical Rehabilitation Guidelines for the Orthopedic Clinician*. We are honored to be a part of your journey as we work together for the ultimate goal of providing the best possible rehabilitative care.

Contributors

Emily Altman, PT, DPT, CHT
Staff Physical Therapist
Hand Therapy
Department of Rehabilitation
Hospital for Special Surgery
New York, New York

Loretta Amoroso, DPT
Staff Physical Therapist
Pediatric Rehabilitation
Department of Rehabilitation
Hospital for Special Surgery
New York, New York

Amy Barenholtz-Marshall, OTR, CHT
Advanced Clinician
Hand Therapy
Department of Rehabilitation
Hospital for Special Surgery
New York, New York

Janet B. Cahill, PT, CSCS
Section Manager
Inpatient Therapy
Department of Rehabilitation
Hospital for Special Surgery
New York, New York

John T. Cavanaugh, PT, MEd, ATC
Advanced Clinician
Sports Medicine Performance and
    Research Center
Department of Rehabilitation
Hospital for Special Surgery
New York, New York

Theresa A. Chiaia, PT
Section Manager
Sports Medicine Performance and
    Research Center
Department of Rehabilitation
Hospital for Special Surgery
New York, New York

Heather M. Cloutman, PT, MSPT, CSCS
Staff Physical Therapist
Pediatric Rehabilitation
Department of Rehabilitation
Hospital for Special Surgery
New York, New York

Deborah Corradi-Scalise, PT, DPT, MA
Section Manager
Pediatric Rehabilitation
Department of Rehabilitation
Hospital for Special Surgery
New York, New York

Amie Diamond, PT
Staff Physical Therapist
Inpatient Therapy
Department of Rehabilitation
Hospital for Special Surgery
New York, New York

Jaime Edelstein, PT, MSPT, CSCS
Advanced Clinician
Sports Medicine Performance and
    Research Center
Department of Rehabilitation
Hospital for Special Surgery
New York, New York

Greg Fives, PT, MSPT, SCS
Staff Physical Therapist
Sports Medicine Performance and
   Research Center
Department of Rehabilitation
Hospital for Special Surgery
New York, New York

Nicole Fritz, PT, DPT
Staff Physical Therapist
Inpatient Therapy
Department of Rehabilitation
Hospital for Special Surgery
New York, New York

Todd Gage, PT, CSCS
Staff Physical Therapist
Joint Mobility Center
Department of Rehabilitation
Hospital for Special Surgery
New York, New York

Kara Gallagher, MS, OTR/L, CHT
Staff Physical Therapist
Hand Therapy
Department of Rehabilitation
Hospital for Special Surgery
New York, New York

Sandy B. Ganz, PT, DSc, GCS
Director
Amsterdam Nursing Home
Department of Rehabilitation
Hospital for Special Surgery
New York, New York

Coleen T. Gately, PT, DPT, MS
Advanced Clinician
Hand Therapy
Department of Rehabilitation
Hospital for Special Surgery
New York, New York

Charlene Hannon, PT, MBA
Clinical Supervisor
Joint Mobility Center
Department of Rehabilitation
Hospital for Special Surgery
New York, New York

Lisa M. Kosman, PT, MSPT
Section Manger
Joint Mobility Center
Department of Rehabilitation
Hospital for Special Surgery
New York, New York

Michael Levinson, PT, CSCS
Clinical Supervisor
Sports Medicine Performance and
   Research Center
Department of Rehabilitation
Hospital for Special Surgery
New York, New York

Jennifer P. Lewin, OTR/L
Advanced Clinician
Pediatric Rehabilitation
Department of Rehabilitation
Hospital for Special Surgery
New York, New York

Robert A. Maschi, PT, DPT, CSCS
Advanced Clinician
Sports Medicine Performance and
   Research Center
Department of Rehabilitation
Hospital for Special Surgery
New York, New York

Dennis J. Noonan, ATC, CMT
Massage Therapist
Sports Medicine Perfomance and
   Research Center
Department of Rehabilitation
Hospital for Special Surgery
New York, New York

Carol Page, PT, DPT, CHT
Clinical Supervisor
Hand Therapy
Department of Rehabilitation
Hospital for Special Surgery
New York, New York

Kataliya Palmieri, PT, MPT
Advanced Clinician
CQI Coordinator
Department of Rehabilitation
Hospital for Special Surgery
New York, New York

Adam Pratomo, PT, MSPT
Advanced Clinician
Integrative Care Center
Department of Rehabilitation
Hospital for Special Surgery
New York, New York

Matthew D. Rivera, PT, MPT, CSCS
Advanced Clinician
Inpatient Therapy
Department of Rehabilitation
Hospital for Special Surgery
New York, New York

Lee Rosenzweig, PT, DPT, CHT
Advanced Clinician
Hand Therapy
Department of Rehabilitation
Hospital for Special Surgery
New York, New York

Holly Rudnick, PT, Cert MDT
Advanced Clinician
Sports Medicine Performance and
   Research Center
Department of Rehabilitation
Hospital for Special Surgery
New York, New York

Kelly Ann Sindle, PT
Staff Physical Therapist
Pediatric Rehabilitation
Department of Rehabilitation
Hospital for Special Surgery
New York, New York

Amanda R. Sparrow, PT
Advanced Clinician
Pediatric Rehabilitation
Department of Rehabilitation
Hospital for Special Surgery
New York, New York

Carmen Young Tucker, PT
Director
Inpatient Division
Department of Rehabilitation
Hospital for Special Surgery
New York, New York

Cathi Wagner, PT, MBA
Associate Director
Rehabilitation Services
Department of Rehabilitation
Hospital for Special Surgery
New York, New York

Heather A. Williams, PT, DPT
Staff Physical Therapist
Joint Mobility Center
Department of Rehabilitation
Hospital for Special Surgery
New York, New York

Aviva Wolff, OTR/L, CHT
Section Manager
Hand Therapy
Department of Rehabilitation
Hospital for Special Surgery
New York, New York

Contents

SECTION III
PEDIATRIC REHABILITATION
Deborah Corradi-Scalise, PT, DPT, MA

SECTION IV
SPINE REHABILITATION
Holly Rudnick, PT, Cert MDT

Section V

SPORTS MEDICINE REHABILITATION

John T. Cavanaugh, PT, MEd, ATC

Chapter *1*

Total Hip Arthroplasty

Carmen Young Tucker, PT
Amie Diamond, PT

Total hip arthroplasty (THA) is one of the most common surgical procedures for the treatment of advanced hip arthritis. More than 254,000 THAs are performed annually. This represents 92 out of 100,000 Americans. The Hospital for Special Surgery (HSS) performs approximately 7000 total joint arthroplasties each year, of which approximately 30% are THA. The primary goals of THA are relief of pain arising from destructive arthritis and improvement in functional mobility. Postoperative rehabilitation is an essential component in the achievement of these goals. The HSS rehabilitation guidelines following THA, which are presented in this chapter, were developed using an evidence-based approach and the clinical expertise of the rehabilitation department's physical therapist.

Surgical Overview

- The successful outcome of a THA is based on several factors: patient selection, type of implant, method of fixation, and surgical technique.
- The determination of implant selection is individualized and based on specific patient characteristics (i.e., level of

activity and bone quality) in addition to the experience of the surgeon.

- There is a wide variety of implant designs and materials available. The materials most commonly used for implants are cobalt-chromium and titanium.
- Implant surfaces can have different finishes, such as porous-coated, plasma-sprayed surfaces, roughened titanium surfaces, and hydroxyapatite-coated surfaces. The different surfaces may enhance the strength between the implant and cement or fixation of implant to bone.
- The type of implant component selected depends on whether the THA will be cemented, porous, or a hybrid.
- The profile of the most common THA performed at HSS is a hybrid THA that combines an uncemented acetabular component and a cemented femoral component. This hybrid combination provides excellent results and is more popular in North America.
- In addition to the standard THA procedure, HSS is currently using minimally invasive surgery (MIS) on a select group of patients to perform hip arthroplasties.
  1. The minimally invasive total hip arthroplasty surgery is a modification of the standard surgical technique performed for THA.
  2. An article by Sculco et al. states that "with modern techniques, implants, and instrumentation, THA could be performed safely and reproducibly through smaller incisions with increased patient satisfaction and without adversely affecting outcome."
  3. The advantages are less soft tissue damage and blood loss.
- Several surgical exposures are used for THA.
  1. The posterior lateral approach is the predominant choice at HSS.
  2. This approach spares the abductors, and a postoperative limp is uncommon.
- It has been demonstrated that adequate repair of the capsule and the short external rotator hip muscles reduces the risk of hip dislocation after a posterior approach.
- Longevity of the implant depends on activity level of the patient, implant type, method of fixation, and technique of insertion.

- At the authors' institution, patients undergoing THA are given a combination of spinal/epidural anesthesia, and a few surgeons combine the spinal/epidural anesthesia with a psoas block for enhanced postoperative pain control. A patient-controlled analgesia (PCA) pump attached via a catheter is used to control pain for the initial 24 to 48 hours.

Rehabilitation Overview

- The measurement of patient progress addressing functional limitations has been documented in the acute care setting following elective THA.
  1. At HSS, the patient's functional progress is documented on the HSS Rehabilitation Department Functional Milestones Form. This form was developed to measure functional progression of patients with joint replacements during their hospitalization and has been proven to be statistically valid and reliable.
  2. The rehabilitation department has been using the Functional Milestones Form to collect outcome data on the total joint arthroplasty patient population for more than 2 decades.
  3. In the early 1990s, the THA clinical pathway and rehabilitation guidelines for phase I were developed using data generated from the Functional Milestones Forms and with the collaboration of HSS surgeons and members of an interdisciplinary team.
  4. Phases II and III are progressive phases based on each patient's functional mobility, strength, flexibility, gait, and balance, which are objectively measured and assessed by the physical therapist.
- Physical therapy management of patients who have undergone a THA is based on the theoretical framework of the disablement model addressing pathology, impairment, functional limitation, and disability.
- The most common impairments seen following THA are:
  1. Functional strength deficits in the hip musculature,
  2. Decreased hip range of motion (ROM),
  3. Decreased standing balance and proprioception,
  4. Decreased functional activity tolerance, and
  5. Increased pain during mobility activities.

- Functional limitations typically affect gait, transfers, stair negotiation, driving, and performing basic activities of daily living (ADL).
- The disabilities that result are in the areas of self-care, social activities, sporting activities, and work.
- Physical therapy treatment approaches following THA are impairment based and focused on reducing pain, increasing strength and flexibility, restoring mobility, teaching adherence to precautions, addressing ADL, and educating the patient and family.

Postoperative Phase I: Acute Care (Days 1 to 4)

GOALS
- Transfer unassisted and safely in and out of bed/chair/toilet
- Unassisted ambulation with cane(s) or crutches on level surfaces and stairs
- Independently perform home exercise program
- Demonstrate knowledge and adherence of total hip replacement precautions
- Independent with basic ADL

PRECAUTIONS
- Avoid hip flexion greater than 90 degrees, adduction past midline, and internal rotation of hip past neutral (for posterior-lateral approach)
- Avoid lying on operated side
- Avoid pillow(s) under knee to prevent hip flexion contracture
- Use abduction pillow when lying supine
- Reduce weight-bearing to 20–30% if concomitant osteotomy performed

TREATMENT STRATEGIES
- Instruct in strengthening exercise to include quadriceps and gluteal isometrics, ankle pumps, hip flexion to 45 degrees in supine; sitting knee extension and hip flexion with hip angle less than 90 degrees; standing hip extension and abduction and knee flexion
- Progressive ambulation with assistive device—walker to cane or crutches

- Emphasize symmetrical lower extremity weight-bearing and reciprocal gait pattern using an assistive device
- Non-reciprocal stair negotiation
- Review/instruct in hip precautions
- ADL instruction/assess equipment needs
- Cryotherapy

CRITERIA FOR ADVANCEMENT
- Progression from walker to cane or crutches when patient can demonstrate symmetrical weight-bearing and a step through non-antalgic gait pattern

Postoperative Phase II: Early Flexibility and Strengthening (Weeks 2 to 8)

GOALS
- Minimize pain
- Normalize gait without assistive device
- Hip extension 0–15 degrees
- Control edema
- Independence with ADLs

PRECAUTIONS
- Avoid hip flexion greater than 90 degrees, adduction past neutral, and internal rotation past neutral (for posterior-lateral approach)
- Avoid heat
- Avoid sitting for prolonged intervals (>1 hour)
- Avoid pain with therapeutic exercise and functional activities
- Avoid reciprocal stair climbing until both ascending and descending step progression has been accomplished

TREATMENT STRATEGIES
- Continuation and progression of advanced home exercise program (HEP)
- Ice
- Prone exercises
- Short crank ergometry (90 mm)
- Gait training

Continued

Postoperative Phase II: Early Flexibility and Strengthening (Weeks 2 to 8)—Cont'd

- Retro treadmill
- Proximal hip strengthening progression
- CKC: leg press/eccentric leg press
- Forward step-up progression (4" to 6" to 8")
- Proprioception/balance training: bilateral dynamic activities and unilateral static stance
- ADL training
- Pool therapy
- Determine baseline measurements for functional reach, TUG, unilateral stance time

CRITERIA FOR ADVANCEMENT
- MD script clearing hip precautions after 6–8 weeks postop visit
- Edema and pain controlled
- Hip extension 0–15 degrees
- Normalized gait pattern without assistive device
- Ascend a 4" step
- Independence with ADLs

Note—This phase continues until precautions are cleared by the surgeon and is based on a general THA population that is WBAT and ambulatory before surgery.

Postoperative Phase III: Advanced Strengthening and Return to Function (Weeks 8 to 14)

GOALS
- Ascending/descending stairs reciprocally
- Ability to independently perform lower extremity dressing, including donning/doffing shoes and socks
- Functional reach, TUG, single leg stance times, all within age-appropriate norms
- Ability to return to patient-specific functional activities

PRECAUTIONS
- Avoid pain with ADL and therapeutic exercise
- Monitor volume with activity

TREATMENT STRATEGIES
- Stationary bike (170mm)
- Treadmill
- Lower extremity stretching
- CKC exercises
- Continue forward step-up
- Initiate forward step-down progression
- Progressive resistive exercises of the lower extremity
- Contralateral hip exercises
- Advanced proprioception and balance activities
- Proximal PRE machines
- Pool therapy
- Reassessment of functional reach, TUG, single limb stance times
- Activity-specific training

CRITERIA FOR DISCHARGE
- Reciprocal stair climbing
- Independent donning/doffing of shoes and socks without aid
- Functional reach, TUG, single leg stance times, within age-appropriate limits
- Patient return to sport or advanced functional activities

Bibliography

American Physical Therapy Association. Guide to Physical Therapist Practice. *Phys Ther* 2001;77:1163-1650.

Berry, D.J. Primary Total Hip Arthroplasty. In Chapman, M.W. (Ed). Chapman's Orthopaedic Surgery. Lippincott Williams & Wilkins, Philadelphia, 2001, pp. 5-10.

Berry, D.J. Primary Total Hip Arthroplasty. In Chapman, M.W. (Ed). Chapman's Orthopaedic Surgery. Lippincott Williams & Wilkins, Philadelphia, 2001, pp. 13, 17.

Ganz, S. A Historic Look at Functional Outcome Following Total Hip and Knee Arthroplasty. *Top Geriatr Rehabil* 2004; 20:236-252.

Harkess, J.W. Arthroplasty of Hip. In Canale, T.P. (Ed). Campbell's Operative Orthopaedics. Mosby, St. Louis, 1998, p. 311.

Kroll, M., Ganz, S., Backus, S., Benick, R., MacKenzie, C., Harris, L. A Tool for Measuring Functional Outcomes after Total Hip Arthroplasty. *Arthritis Care Res* 1994;7:78-84.

Masonis, J.L., Bourne, R.B. Surgical Approach, Abductor Function, and Total Hip Arthroplasty Dislocation. *Clin Orthop Relat Res* 2002;405:46-53.

NIH Concensus Statement. Paper presented at NIH Consensus Development Conference on Total Hip Arthroplasty, September 12-14, 1994, Washington, DC.

Sculco, T.P., Jordan, L.C., William, W.L. Minimally Invasive Total Hip Arthroplasty: The Hospital for Special Surgery Experience. *Orthop Clin North Am* 2004;35:137-142.

U.S. Department of Health and Human Services, Center for Disease Control and Prevention, National Center for Health Statistics. Health Care in America: Trends in Utilization. Available online at http://www.edc.gov/nehs/data/misc/healthcare.pdf. Accessed April 9, 2004.

Total Knee Arthroplasty

Janet B. Cahill, PT, CSCS

Lisa M. Kosman, PT, MSPT

Total knee arthroplasty (TKA) is a common surgical procedure to treat osteoarthritis (OA)/degenerative joint disease (DJD) of the knee joint. More than 300,000 TKAs are performed annually in the United States. The Hospital for Special Surgery (HSS) performs more than 1700 TKAs per year.

Patients with OA of the knee typically present with the following impairments: decreased knee range of motion (ROM), decreased knee strength, gait deviations, decreased balance, and decreased proprioception. These impairments result in functional limitations, including difficulty ambulating because of abnormal biomechanics at the knee joint, difficulty transferring in and out of bed, difficulty ascending and descending stairs, and difficulty with activities of daily living (ADL).

The goal of TKA is to restore soft tissue balance, optimize biomechanics of the knee, maximize function, and relieve pain. Rehabilitation following TKA is a crucial component to the success of the surgery to address all preoperative and postoperative impairments and maximize function. It is imperative that the patient has an understanding of the expectations throughout the continuum of care. The patient's participation in his or her own rehabilitation program is essential. This chapter presents the HSS postoperative rehabilitation guidelines following TKA.

Surgical Overview

- Surgical techniques in TKA have made significant advances in the past 3 decades to treat advanced degenerative arthritis of the knee.

- Technology has allowed surgeons to replace the entire anatomical knee joint or replace either the medial or lateral portions of the knee, known as a unicondylar knee replacement.
  1. Minimally invasive surgery and high-flex knee prostheses are a few of the most recent technological advancements in joint replacement surgery.
  2. Standard TKA designs allow for bicondylar surface replacement, with either a posterior cruciate retaining (PCR) design or posterior cruciate substituting (PCS) design.
  3. Other prosthetic designs are either constrained or semiconstrained, which provide different levels of stability and varying degrees of freedom.
  4. The tibial and femoral components are commonly made of titanium alloy, and the tibial tray and the patella button are made of polyethylene.
- A midline or parapatellar incision is commonly used for joint exposure.
- Osteotomies of the proximal tibia, distal femur, anterior and posterior aspect of the femoral condyles, and retropatellar surface are performed.
- The anterior cruciate ligament (ACL) is resected to provide greater joint exposure during the procedure.
- The posterior cruciate ligament (PCL) may be resected if severe damage from degenerative osteophytes is found or if the surgeon prefers a PCS design.
- The medial and lateral collateral ligaments are retained; however, their anatomical positions may be surgically altered to achieve optimal varus or valgus alignment.
- If a knee flexion contracture is found, posterior condylar osteophytes may be removed, or the posterior capsule may be released.
- Once soft tissue balance is achieved, a trial reduction is performed, and stability and alignment of tibiofemoral and patellofemoral joints are checked in both flexion and extension.

- When optimal joint kinematics are achieved, the components are fixated with methylmethacrylate cement.
- The majority of patients who undergo TKA at HSS receive a combination spinal/epidural anesthesia, with a local femoral nerve block (FNB).
  1. General anesthesia is no longer used routinely at HSS.
  2. Williams-Russo et al. have shown that patients progress at a faster rate, using epidural anesthesia than general.
- Postoperative pain is managed primarily by a patient-controlled analgesia (PCA) pump through the epidural catheter.

Rehabilitation Overview

- The postoperative TKA rehabilitation program at our institution is designed and individually based on functional ability, clinical research, objective measurements, and the clinical expertise of the physical therapist.
- The HSS TKA rehabilitation guideline incorporates three progressive phases of postoperative rehabilitation to maximize patient outcomes. These guidelines include a general timeline of expected goals, which patients may achieve at a faster or slower rate, depending on age, comorbidities, pain, or surgical complications.
  1. Postoperative phase I of the inpatient TKA guideline was developed in part from functional outcome data that have been collected on more than 10,000 patients who have undergone TKA over the past 15 years at the HSS, using a valid and reliable Functional Milestones Form. This valuable information enabled us to benchmark functional status and design treatment interventions and goals in the early postoperative or inpatient phase.
  2. The subsequent postoperative phases II and III of the TKA guideline are based on progression and changes in function, ROM, gait, strength, flexibility, and balance, which are measured objectively.

Postoperative Phase I: Acute Care (Days 1 to 5)

GOALS
- Unassisted transfers
- Unassisted ambulation with appropriate device on level surfaces and stairs
- Ability to perform independent home exercise program
- A/AAROM range of motion:
  active flexion $\geq$80 degrees (sitting)
  extension $\leq$10 degrees (supine)

PRECAUTIONS
- Avoid prolonged sitting, standing, and walking
- Severe pain with walking and ROM exercises

TREATMENT STRATEGIES
- CPM—Initiate at 60 degrees knee flexion and advance as tolerated
- Transfer training
- Gait training weight bearing as tolerated (WBAT) with appropriate assistive device
- ADL training
- Cryotherapy
- Elevation to prevent edema
- HEP to include—Strengthening exercises: quadriceps, gluteal, and hamstring isometrics, SLR, AROM knee extension, sitting hip flexion; ROM exercises: A/AAROM knee flexion in sitting, passive knee extension with towel roll under ankle, stair stretch

CLINICAL CRITERIA FOR ADVANCEMENT
- Patients are discharged home within 5 days when all the inpatient phase I goals are achieved
- Gait progression from rolling walker to cane when patient demonstrates symmetrical step through gait, symmetrical weight-bearing
- CPM is discontinued when AROM is >90 degrees for 2 consecutive days

Note: Patients are discharged to an inpatient rehabilitation facility within 3–4 days if the patient requires progressive and additional rehabilitation to achieve independence with all functional activities.

Postoperative Phase II (Weeks 2 to 8)

GOALS
- Range of motion: active assistive knee flexion ≥ 105 degrees
- Active-assistive knee extension = 0 degrees
- Minimize postoperative edema
- Ascend 4″ step
- Independence in home exercise program
- Normalize gait pattern with/without assistive device
- Independent with ADL

PRECAUTIONS
- Avoid ambulation without assistive device if gait deviation present
- Avoid prolonged sitting and walking
- Avoid pain with therapeutic exercise and functional activities
- Avoid reciprocal stair climbing until adequate strength/control of operated limb is achieved

TREATMENT STRATEGIES
- Passive extension with towel extensions, prone hangs
- Active knee flexion/extension exercise
- AAROM knee flexion: manual, heel slides, wall slides
- Short crank ergometry (90 mm) for ROM >90 degrees
- Cycle ergometry (170 mm) for ROM >110 degrees
- Cryotherapy/elevation/modalities for edema control
- Patellar mobilization (once staples/sutures removed, incision stable)
- Electrical stimulation or biofeedback for quadriceps reeducation
- SLR (all planes) PREs
- CKC: leg press
- Forward step-up progression (2″→4″)
- Proximal resistive exercises: multihip machine
- CKC terminal knee extension exercise
- Balance/proprioceptive training: unilateral static stance, bilateral dynamic activities
- Determine baseline measurements for functional tests: TUG and functional reach as appropriate

Continued

Postoperative Phase II (Weeks 2 to 8)—Cont'd

- Gait training with assistive device: emphasize active knee flexion, extension, heel-strike, reciprocal pattern, symmetrical weight-bearing
- ADL training in/out of tub/shower, car transfers

CRITERIA FOR ADVANCEMENT
- Flexion >105 degrees
- Absence of quadriceps lag
- Normal gait pattern on level surfaces with/without assistive device
- Ascend 4" step

Postoperative Phase III (Weeks 9 to 16)

GOALS
- Range of motion: active assistive knee flexion >115 degrees
- Transfer sit to stand with equal limb symmetry and equal weight-bearing
- Independence with ADLs, including tying shoelaces and putting on socks
- Reciprocal stair negotiation:
  Ascending 6"–8"?
  Descending steps 4"–6"
- Maximize quadriceps/hamstring strength, control, and flexibility to meet the demands of high-level ADL activities
- Functional test scores: Timed get-up and go:
  <15 seconds
  Functional reach: 10"

PRECAUTIONS
- Avoid reciprocal stair negotiation if pain or deviations are present
- No running, jumping, or plyometric activity unless allowed by the doctor

TREATMENT STRATEGIES
- Patella mobilizations/glides
- Cycle ergometry 170mm
- Quadricep stretching
- Hamstring stretching
- Leg press/eccentric leg press/unilateral leg press

- Forward step-up 6"→8"
- Forward step-down 4"→6"
- Ball/wall squats
- Retro treadmill on incline
- Functional ball squats
- Balance/proprioceptive training: bilateral and unilateral dynamic activities

CRITERIA FOR DISCHARGE
- Patient has achieved all goals and functional outcomes
- Functional test measures within age-appropriate parameters
- Ascend 6"–8" forward step up/descend 4"–6" forward step down

Bibliography

Burke, D., O'Flynn, H. Primary Total Knee Arthroplasty. In Chapman, M. (Ed). Chapman's Orthopaedic Surgery. Lippincott Williams & Wilkins, Philadelphia, 2001.

Guyton, J. Arthroplasty of Ankle and Knee. In Canale, T. (Ed). Campbell's Operative Orthopaedics. Mosby, St. Louis, 1998, pp. 232–295.

Insall, J. Historical Development, Classification and Characteristics of Knee Prostheses. In Insall, J.N., Kelly, M.A., Scott, W.N., Anglietti, P. (Eds). Surgery of the Knee. Churchill Livingstone, New York, 1993, pp. 677–717.

Insall, J. Surgical Techniques and Instrumentation in Total Knee Arthroplasty. In Insall, J.N., Kelly, M.A., Scott, W.N., Anglietti, P. (Eds). Surgery of the Knee. Churchill Livingstone, New York, 1993, pp. 739–804.

Kroll, M., Ganz, S., Backus, S., Benick, R., MacKenzie, C., Harris, L. A Tool for Measuring Functional Outcomes After Total Hip Arthroplasty. *Arthritis Care Res* 1994;7:78–84.

Lotke, P. Primary Total Knees: Standard Principles and Techniques. In Lotke, P. (Ed). Knee Arthroplasty. Raven Press, New York, 1995, pp. 65–92.

Statistics, N.C.F.H. Nation Wide Inpatient Survey 1997, UDOHAH Services, Editor. 1997.

Williams-Russo, P., Sharrock, N.E., Haas, S.B., Insall, J., Windsor, R.E., Laskin, R.S., Ranawat, C.S., Go, G., Ganz, S.B. Randomized Trial of Epidural Versus General Anesthesia. *Clin Orthop Relat Res* 1996;331:199–208.

CHAPTER 3

Total Shoulder Arthroplasty

John T. Cavanaugh, PT, MEd, ATC

Janet B. Cahill, PT, CSCS

Total shoulder arthroplasty (TSA) has become the management of choice for many patients with debilitating glenohumeral injury or disease. More than 10,000 shoulder arthroplasties are performed annually in the United States. The primary indication for a total shoulder replacement is pain from an arthritic or incongruous glenohumeral joint that is unresponsive to conservative treatment. Other less common indications may include severe fractures or osteonecrosis. Contraindications for a TSA include paralysis of the deltoid and rotator cuff musculature, active infection, or a patient who is unwilling or unable to participate in the extensive rehabilitation necessary for success.

TSA requires meticulous surgical skill and is a technically challenging operation. The variations in shoulder components (constrained, semiconstrained, unconstrained, and modular designs) provide the surgeon with the flexibility to anatomically restore the shoulder joint. Many factors contribute to the outcome of shoulder arthroplasty, including quality of bone, integrity of soft tissues, underlying etiology of disease, and the rehabilitation program. The Hospital for Special Surgery (HSS) rehabilitation guidelines following TSA are presented.

Surgical Overview

- Many variations exist to the surgical procedure of a TSA. A surgeon's surgical experience and preference, as well as a patient's soft tissue and bone quality, are integral factors to the technique of choice. Described is a surgical overview for patients undergoing primary TSA.

- TSA is performed using either an interscalene regional block or general anesthesia, depending on the surgeon's preference.
- The patient is typically in a beach chair position and passive range of motion (PROM) is assessed under anesthesia, which will enable the surgeon to determine the expected postoperative ROM outcomes.
- A deltopectoral incision is commonly used to attain exposure of the shoulder joint.
- Superficial soft tissue structures are identified and retracted at the level of the deltopectoral interval.
- The cephalic vein can be preserved and retracted with the pectoralis major, or ligated and removed.
- The clavipectoral fascia is incised superiorly to the level of the coracoacromial ligament. This allows medial retraction of the "strap muscles" (the short head of the biceps, coracobrachialis, and pectoralis minor).
- The coracoacromial ligament may be released (assuming there is an intact rotator cuff with good quality tissue) to more effectively expose the rotator interval.
- The superior third of the pectoralis major tendon may be released and tagged for later repair, if necessary, for exposure as well.
- Adhesions between the rotator cuff and deltoid should be released if present.
- The subscapularis is identified, and the surgeon assesses external rotation ROM.
- To obtain greater exposure of the glenohumeral joint, the subscapularis tendon can be divided just medial to its insertion on the lesser tubercle, or a release of the tendon from its insertion into the lesser tuberosity may be performed.
- If an internal rotation (IR) (40 degrees) contracture is present, a lengthening of the tendon may be performed.
- Once soft tissue dissection is complete, the shoulder joint is dislocated; an osteotomy of the humeral head is performed, and degenerative bone and osteophytes are excised from the humerus and glenoid.
- When trial components are fitted and joint mechanics are restored, final components of titanium alloy humeral stem

and head and polyethylene glenoid are cemented with methyl methacrylate.

- The humeral and glenoid versions are restored to provide stability and ROM.
- Appropriate sizing is critical to avoid mechanical impingement or "overstuffing" of the joint and ensure that the stability of the joint is not sacrificed.
- Final components are fitted, the subscapularis tendon is repaired, or reattached, to the humerus and secured with heavy nonabsorbable sutures, and the wound is closed and the patient is placed in a shoulder immobilizer.

Rehabilitation Overview

- Rehabilitation following TSA is a long and arduous course.
- Secondary to the amount of bone dissection during the procedure, pain management becomes an important treatment intervention in the early days and weeks following the procedure.
- Early mobilization is encouraged to prevent shoulder contractures and adhesions from developing.
- Therapeutic interventions are progressed using the guidelines that follow. Each patient, however, is treated individually, because preoperative ROM, bone quality, and soft tissue integrity will have an influence on the progression of the program.
- Communication with the referring orthopedic surgeon to ascertain this information is imperative to ensure a safe and effective response to the rehabilitation program.
- A surgeon's prognosis, determined by the success of the procedure, should be considered when establishing rehabilitation goals.
- ROM, flexibility, and strengthening exercises are progressed via a criteria based approach, based on basic science principles, healing response of surgically repaired tissues, and rehabilitative experience.
- Patient education is essential throughout the rehabilitative course.
- Compliance to home therapeutic exercises as well as functional restrictions should be continually reinforced.

- Goals following TSA include maximizing ROM, flexibility, and muscle strength necessary for the pain-free performance of activities of daily living (ADL).

Preoperative Phase

GOALS
- Patient education
- Independence with donning and doffing sling
- Independence with home exercise program and precautions

TREATMENT STRATEGIES
- Measure for postoperative sling
- Instruct patient in donning and doffing the sling
- Instruct patient in necessary ADL (dressing, cooking, and self-care)
- Instruct patient in and provide with written precautions
- Instruct patient in cryotherapy application
- Instruct patient in appropriate exercises (physician-specific) to address ROM and strength deficits

Postoperative Phase I (Weeks 0 to 4)

GOALS
- Pain and edema control
- ROM to 120 degrees of elevation, ER to 30 degrees
- Independent home exercise program (HEP)
- Independent light ADL

PRECAUTIONS
- Avoid unnecessary lifting beyond normal ADL
- Avoid ranges of motion beyond physician direction

TREATMENT STRATEGIES
- Sling immobilization except for light ADL and therapeutic exercises
- Codman/pendulum exercise
- Passive ROM exercises
- Active-assisted ROM exercises
- External rotation (supine with wand, in the plane of the scapula, physician-directed ROM limit)
- Forward flexion (supine with contralateral limb)
- Scapulothoracic mobilization

Continued

Postoperative Phase I (Weeks 0 to 4)—Cont'd

- Scapula strengthening
- Side-lying active range of motion → active manual resistive strengthening
- Scapula retraction (sitting)
- Distal active ROM exercises (elbow, wrist, hand)
- Cryotherapy/transcutaneous electrical nerve stimulation as needed

CRITERIA FOR ADVANCEMENT
- Pain controlled
- ROM, elevation to 120 degrees, external rotation to 30 degrees
- Independent light ADL
- Independent home exercise program

Postoperative Phase II (Weeks 4 to 10)

GOALS
- Pain control 0/10 with ADL
- Passive ROM
  1. Elevation to 150 degrees
  2. External rotation to 45 degrees
- Independent HEP

PRECAUTIONS
- Avoid painful activities in ADL
- Avoid ranges of motion beyond doctor direction

TREATMENT STRATEGIES
- Passive ROM exercises
- Active-assisted ROM exercises
  1. ER wand
  2. Advance forward flexion to using wand in neutral rotation
  3. Pulleys (ROM >120 degrees/good humeral head control)
- Active ROM
  1. Forward flexion (supine)
  2. Internal rotation at 6 weeks (towel pass)
- Humeral head control exercises
  1. ER/IR (supine/scapular plane)
  2. Elevation at 100 degrees

- Hydrothorapy
  1. Pool exercises: forward flexion (scapular plane), horizontal abduction/adduction
- Isometrics
  1. Deltoid in neutral
  2. ER (modified neutral) ROM >30 degrees
  3. Internal rotation (IR) (modified neutral) at 6 weeks
- Closed kinetic chain exercises
  1. Ball stabilization, weight shifting
- Scapular retraction with elastic bands
- Extension with elastic bands
- Airdyne or upper body ergometry
- Modalities as needed
- Modify home exercise program as appropriate

CRITERIA FOR ADVANCEMENT
- 0/10 pain with ADL
- ROM (150 degrees elevation, 45 degrees external rotation)
- Good humeral head control
- Independent home exercise program

Postoperative Phase III (Weeks 10 to 16)

GOALS
- Pain control 0/10 with advanced ADL
- Passive ROM
  1. Elevation to 160 degrees
  2. External rotation to 60 degrees
- Internal rotation to T12
- Restore normal scapulohumeral rhythm <90-degree elevation
- Improve muscle strength 4/5
- Independent in current HEP

PRECAUTIONS
- Avoid painful activities in ADL
- Avoid ROMs that encourage scapular hiking, poor biomechanics

TREATMENT STRATEGIES
- Progress range of motion as tolerated
- Flexibility exercises: towel stretch, posterior capsule stretch
- Hydrotherapy exercises

Continued

Postoperative Phase III (Weeks 10 to 16)— Cont'd

- Isometrics
  1. Deltoid away from neutral
- Scapular stabilization
- Rhythmic stabilization
- Progressive resistive exercises (PREs) for scapula, elbow (biceps/triceps)
- Forward flexion (scapular plane)
- Airdyne/upper body ergometry
- Progressive resistive equipment: row, chest press (light weight)
- Modalities as needed
- Modify HEP

CRITERIA FOR ADVANCEMENT
- Pain control 0/10 with advanced ADL
- Passive ROM
  1. Elevation to 160 degrees
  2. External rotation to 60 degrees
- Internal rotation to T12
- Restore normal scapulohumeral rhythm <90-degree elevation
- Muscle strength 4/5
- Independent in current HEP

Postoperative Phase IV (Weeks 16 to 22)

GOALS
- Maximize ROM
- Achieve adequate strength and flexibility to meet demands of ADL
- Functional muscle strength throughout the involved upper extremity
- Normal scapulohumeral rhythm >100-degree elevation
- Independent in home and gym therapeutic exercise programs

PRECAUTIONS
- Avoid painful activities in ADL
- Avoid lifting heavy objects

TREATMENT STRATEGIES
- Assess and address any remaining deficits in ROM, flexibility, and strength
- Active, active-assisted, and passive ROM exercises
- Flexibility program
  1. Posterior capsule stretching
  2. Towel stretch (IR)
- Progressive resistive exercises program
  1. Dumbbells
- Progressive resistive equipment
  1. Elastic band IR/ER (modified neutral)
- Rhythmic stabilization
- Proprioceptive neuromuscular facilitation patterns
- Modalities as needed
- Modify home exercise program
- Individualize program to meet the specific needs of the patient
  1. Sports-specific training
- Discharge planning for maintenance and advancement of gains achieved during rehabilitation

CRITERIA FOR DISCHARGE
- Maximize ROM
- Full independence in ADL
- Normal scapulohumeral rhythm > 100-degree elevation
- Functional muscle strength throughout the involved upper extremity

Bibliography

Fenlin, J.M., Frieman, B.G. Indications, Technique and Results of TSA in Osteoarthritis. *Orthop Clin North Am* 1998;29:423–434.

Marx, R.G., Craig, E.V. Primary Arthroplasty of the Shoulder. In Chapman, M.W. (Ed) Chapman's Orthopedics. Lippincott Williams & Wilkins, Philadelphia, 2001, pp. 2630–2664.

Matsen, F.A., Rockwood, C.A., Wirth, M.A., Lippitt, S.B. Glenohumeral Arthritis and its Management. In Rockwood, C.A., Matsen, F.A. (Eds). The Shoulder, 2nd ed. WB Saunders, Philadelphia, 1998, pp. 840–964.

Personal communication, F. Cordasco, December 2004.

CHAPTER 4

Total Elbow Arthroplasty

Aviva Wolff, OTR/L, CHT

The primary goal of total elbow arthroplasty (TEA) is pain relief with restoration of stability and functional motion (arc of 30 to 130 degrees). An elbow replacement is considered when the joint is painful, is restricted in motion, and has destroyed articular cartilage. Patients who are elderly or have low demands that present with rheumatoid arthritis, advanced posttraumatic arthritis, advanced degenerative arthritis or nonunion, and comminuted, distal humeral fractures are good candidates for this surgery. A total elbow replacement is contraindicated in situations where there is active sepsis in the joint, previous infection or open wounds at the elbow, poor soft tissue envelope, skeletal immaturity, and paralysis of biceps or triceps. Complications of this surgery include delayed wound healing, infection, ulnar neuritis, triceps insufficiency, instability, and mechanical failure.

Surgical Overview

- TEA includes three types of implants: constrained, nonconstrained, and semiconstrained.
  1. The first prosthesis developed was rigid and fully constrained. It had a metal-to-metal interface and provided immediate stability, but had a high failure rate with loosening occurring after several years.
  2. This was followed by a nonconstrained implant, which is composed of two separate units and is a resurfacing of the distal humerus and proximal ulna.
     - This design requires strong ligaments, good bone quality, and adequate soft tissue support and is therefore only indicated in a select group of patients.

- Examples include capitellocondylar, Kudo, and Souter implants.
3. The latest semiconstrained design, referred to as a "sloppy hinge," is the most popular.
   - Although it provides stability similar to the constrained implant, its "toggle" characteristic allows for varus–valgus play and axial rotation.
   - This type of design reduces some of the problems related to the constrained device.
   - Examples include the Coonrad-Morrey and GSB 3 (Gschwend) implants.
- The choice for a specific implant is based on the extent and cause of the disease, the specific needs of the patient, and the surgeon's preference.
- At the Hospital for Special Surgery (HSS), the Coonrad-Morrey semiconstrained total elbow prosthesis (Zimmer, Warsaw, IN) is most frequently used. When a nonconstrained implant is indicated, the capitellocondylar implant is most often used.

Rehabilitation Overview

- Progression of therapy is based on the stages of wound healing and is affected by implant type, skin integrity, rate of healing, and the preoperative and postoperative condition of the triceps.
- Timeframes may be delayed to allow for wound closure and adequate healing of the triceps in patients with poor soft tissue quality, as is common in rheumatoid arthritis (RA).
- Each surgeon has different preferences in the type of implant, surgical technique, and postoperative treatment. The referring surgeon is consulted for specific range of motion (ROM) restrictions and time frames.
- The guidelines below are for semiconstrained total elbow replacements performed with the triceps sparing approach.
  1. This technique was developed to avoid complications such as triceps avulsion, triceps weakness, and wound healing problems.
  2. Notes in italic refer to guideline modifications for nonconstrained TEA. Timeframes may be delayed in these implants to allow for adequate stability.

Postoperative Phase I: Inflammation/Protection (Weeks 0 to 2)

GOALS
- Protective immobilization
- Wound healing and closure
- Control of edema and inflammation
- Full ROM of proximal and distal joints
- Full elbow ROM within protected arc

PRECAUTIONS
- Monitor wound carefully (increased potential for delayed wound healing and infection in RA)
- Triceps precautions: active elbow flexion to 90 degrees, passive elbow extension (gravity assist)
- Nonconstrained implants: no combined shoulder abduction and elbow extension (may lead to implant dislocation); extension limited to 30 degrees

TREATMENT STRATEGIES
Immobilization Options
- Bledsoe brace
- Static posterior elbow splint: custom molded at 90 degrees
- Static anterior elbow splint
- Sling

Wound Care
- Monitor wound, dressing changes (no bulky dressings that restrict motion)

Edema Control
- Cold packs/ice, elevation, retrograde massage, light Ace wrapping, Isotoner glove; avoid tight elastic sleeves

Proximal and Distal ROM
- A/AAROM of digits, wrist, and shoulder
- No shoulder abduction with elbow extension in nonconstrained implants

Protected Elbow ROM (Begin POD 2 with Doctor's Approval)
- Active/gentle active-assisted elbow flexion to 90 degrees
- Elbow extension passively via gravity
- Gentle active pronation and supination
  1. *Elbow flexed at 90 degrees with arm at side to maintain stability in nonconstrained implants*

- CPM if patient is unable to perform exercises: 30 to 90 degrees, 2 consecutive hours, three times daily

CRITERIA FOR ADVANCEMENT
- Wound closure
- Sufficient healing of triceps and stability of implant to withstand greater stresses

Postoperative Phase II: Fibroplasia (Weeks 2 to 6)

GOALS
- Maximum active elbow ROM
- Minimal adhesion formation and decreased scar development
- Isolated active triceps muscle contraction
- Functional use of the extremity

PRECAUTIONS
- Obtain doctor approval before discharge of triceps precautions
- No forceful active elbow extension, including during ADL (i.e., pushing up from a chair)
- No lifting more than 1 pound or other ADL stressful to elbow
- No resistive exercises
- *Avoid varus-valgus stress in unconstrained implants*

TREATMENT STRATEGIES
ROM/Isometrics
- A/AAROM
  1. Progress elbow flexion to tolerance
  2. Active extension with gravity assist, gradually progressing to other planes
  3. Place and hold exercises at comfortable end range
- Submaximal isometrics to isolate triceps throughout range
- Education to avoid compensatory motions (shoulder shrug, protraction)

Modalities
- Massage, moist heat to biceps and triceps to inhibit co-contraction
- Biofeedback to inhibit co-contraction and isolate triceps
- Cold packs and other edema reduction measures

Continued

Postoperative Phase II: Fibroplasia (Weeks 2 to 6)—Cont'd

Scar Management
- Scar massage when sutures/staples have been removed and incision is dry and closed
- Soft tissue mobilization and cross-friction massage to triceps tendon insertion
- Silicone/otoform insert with light compression for night use

Functional Use
- Gradually wean splint and promote performance of light ADL/self-care

CRITERIA FOR ADVANCEMENT
- Sufficient stability and soft tissue healing to withstand light resistive exercise and static progressive/serial static splinting

Postoperative Phase III: Scar Maturation (Week 6 to Month 6)

GOALS
- Maximum stable passive elbow ROM
- Adequate strength required for elbow active ROM to equal passive ROM
- Functional strength required for independent use of upper extremity for ADL, work, and leisure
- Awareness of lifetime precautions and potential complications

PRECAUTIONS
- No aggressive stretching; no joint mobilizations
- Avoid dynamic splints (these apply to excessive, uncontrolled force to elbow)
- Do not sacrifice stability to gain ROM
- Lifetime precautions:
  1. Five-pound maximum for lifting or carrying
  2. No weight-bearing on extended elbow
  3. No impact sports, such as golf or tennis

TREATMENT STRATEGIES
Splinting/PROM for maximum stable ROM
- Static progressive elbow flexion: worn intermittently during the day
- Serial static extension splint: worn at night and/or intermittently during the day
- Alternative to splints previously mentioned: Universal Mayo Clinic Elbow Brace (Aircast)
- PROM/gentle stretching at end range

Gentle Strengthening
- Elbow extension exercises against gravity (overhead)
- Isometrics
- Light resistive exercises for triceps, biceps, and scapular muscles: light Thera Band (mid-range), 1-pound free weights, or cable column
- Neuromuscular electrical stimulation to triceps if weakness and adhesions persist

Restoration of Function
- Encourage resumption of functional activities while observing lifetime precautions

CRITERIA FOR DISCHARGE
- Achievement of functional ROM and strength for all light ADL
- Independence in home exercise program, joint protection, and awareness of precautions

Bibliography

Bryan, R.S., Morrey, B.F. Extensive Posterior Approach of the Elbow: A Triceps Sparing Approach. *Clin Orthop Relat Res* 1982;166: 188-192.

Cooney, W. Elbow Arthroplasty: Historical Perspective and Current Concepts. In Morrey, B.F. (Ed). The Elbow and Its Disorders, 3rd ed. WB Saunders, Philadelphia, 2000.

Ewald, F. Total Elbow Replacement. *Orthop Clin North Am* 1975;6:685.

Ferlic, D. Total Elbow Arthroplasty for Treatment of Elbow Arthritis. *J Elbow Shoulder Surg* 1999;75:367-378.

Gschwend, N., Lowhr, J., Ivosevic-Radovanovic, D., Scheler, H. Semi-constrained Elbow Prosthesis with Special Reference of the GBS III Prosthesis. *Clin Orthop Relat Res* 1988;232:104.

Kudo, H., Iwano, K., Watanabe, S. Total Replacement of the Rheumatoid Elbow with a Hingeless Prosthesis. *J Bone Joint Surg* 1980;62A:277.

Morrey, B. Complications of Elbow Replacement Surgery. In Morrey, B. (Ed). The Elbow and Its Disorders, 2nd ed. WB Saunders, Philadelphia, 2000.

Morrey, B.F., Adams, R.A., Bryan, R.S. Total Replacement for Post-traumatic Arthritis of the Elbow. *J Bone Joint Surg* 1991;73: 607–612.

Pierce, T.D., Herndon, J.H. The Triceps Preserving Approach to Total Elbow Arthroplasty. *Clin Orthop Relat Res* 1998;354:144–152.

Souter, W.A. Arthroplasty of the Elbow: With Particular Reference to Metallic Hinge Arthroplasty in Rheumatoid Patients. *Orthop Clin North Am* 1973;4:395.

CHAPTER 5

Metacarpophalangeal Joint Arthroplasty

Carol Page, PT, DPT, CHT

Rheumatoid arthritis (RA) is a chronic, progressive, autoimmune disease that causes joint destruction. It affects women more than men and increases in prevalence with aging. An estimated 0.5% to 1% of adults are affected.

Unlike osteoarthritis and traumatic arthritis, which rarely affect the metacarpophalangeal (MP) joints of the fingers, RA commonly affects these joints. Soft tissue and bony destruction lead to deformities that are often severe. Ulnar drift of the fingers at the MP joint level results from attenuation of the radial collateral ligament and joint capsule, with ulnar dislocation of the extensor tendon. The ulnar collateral ligament, capsule, and intrinsic muscles become contracted. The metacarpal heads are usually subluxed palmarly.

Anatomic and Surgical Overview

- Although arthrodesis may be indicated for deformities of the proximal and distal interphalangeal (IP) joints, arthrodesis is rarely indicated for MP joint deformities because it is so functionally limiting.
- Arthroplasty is the treatment of choice. Surgery consists of a replacement of the MP joint with an implant (typically made of silicone) and soft tissue rebalancing.
  1. MP joint arthroplasty necessitates excision of the head of the metacarpal, the hypertrophied synovium, and the base of the proximal phalanx.
  2. The medullary canals of the metacarpal and proximal phalanx are reamed and trial implants inserted to determine the best fit.
  3. Soft tissue releases are performed to correct ulnar deviation, palmar subluxation, and ulnar intrinsic tightness.

4. Residual laxity of the radial structures is corrected and the extensor tendon centralized over the MP joint.

- Many approaches to MP arthroplasty have been taken, including joint resurfacing and hinged, semiconstrained, and constrained implants.
- Awareness of the particular implant used is helpful to the therapist in setting goals for motion.
  1. Silicone arthroplasty is currently the most commonly performed procedure.
  2. The Swanson (Dow Corning, Midland, MI), NeuFlex (Depuy Inc., Warsaw, IN), and Avanta (Avanta Orthopedics, San Diego, CA) MP implants are all one-piece, flexible prostheses of this type. However, differences between them may result in different, potential motion ranges.
  3. Because the NeuFlex MP joint prosthesis rests in 30-degree flexion, greater flexion may result than with use of the Swanson MP implant, which rests in 0-degree extension.
  4. The Avanta MP implant, unlike the Swanson and Neu-Flex implants, has a volar axis designed to increase potential for MP flexion.

Rehabilitation Overview

- The primary purpose of rehabilitation is to promote functional motion of the implanted MP joints while preserving correct alignment as healing occurs.
- Stability of the implanted MP joints depends on the formation of a fibrous pseudo-capsule around the implants, a process known as encapsulation.
- Protection is provided both through splinting and through patient education, in avoidance of deforming forces during exercises and functional activities.
- Lifelong adherence to joint protection principles is critical to preserve the implants and maximize joint stability.
- MP joint arthroplasty is widely considered to be effective in improving motion, cosmesis, function, and pain. However, implant fracture and deformation have been shown to be common with long-term follow-up, performed at an average of 14 years postoperatively.

Postoperative Phase I: Inflammation/ Protection (Weeks 0 to 3)

GOALS
- Provide correct protective splinting
- Protect repaired structures
- Reduce edema and pain
- Achieve full wound closure
- Protective mobilization of involved joints
- Maintain active range of motion (AROM) of uninvolved joints, including wrist and thumb

PRECAUTIONS
- No use of involved digits for functional activities
- Protect MP joints from ulnar deviation forces
- No forceful passive ROM (PROM), stretching, or resistance
- Never attempt to perform joint mobilizations on implants
- Modify treatment for additional surgeries performed, such as fusions of the thumb MP and IP joints, and finger IP joints

TREATMENT STRATEGIES
- Splinting options
  1. Dynamic MP extension outrigger splint: MP joints extended to neutral with 10 degrees radial deviation, wrist extended 15 degrees
  2. Static MP extension splint: MP joints extended to neutral with 10 degrees radial deviation, IP joints extended, wrist extended 15 degrees
  3. Static MP flexion splint: MP joints flexed to a maximum of 70 degrees with 10-degree radial deviation, IP joints extended, wrist extended 15 degrees
- Edema and pain reduction: instruct patient in elevation, cold modalities, retrograde massage (avoiding surgical incision until fully closed)
- Wound care: Change dressings, monitor surgical incision
- A/AAROM of involved digits: Tendon gliding, thumb opposition to index and middle fingers, radial digit walking
- Gentle PROM by therapist: MP flexion, avoiding ulnar deviation; gentle intrinsic stretching

Continued

Postoperative Phase I: Inflammation/ Protection (Weeks 0 to 3)—Cont'd

- ROM exercises for uninvolved joints: Thumb, wrist, elbow, forearm, shoulder

CRITERIA FOR ADVANCEMENT
- Edema and pain well controlled
- Surgical incision fully closed
- MP joint stability

Postoperative Phase II: Fibroplasia (Weeks 3 to 6)

GOALS
- Protect MP arthroplasties through continued splinting and activity modification
- Reduce residual edema and pain
- Minimize scar adhesions
- Achieve functional AROM of MP joints
- Perform light functional activities while adhering to joint protection principles

PRECAUTIONS
- No resistive activities or exercises
- Protect MP joints from ulnar deviation forces

TREATMENT STRATEGIES
- Splinting
  1. Continue protective splinting
  2. Serial static or static progressive MP flexion splinting as necessary to regain functional flexion
- Continue phase 1 edema treatments, adding light compression wrapping if necessary (avoiding overly tight application)
- Precondition soft tissues with superficial heat modalities before ROM and scar techniques
- Scar management when incision has healed: Scar massage, silicone pad
- A/AA/PROM: Digits (avoiding ulnar deviation of MP joints), wrist
- Light functional activities while adhering to joint protection principles

CRITERIA FOR ADVANCEMENT
- Minimal pain with light activities and motion exercises
- Patient cleared by physician for strengthening exercises

Postoperative Phase III: Scar Maturation (Weeks 6 to 12)

GOALS
- Maximize stable digital AROM and PROM
- Achieve functional hand strength
- Preserve correct digital alignment
- Promote safe hand function with awareness of joint protection principles
- Restore independent activities of daily living while maintaining joint protection

PRECAUTIONS
- MP joint stability should not be sacrificed to maximize ROM
- Resistive exercises must be used with caution
- Lateral pinch and other activities that promote MP radial deviation are avoided
- Patient must adhere to lifetime joint protection principles, with avoidance of all excessive forces to the implants, especially into ulnar deviation

TREATMENT STRATEGIES
- Gradually wean from splint during day at 6–8 weeks postoperatively with concurrence of a doctor
- Continue static MP extension splint at night for ongoing joint protection
- Consider neoprene anti-ulnar deviation splint for use during functional activities
- Continue edema control and modalities as needed
- Continue scar management until scar is mature
- Maximize stable AROM and PROM through therapeutic exercise, gentle stretching, and addition of flexion splinting if needed (serial static or static progressive), protecting MP joints from ulnar deviation

Continued

Postoperative Phase III: Scar Maturation (Weeks 6 to 12)—Cont'd

- Light resistance for grip and three point-pinch strengthening; avoid lateral pinch
- Reinforce patient education in joint protection principles
- Promote independence in safe performance of functional activities

CRITERIA FOR DISCHARGE

- Independence in home program of splinting, scar management, joint protection, and therapeutic exercise
- Understanding and application of joint protection principles
- Functional hand ROM and strength
- Independence in light activities of daily living with adherence to joint protection principles

Bibliography

Berger, R.A., Beckenbaugh, R.D., Linscheid, R.L. Arthroplasty in the Hand and Wrist. In Green, D.P., Hotchkiss, R.N., Pederson, W.C. (Eds). Green's Operative Hand Surgery, 4th ed. Churchill Livingstone, New York, 1999, pp. 156-161.

Chung, K.C., Kowalski, C.P., Kim, H.M., Kazmers, I.S. Patient Outcomes Following Swanson Silastic Metacarpophalangeal Joint Arthroplasty in the Rheumatoid Hand: A Systemic Overview. *J Rheumatol* 2000;27:1395-1402.

Goldfarb, C.A., Stern, P.J. Metacarpophalangeal Joint Arthroplasty in Rheumatoid Arthritis. A Long-term Assessment. *J Bone Joint Surg* 2003;85A:1869-1878.

Kvien, T.K. Epidemiology and Burden of Illness of Rheumatoid Arthritis. *Pharmacoeconomics* 2004;22(Suppl 1):1-12.

Stirrat, C.R. Metacarpophalangeal Joints in Rheumatoid Arthritis of the Hand. *Hand Clin* 1996;12:515-529.

Swanson, A.B. Flexible Implant Arthroplasty for Arthritic Finger Joints. *J Bone Joint Surg* 1972;54A:435-455.

The Avanta Soft Skeletal Hand Implant System. Available online at http://www.avanta.org/arthroplasty/hand.htm. Accessed 20 Jan, 2006.

CHAPTER 6

Hip Fractures

Sandy B. Ganz, PT, DSc, GCS

Hip fractures are associated with significant morbidity and mortality in the United States, resulting in 350,000 hospitalizations annually. This number is an increase of 23% from 1988. Census trends indicate that the fastest rate of growth occurs in those populations over age 85 and those most susceptible to sustain a hip fracture. It is estimated that by 2040, the annual number of hip fractures will surpass 500,000, and that one in four women and one in eight men will sustain a hip fracture by age 90.

Since the inception of the prospective payment system (PPS), the care of elderly patients who have sustained a hip fracture has changed dramatically. Hospital length of stay for Medicare recipients decreased from 21.9 days in 1981 to 12.4 days in 1986, and patients enrolled in managed care programs had a hospital length of stay of 7.3 days. Discharge to skilled nursing facilities for short-term rehabilitation rose from 38% to 60%.

For those individuals who have sustained a hip fracture, returning to their prefracture functional status is a primary goal. Rehabilitation following hip fracture occurs along a continuum. Patients improve along a line of increasing functional status and may transition from the acute care setting to a free-standing rehabilitation hospital or a subacute facility, such as a nursing home for short-term rehabilitation where physical therapy services are provided daily. Patients may be discharged directly home following surgery and receive physical therapy services at home, or they are discharged home and receive physical therapy services in an outpatient facility.

The rehabilitation program following hip fracture is begun immediately following surgery. The clinician must take into consideration the type of surgical repair—whether it is an open or closed reduction and internal fixation or type of total hip arthroplasty (THA) or hemiarthroplasty—and surgical approach used (i.e., anterior/posterior approach) to set realistic short- and long-term goals and deliver appropriate postoperative care. The choice of settings in which rehabilitation is provided following hip fracture is most often determined by the physician, insurance coverage, patient factors, and the health care delivery system. Patients improve along a continuum. It is not uncommon for patients to receive therapy up to 6 months following fracture, and it is crucial for physical therapists to know the expected rate of recovery throughout this continuum of care. The purpose of this chapter is to describe the postoperative rehabilitation following internal fixation after hip fracture along a trajectory.

Surgical Overview

- Rehabilitation following femoral neck, intertrochanteric, and subtrochanteric hip fractures that were surgically repaired using an open/closed reduction and internal fixation is discussed in this chapter.
- The femoral neck fracture is a fracture that occurs proximal to the intertrochanteric line in the intracapsular region of the hip and is classified as nondisplaced or minimally displaced.
  1. Nondisplaced or minimally displaced femoral neck fractures are commonly repaired using cannulated screws.
  2. Cannulated (hollow) screws are typically inserted through fluoroscopy-aided placement for nondisplaced or minimally displaced fractures through a limited or percutaneous lateral approach.
     - The hollow screws are placed over thin wires, which are removed from the screws after bone alignment has been made.
     - Using this approach, the subcutaneous fat, vastus lateralis, and deep fascia of the fascia lata are affected.
- An intertrochanteric fracture is a fracture that occurs between the greater and lesser trochanter along the intertrochanteric line outside the capsule and is classified as stable or unstable.

1. The intertrochanteric region connects the femoral shaft and femoral neck at an angle of about 130 degrees. This angular moment created by weight bearing is greatest at this angle.
2. The most common instrumentation used for a stable intertrochanteric fracture is a sliding compression screw and side plate.
3. The instrumentation holds the bone fragments in their proper position while fracture healing occurs.
   - A lateral approach is used, violating skin, subcutaneous tissue, fascia lata, vastus lateralis fascia, and muscle belly.
   - Using this type of instrumentation, the distance is shortened between the insertion of the hip abductors in the greater trochanter and the center of rotation of the hip, which creates a mechanical disadvantage for the abductors. This may lead to a Trendelenburg gait pattern.
- A subtrochanteric fracture is a fracture that occurs between the lesser trochanter and the adjacent proximal third of the femoral shaft and may extend proximally to the intertrochanteric region.
  1. Subtrochanteric fractures have been extremely difficult to fix because of the extreme angular force in the subtrochanteric region.
  2. The bone type in the subtrochanteric region is cortical. Cortical bone has poor blood supply and decreased osteogenic activity; therefore, the two preferred methods of fixation are an extended compression screw device and intermedullary nail.
  3. Fixation using a Richards compression screw-plate device is to repair a subtrochanteric fracture.
- The type of surgical intervention is determined by the severity, type, and location of the hip fracture.
  1. Four types of instrumentation are commonly used in surgical intervention following hip fracture.
  2. Internal fixation may be either open (ORIF) or closed (CRIF), bipolar hemiarthroplasty, hemiarthroplasty, or THA.
- Rehabilitation following THA was discussed in Chapter 1. This chapter focuses on the rehabilitation management of a hip fracture following open reduction and internal fixation.

- It is important for physical therapists to have an understanding of the phases of bone healing, as well as an understanding of the types of instrumentation and the principles of the fixation devices used in the surgical management of patients who have sustained a hip fracture. These concepts are pivotal because rehabilitation is guided by the phases of bone healing, type of fracture, and surgical procedure performed.
- Fixation devices used in fracture repair are either stress-sharing or stress-shielding devices.
  1. Stress sharing implies that the fixation device permits partial transmission of a load across the fracture site, and micromotion occurs at the fracture site, which induces secondary bone healing with callus formation.
  2. Examples of stress-sharing devices are rods, pins, and screws.
     - A dynamic hip screw was used in the repair of an intertrochanteric fracture.
     - The dynamic hip screw slides, causing micromotion at the fracture site and inducing secondary fracture healing.
     - Cannulated screws were used in the repair of a femoral neck fracture.
  3. Stress-shielding devices, such as the Gamma nail or Richards intermedullary hip screw, shield the fracture site from stress and transfer the stress to the rod, and primary bone healing occurs without callus.
- Regardless of the type of hip fracture or internal fixation performed, the principles of both fracture healing and rehabilitation are the same.

Rehabilitation Overview

- The rehabilitation goals following hip fracture are to have a successful outcome. A successful outcome is often defined as the return to prefracture level of function. This is a daunting task, because less than 50% of patients who have sustained a hip fracture do not return to their prefracture level of function.
- Following hip fracture, the following impairments are commonly seen: functional strength deficits, functional activity intolerance, impaired balance and coordination, decreased

walking speed, and decreased ability to perform activities of daily living (ADL).

- The goals of rehabilitation following hip fracture are to increase muscle strength, endurance, and balance coordination, in an effort to improve the ability to transfer, walk, stair climb, and perform ADL.

- According to the guide to physical therapist practice, for the practice pattern 4G: Impaired joint mobility, muscle performance, and range of motion (ROM) associated with fracture; and 4H: Impaired joint mobility, motor function, muscle performance, and ROM associated with joint arthroplasty relating to the International Classification of Disease 9 code 820 (fracture of the neck or femur), the expected numbers of therapy visits throughout the continuum of care range from 6 to 70 visits.

Postoperative Phase I: Hospitalization (Days 1 to 7)

GOALS
- Assisted transfers in and out of bed
- Assisted ambulation with walker
- Assisted lower body dressing
- Unassisted upper body dressing
- Ability to cover a distance of 100 feet with walker in 6 minutes
- Ability to score 5/28 on Tinetti gait and balance
- Gait speed of 0.60 feet per second
- A score of 75 seconds on the timed "get-up and go" test
- Independent with bedside exercise program

PRECAUTIONS
- Femoral neck
  1. Protected weight bearing, if fracture is unstable
  2. Avoid passive ROM on fractures that have been reduced
- Intertrochanteric fracture
  1. Protected weight bearing, if fracture is unstable
  2. Avoid passive ROM on fractures that have been reduced
  3. Avoid strengthening the adductors because of increased stress at the fracture site
- Subtrochanteric
  1. Protected weight bearing, if fracture is unstable

Continued

Postoperative Phase I: Hospitalization (Days 1 to 7)—Cont'd

2. Avoid passive ROM on fractures that have been reduced
3. Avoid active adduction/abduction because of increased stress (torque on fracture site)
4. No isometric exercises to quadriceps or hamstrings (1 week)

TREATMENT STRATEGIES
- Bed mobility training
- Transfer training in and out of bed, on and off toilet
- Gait training with walker
- Regaining muscle control of the operated limb through hip, knee, and active ankle ROM; isometric exercises such as quadriceps and gluteal sets
- Prevention of pressure ulcers, specifically on the heel, through positioning or pressure-relieving device
- Upper extremity strengthening
- ADL retraining

CLINICAL CRITERIA FOR ADVANCEMENT
- Patients are typically discharged to a subacute facility when independence in bed mobility, transfers, and ambulation have not been achieved.
- Gait progression from assisted ambulation with rollator walker to unassisted ambulation with rollator walker
- Weight bearing is advanced, depending on stability of fracture.

Postoperative Phase II: Patients Who Remain on a Walker and Do Not Advance to a Cane (Weeks 2 to 6)

GOALS
- Independent transfers in and out of bed
- Independent transfers on and off toilet
- Independent ambulation with wheeled walker
- Independent lower body dressing
- Increase active ROM (AROM) of hip to 90 degrees (for sitting)
- Independent with bedside exercise program

(Week 2)

Ability to ambulate 150 feet with wheeled walker during six-minute walk test

Ability to score 7/28 on Tinetti gait and balance

Gait speed of 0.46 feet per second

Timed "up and go" test of 60 seconds

(Week 3)

Ability to ambulate 225 feet with wheeled walker during 6-minute walk test

Ability to score 9/28 on Tinetti gait and balance

Gait speed of 0.63 feet per second

Timed "up and go" test of 55 seconds

(Week 4)

Ability to ambulate 270 feet with wheeled walker during 6-minute walk test

Ability to score 12/28 on Tinetti gait and balance

Gait speed of 0.75 feet per second

Timed "up and go" test of 49 seconds

(Week 5)

Ability to ambulate 340 feet with wheeled walker during 6-minute walk test

Ability to score 14/28 on Tinetti gait and balance

Gait speed of 0.94 feet per second

Timed "up and go" test score of 43 seconds

(Week 6)

Ability to ambulate 500 feet with wheeled walker during 6-minute walk test

Ability to score 16/28 Tinetti gait and balance

Gait speed of 1.40 feet per second

Timed "up and go" test score of 32 seconds

PRECAUTIONS
- Femoral neck fracture
  1. Passive hip ROM for 6 to 8 weeks
- Intertrochanteric fracture
  1. Muscle strengthening of the adductors causes stress to the fracture siteimplant: avoid strengthening until fracture is stable
  2. Torsion or twisting at the fracture site (6 weeks)
  3. Passive hip ROM (6 to 8 weeks)
  4. *Caution should be used when prescribing strengthening exercises to patients who are not full weight bearing.*

Continued

Postoperative Phase II: Patients Who Remain on a Walker and Do Not Advance to a Cane (Weeks 2 to 6)—Cont'd

- Subtrochanteric fracture
  1. No adduction/abduction to hip (2 weeks)

TREATMENT STRATEGIES
- Stair training using bilateral upper extremity support nonreciprocally
- Outdoor ambulation on variable surfaces using wheeled walker
- Gait speed >1.18 feet per second to cross 33 feet of city street
- AROM of hip in supine, standing, side-lying, and prone if tolerated
- Strengthening exercises using cuff weights (1 repetition max.—60%)
- Strengthening exercises using elastic tubing exercises in supine, sitting
- Balance retraining/perturbation activities on unleveled surfaces (foam/carpet) with bilateral upper extremity support
- Isotonic exercise machines
- Kinetron, Nu-Step
- KAT, balance board with bilateral upper extremity support
- Progressive resistive exercises and functional activities

Postoperative Phase II: Patients Who Advance to a Cane (Weeks 2 to 6)

GOALS
- Independent transfers in and out of bed
- Independent transfers on and off toilet
- Independent ambulation with cane on level surfaces
- Independent ambulation with cane on variable surfaces
- Independent lower body dressing
- Increase AROM of hip to 90 degrees (for sitting)
- Independent with bedside exercise program

(Week 2)

Ability to ambulate 260 feet with cane during 6-minute walk test

Gait speed of 0.72 feet per second
Timed "up and go" test score of 36 seconds
Tinetti gait and balance score of 10/28
(Week 3)
Ability to ambulate 400 feet with cane during 6-minute walk test
Gait speed of 1.11 feet per second
Timed "up and go" test score of 34 seconds
Tinetti gait and balance score of 12/28
(Week 4)
Ability to ambulate 410 feet with cane during 6-minute walk test
Gait speed of 1.14 feet per second
Timed "up and go" test score of 30 seconds
Tinetti gait and balance score of 15/28
(Week 5)
Ability to ambulate 460 feet with cane during 6-minute walk test
Gait speed of 1.28 feet per second
Timed "up and go" test score of 27 seconds
Tinetti gait and balance score of 17/28
(Week 6)
Ability to ambulate 550 feet with wheeled walker during 6-minute walk test
Gait speed of 1.53 feet per second
Timed "up and go" test score of 24 seconds
Tinetti gait and balance score of 19/28

PRECAUTIONS
- Femoral neck fracture
  1. Passive hip ROM for 6 to 8 weeks
- Intertrochanteric fracture
  1. Muscle strengthening of the adductors causes stress to the fracture site and implant: avoid strengthening until fracture is stable
  2. Torsion or twisting at the fracture site (6 weeks)
  3. Passive hip ROM (6 to 8 weeks)
  4. *Caution should be used when prescribing strengthening exercises to patients who are not full weight bearing.*
- Subtrochanteric fracture
  1. No adduction/abduction to hip (2 weeks)

Continued

Postoperative Phase II: Patients Who Advance to a Cane (Weeks 2 to 6)—Cont'd

TREATMENT STRATEGIES
- Stair training using unilateral upper extremity support and cane reciprocally
- Outdoor ambulation on variable surfaces using cane
- Gait speed >1.18 feet per second to cross 33 feet of city street
- AROM of hip in supine, standing, side-lying, and prone if tolerated
- Strengthening exercises using cuff weights (1 repetition max.—60%)
- Strengthening exercises using elastic tubing exercises in standing
- Balance retraining/perturbation activities on unleveled surfaces (foam/carpet) with unilateral upper extremity support
- Isotonic exercise machines
- Kinetron
- Nu-Step
- Kinesthetic awareness trainer with unilateral upper extremity support
- Heel rises
- Progressive resistive exercises and functional activities

CLINICAL CRITERIA FOR ADVANCEMENT
- Independent ambulation without a device on leveled and variable surfaces
- Able to perform balance activities without external support

Postoperative Phase III (Weeks 12 to 26)

GOALS
(Week 12)
Ability to ambulate 862 feet during 6-minute walk test
Timed "up and go" score of 16 seconds
Gait speed of 2.4 feet per second
Functional reach test score of 9 inches

(Week 28)
Ability to ambulate 980 feet during 6-minute walk test
Gait speed of 2.7 feet per second
Timed "up and go" test score <13 seconds
Functional reach test score of 10 inches

PRECAUTIONS
If femoral neck, intertrochanteric, subtrochanteric fractures are generally healed, precautions are lifted.

TREATMENT STRATEGIES
- Stair training without upper extremity support nonreciprocally
- Outdoor ambulation on variable surfaces without device
- Gait speed >1.74 feet per second
- Stationary bicycle
- Isotonic hip and knee machines
- Isokinetic machines
- Kinetron
- Nu-Step
- Balance Master
- Progressive resistive exercises and functional activities in preparation for return to sport

Bibliography

Alarcon, T., Gonzalez-Montalvo, J.I., Barcena, A., Saez, P. Further Experience of Nonagenarians with Hip Fractures. *Injury* 2001; 32:555-558.

Clancy, T., Kitchen, S., Churchill, P., Covingto, D., Hundley, J., Maxwell, J.G. DRG Reimbursement: Geriatric Hip Fractures in the Community Hospital Trauma Center. *South Med J* 1998;91: 457-461.

Coleman, E.A., Kramer, A.M., Kowalsky, J.C., Eckhoff, D., Lin, M., Hester, E.J., Morgenstern, N., Steiner, J.F. A Comparison of Functional Outcomes After Hip Fracture in Group/Staff HMOs and Fee-for-Service Systems. *Eff Clin Pract* 2000;3:229-239.

Eastwood, E.A., Magaziner, J., Wang, J., Silberzweig, S.B., Hannan, E.L., Strauss, E., Siu, A.L. Patients with Hip Fracture: Subgroups and Their Outcomes. *J Am Geriatr Soc* 2002;50:1240-1249.

Fitzgerald, J., Moore, P., Dittus, R. The Care of Elderly Patients with Hip Fracture: Changes Since Implementation of the Prospective Payment System. *N Engl J Med* 1988;319:1392-1397.

Guccione, A.A., Fagerson, T.L., Anderson, J.J. Regaining Functional Independence in the Acute Care Setting Following Hip Fracture. *Phys Ther* 1996;76:818-826.

Guide to Physical Therapist Practice. *Phys Ther* 2001;77: 1163-1650.

Harada, N.D., Chun, A., Chiu, V., Pakalniskis, A. Patterns of Rehabilitation Utilization After Hip Fracture in Acute Hospitals and Skilled Nursing Facilities. *Med Care* 2000;38:1119-1130.

Jette, A.M., Harris, B.A., Cleary, P.D., Campion, E.W. Functional Recovery After Hip Fracture. *Arch Phys Med Rehabil* 1987; 68:735-740.

McRae, R. Practical Fracture Treatment, 3rd ed. Churchill Livingstone, New York, 1994.

Morris, A., Zuckerman, J. National Consensus Conference on Improving the Continuum of Care for Patients with Hip Fracture. Washington, DC, 2001.

National Center for Health Statistics. Health, United States, with Health and Aging Chartbook. Hyattsville, MD, National Center for Health Statistics, 1999.

Ray, W., Griffin, M., Baugh, D. Mortality Following Hip Fracture Before and After Implementation of the Prospective Payment System. *Arch Intern Med* 1990;150:2109-2114.

Studenski, S., Duncan, P.W. Measuring Rehabilitation Outcomes. *Clin Geriatr Med* 1993;9:823-830.

Wheeless' Textbook of Orthopaedics. Available online at http://www.medmedia.com/oo1/238.htm. Accessed 23 Jan, 2006.

CHAPTER *7*

Elbow Fractures and Dislocations

Aviva Wolff, OTR/L, CHT

The elbow joint consists of three bones: the distal humerus, olecranon, and radial head. Elbow trauma can result in a simple one-bone fracture or a complex fracture/dislocation involving a combination of bones. These injuries vary by the bones and structures involved and the extent of the injury. Elbow dislocations occur in isolation or along with a fracture. Both fractures and dislocations often include concomitant soft tissue injury, such as ligament, muscle, or nerve.

Seven percent of all fractures are elbow fractures, and one third of those involve the distal humerus. The mechanism of injury is a posterior force directed at the flexed elbow, often a fall to an outstretched hand, or axial loading of an extended elbow.

Thirty-three percent of all elbow fractures occur in the radial head and neck by axial loading on a pronated forearm, with the elbow in more than 20 degrees of flexion. Radial head fractures are often associated with ligament injuries. Radial head fractures that are associated with interosseous membrane disruption and distal radial ulnar joint dislocation are termed *Essex-Lopresti lesions.*

Twenty percent of elbow fractures occur in the olecranon as a result of direct impact or a hyperextension force. When the

49

radial head dislocates anteriorly along with an ulnar fracture, the result is a *Monteggia* fracture. Another common fracture location along the proximal ulna is the *coronoid process.*

Anatomic Overview

- The elbow joint is composed of three complex articulations: ulna-humeral, radio-capitellar, and proximal radio-ulnar.
- The joint capsule is thin, translucent, and has an exaggerated response to injury.
- The radial head, along with the medial and lateral ligaments, plays a major role in the stability of the elbow joint by preventing dislocation.
- The joint is highly congruent and has limited joint play.
- The elbow is particularly prone to contracture and stiffness because of the high congruity, multiple articulations, and the close relationship of ligaments and muscle to the joint capsule.
- Types of fixation range from rigid to tenuous.
  1. *Rigid* fixation allows early active and passive motion with minimal pain.
  2. *Stable* fixation allows early protected motion.
  3. *Tenuous* fixation requires delayed protected mobilization.

Rehabilitation Overview

- General rehabilitation goals are to restore motion and strength for optimal function while protecting injured and repaired structures and preventing joint stiffness.
  1. The trend in rehabilitation has been toward early mobility with less immobilization.
  2. The greatest challenge facing therapists is determining the balance between mobility and stability.
  3. Often, attention is given to mobility and strength at the expense of stability and comfort, but clinicians must consider mobility and stability of equal importance and not strive for progress in one while sacrificing gains in the other.
- Range of motion (ROM) is initiated as early as possible within safe parameters to prevent the development of stiffness.

1. In cases where fractures and dislocations are considered unstable, ROM should not be ignored, but rather delayed or performed in a protective position.

• The following guideline outlines appropriate treatment to restore joint motion and function after elbow fractures, while avoiding damage to repaired and injured structures. The phases of wound healing are correlated to treatment so that techniques are used appropriately to augment healing and avoid inflammation.

Postoperative Phase I: Inflammation/Protection (Weeks 0 to 2)

GOALS
• Protective immobilization
• Edema and pain control
• Full ROM in uninvolved joints
• Active/active assisted ROM (A/AAROM) of elbow within safe parameters
• Awareness and understanding of repair process and precautions
• Independence in home exercise program (HEP)

PRECAUTIONS
• Exercise only within safe prescribed arc
• Monitor pressure areas over posterior aspect of elbow from prolonged splinting
• No passive manipulation or stretching
• No aggressive motion, which can cause inflammation and pain
• Avoid neurovascular compromise

TREATMENT STRATEGIES
Protection Options
• Custom thermoplastic splint
  1. Adequate padding over the olecranon, medial/lateral epicondyles, and ulnar styloid
Pin and Wound Care for Open Reduction, Internal Fixation and Closed Reduction, External Fixation
• Solution of 50% hydrogen peroxide and sterile water daily to pin sites
• Standard sterile wound care procedures to open reduction, internal fixation

Continued

Postoperative Phase I: Inflammation/ Protection (Weeks 0 to 2)—Cont'd

- Use of nonadherent dressing with minimal bulk to allow for early motion

Edema/Pain Management

- Elevation, correct positioning, cryotherapy, light compression wrap (Ace bandage), safe early active ROM

Uninvolved Joint ROM

- Hand: tendon gliding (full composite flexion to distal palmar crease), thumb all planes
- Wrist: physician approval required, gravity eliminated flexion, extension, deviation
- Shoulder: in supine, wearing splint, AAROM exercises— all planes
- Avoid use of sling or posturing in the sling position

Elbow ROM

Only appropriate for stable fractures/dislocations and within limits of repaired structures

- Removal of splint to allow early AAROM exercises
- Exercise only in safe prescribed arc, in gravity-eliminated or gravity-assisted positions
- Forearm pronation/supination if permitted

CRITERIA FOR ADVANCEMENT

- Clinical union at fracture site or stability via surgical fixation
- Joint stability throughout full arc of motion at ulna/ humeral and radio-ulnar joints

Postoperative Phase II: Fibroblastic/ Fracture Stability (Weeks 2 to 8)

GOALS

- Maximize active/passive ROM of the elbow and forearm in a pain-free range
- Control of edema and inflammation
- Decrease scar adherence
- Increase distal strength and proximal stabilization strength
- Improved muscle-tendon unit length
- Return to light, functional tasks with use of involved extremity

PRECAUTIONS
- Full arc active/passive ROM with doctor approval
- Monitor response to ROM: avoid inflammatory episodes and/or exacerbation of pain
- No dynamic elbow splinting
- Monitor for early forearm and/or elbow joint contractures
- No grade III or IV joint mobilization
- No resistive exercises or activities

TREATMENT STRATEGIES

Protection
- Use thermoplastic splint for travel, sleep, or at-risk activities
- D/C sling, avoid posturing in "sling" position

ROM Program
- Active, active-assisted, and gentle passive ROM exercises, against gravity
- Emphasize total end range time over several repetitions
- Gentle distraction, grades I and II joint mobilizations only
- Use of moist heat before exercising, heat on stretch
- Contract/relax exercises
- Biofeedback and/or neuromuscular electrical stimulation

Edema Control
- Cold pack, retrograde massage, moist heat before retrograde massage, light compression wrapping or sleeve, overhead ROM exercises

Scar Management
- Scar massage and silicone gel sheeting following removal of sutures/staples and complete closure of the wound
- Decrease scar adherence with cross-friction massage at scar interface
- Deep muscle massage to flexor/extensor muscle groups
- Compression sleeves (Tubigrip) to minimize hypertrophic scarring

Light, Functional Activities
- Restoration of normal movement patterns and encouraged use of extremity for light activities of daily living
- Encourage functional splinting (holding phone to increase flexion, swinging arm while walking, and/or using keyboard)
- Proprioceptive neuromuscular facilitation patterns encouraged

Continued

**Postoperative Phase II: Fibroblastic/
Fracture Stability (Weeks 2 to 8)—Cont'd**

CRITERIA FOR ADVANCEMENT
• Evidence of radiographic union or confirmation by doctor
  of fracture, joint, and repaired structures to withstand
  resistance/stress

**Postoperative Treatment Phase III: Scar
Maturation and Fracture Consolidation
(Week 8 to Month 6)**

GOALS
• Full functional ROM
• Full functional strength and endurance
• Full participation in all functional activities, work, and
  leisure

PRECAUTIONS
• Hard end feel indicating a bony or hardware block; notify
  physician
• Failure of hardware, joint incongruity
• Nonunion or malunion
• Progressive resistive exercise (PRE) is contraindicated if
  patient is unable to isolate specific muscle group

TREATMENT STRATEGIES
Strategies
ROM Program
• Focus on end range parameters and quality of motion
• Continue previous exercises; goal: passive ROM=active
  ROM
Strength and Endurance
• PRE to all muscle groups
• Free weights, wall pulleys, Thera-Band, weight well,
  multi-upper limb exercises (MULEs), Baltimore
  therapeutic equipment, proprioceptive neuromuscular
  facilitation patterns with resistance
Splinting Program
• Continue splinting program overnight and intermittently
  during the day
• Upgrade splint parameters to passive end range
  position
• Continue functional splinting throughout the day

Return to Function
- Encourage return to activities of daily living, work, and leisure activities
- Activity analysis
- BTE

CRITERIA FOR DISCHARGE
- Achieved full or functional ROM and strength
- Returned to previous level of function
- Independence in home exercise program and splinting program
- Progress has plateaued, and status has not changed over 6 weeks

Bibliography

Barenholtz, A., Wolff, A. Elbow Fractures and Rehabilitation. *Orthop Phys Ther Clin North Am* 2001;10:525-539.

Cabanela, M.F., Morrey, B. Fractures of the Olecranon. In Morrey, B. (Ed). The Elbow and Its Disorders, 3rd ed. WB Saunders, Philadelphia, 2000, p. 365.

Hotchkiss, R. Fractures and Dislocations of the Elbow. In Rockwood, C., Green, D.P. (Eds). Rockwood and Green's Fractures in Adults, 4th ed. Lippincott-Raven, Philadelphia, 1996, p. 929.

Hotchkiss, R., Davila, S. Rehabilitation of the Elbow. In Morrey, B., Nickel, V.N. (Eds). Orthopedic Rehabilitation. Churchill Livingstone, New York, 1992, p. 157.

Jupiter, J., Morrey, B. Fractures of the Distal Humerus in Adults. In Morrey, B. (Ed). The Elbow and Its Disorders, 3rd ed. WB Saunders, Philadelphia, 2000, p. 293.

Morrey, B. Anatomy of the Elbow Joint. In Morrey, B. (Ed). The Elbow and Its Disorders, 3rd ed. WB Saunders, Philadelphia, 2000, p. 13.

Morrey, B. Radial Head Fractures. In Morrey, B. (Ed). The Elbow and Its Disorders, 3rd ed. WB Saunders, Philadelphia, 2000, p. 341.

Regan, W. Coronoid Process and Monteggia Fractures. In Morrey, B. (Ed). The Elbow and Its Disorders, 3rd ed. WB Saunders, Philadelphia, 2000, p. 396.

CHAPTER 8

Radial Head Replacement

Aviva Wolff, OTR/L, CHT

Elbow Stability

In the normal elbow, stability is provided by the bony anatomy, ligaments, and muscle forces surrounding the joint. The joint surfaces are highly congruent, thus contributing to the overall stability. The biceps and brachialis create a posterior force vector at the elbow, which is counteracted by the coronoid and radial head creating a joint reaction force at the elbow. Stability is further provided by the medial and lateral ligament complexes and the anterior capsule. Historically, much attention has been devoted to the role of the medial collateral ligament, but in recent years, descriptions of the anatomy of the lateral ligament complex have been discussed, expanded, and studied. Sojberg et al. have further studied the role of the lateral ligament complex in elbow stability. The findings of these investigators indicate that the lateral ligament complex, specifically the lateral ulnar collateral ligament, is a major stabilizer of the elbow joint. Elbow instability results when these structures are injured or disrupted.

Elbow Instability

Elbow instability results from a dislocation of the ulnohumeral joint and injury to the varus and valgus stabilizers of the elbow and the radial head. This injury often results from a forceful fall on an outstretched hand. The impact drives the head of the radius into the capitellum of the humerus, which may result in radial head and coronoid process fracture, medial collateral, posterolateral, and/or lateral collateral ligament disruption. When all of the previous structures are injured, the condition is described as the "terrible triad."

Surgical/Medical Management

- The surgical treatment of complex unstable elbow injuries may include titanium radial head replacement, open reduction internal fixation to the radial head, primary repair of the posterolateral ligament, and open reduction internal fixation to the ulnohumeral joint.
- Nonsurgical treatment in the form of immobilization may be appropriate in less complex injuries.
- Radial head excision vs radial head replacement has long been debated among surgeons.
  1. Radial head replacements have evolved over the years to include a metallic head, silicone head, allograft head, and most recently the titanium head replacement.
  2. The titanium head replacement has been used effectively in the treatment of complex radial head fractures and fracture dislocations.
- The annular ligament is repaired surgically to reinforce lateral stability of the elbow.

Postoperative Phase I: Inflammation/ Protection (Weeks 0 to 3)

GOALS
- Maintain stability of the elbow in a *safe position* elbow splint
- Begin early, protective range of motion (ROM) exercises to the elbow and forearm in a *safe overhead position* to avoid joint stiffness
- Minimize edema of the hand
- Maintain active ROM (AROM) of the uninvolved joints

PRECAUTIONS
- Maintain the shoulder position in neutral to external rotation and the forearm in pronation to avoid stress to the lateral elbow when the patient is not in the splint or performing the specific exercises described below

Continued

Postoperative Phase I: Inflammation/ Protection (Weeks 0 to 3)—Cont'd

TREATMENT STRATEGIES
Protective Immobilization
- Choice is based on surgeon's preference, therapists, experience, and specific injury
- Posterior elbow shell or Bledsoe brace

Early Protected Motion
- Protected active and active-assisted elbow and forearm ROM exercises performed in a supine overhead position
- Protected forearm supination
- Protected elbow extension: maintain full pronation throughout ROM at the elbow

ROM Exercises
- AROM exercises to the uninvolved joints
- Active and active-assisted ROM shoulder forward flexion and abduction are performed in supine with the splint on
- Active and active-assisted wrist ROM exercises and hand tendon gliding exercises

Edema Control and Wound Care
- Standard wound care procedures and edema management is followed

CRITERIA FOR ADVANCEMENT
- Joint stability determined by the surgeon

Postoperative Phase II: Fibroplastic/Early Remodeling (Weeks 3 to 6)

GOALS
- Wean from splint over a 2- to 6-week time period
- Initiate scar management
- Achieve full AROM of the elbow and forearm
- Begin gentle grip and wrist strengthening
- Initiate light activities of daily living (ADL)

PRECAUTIONS
- The shoulder is positioned in slight external rotation during exercises to avoid stress to the lateral ligaments of the elbow
- Passive ROM for elbow extension and for forearm supination is avoided

TREATMENT STRATEGIES
Splint Adjustment and Management
- The posterior elbow shell splint is adjusted to 90 degrees of flexion and the forearm in neutral rotation
- The splint is weaned from the patient during the day for self-care and light ADL
- Splinting is continued for sleeping and for protection

Scar Management
- Scar massage is initiated when the wound is fully healed
- Silicone gel sheet or otoform is provided for use at night

Active/Active-Assisted and Passive ROM Exercises
- Phase II ROM exercises are performed in sitting or standing
- Active and active-assisted ROM for elbow extension and forearm pronation is progressed as tolerated

Gentle Grip and Wrist-Strengthening Exercises
- Wrist PREs using 1-pound and 2-pound weights for forearm pronation and elbow flexion at 4 weeks
- Grip strengthening: isometrics, putty, and hand-helper exercises may be initiated gradually

CRITERIA FOR ADVANCEMENT
- Joint stability determined by surgeon

Postoperative Phase III: Scar Maturation (Weeks 6 to 12)

GOALS
- To achieve full active and passive elbow and forearm ROM
- To achieve functional upper extremity strength
- Independence in ADL and other activities

TREATMENT STRATEGIES
ROM Exercises
- Prolonged end range stretching for elbow flexion and extension, forearm supination, and pronation
- Combined elbow extension and forearm supination active and passive ROM exercises
- Static progressive elbow and forearm splints to achieve end ROM

Continued

**Postoperative Phase III: Scar Maturation
(Weeks 6 to 12)—Cont'd**

Progressive Resistive Exercises
- Elbow flexion/extension: Thera-Band exercises, dumbbell progressive resistive exercises
- Wrist and forearm: Thera-Band and dumbbell progressive resistive exercises
- Grip strengthening: hand-helper and putty exercises

Functional and Sports-Specific Activities Training

Bibliography

An, K., Morrey, B.F. Biomechanics of the Elbow. In Morrey, B.F. (Ed). The Elbow and Its Disorders. WB Saunders, Philadelphia, 2000.

Beredjiklian, P.K., Nalbantoglu, U., Potter, H.G., Hotchkiss, R.N. Prosthetic Radial Head Components and Proximal Radial Morphology: A Mismatch. *J Shoulder Elbow Surg* 1999;8:471-475.

Birkedal, J.P., Deal, D.N., Ruch, D.S. Loss of Flexion After Radial Head Replacement. *J Shoulder Elbow Surg* 2004;13:208-213.

Frankle, M.A., Koval, K.J., Sanders, R.W., Zuckerman, J.D. Radial Head Fractures Associated with Elbow Dislocations Treated by Immediate Stabilization and Early Motion. *J Shoulder Elbow Surg* 1999;8:355-360.

Furry, K.L., Clinkscales, C.M. Comminuted Fractures of the Radial Head: Arthroplasty versus Internal Fixation. *Clin Orthop Relat Res* 1998;353:40-42.

Gupta, G.G., Lucas, G., Hahn, D.L. Biomechanical and Computer Analysis of Radial Head Prostheses. *J Shoulder Elbow Surg* 1997;6:37-48.

Hotchkiss, R.N. Fractures and Dislocations of the Elbow. In Rockwood, C.A., Green, D.P., Bucholz, R.W., Heckman, J.D. (Eds). Rockwood and Green's Fractures in Adults. Lippincott, Philadelphia, 1996.

Hotchkiss, R.N., Kai-Nan, A., Sowa, D.T., Basta, S., Weiland, A.J. An Anatomic and Mechanical Study of the Interosseous Membrane of the Forearm: Pathomechanics of Proximal Migration of the Radius. *J Hand Surg* 1989;14A:256-261.

Morrey, B.F., An, K.N. Functional Anatomy of the Ligaments of the Elbow. *Clin Orthop* 1985;201:84.

O'Driscoll, S.W. Elbow Dislocations. In Morrey, B.F. (Ed). The Elbow and Its Disorders. WB Saunders, Philadelphia, 2000.

Sojberg, J.O., Ovesen, J., Nielsen, S. Experimental Elbow Stability After Transection of the Annular Ligament. *Arch Orthop Trauma Surg* 1987;106:248.

CHAPTER 9

Contracture Release of the Elbow

Aviva Wolff, OTR/L, CHT

Emily Altman, PT, DPT, CHT

Elbow contractures have many causes. The choice of intervention for the stiff elbow is dictated by the cause of stiffness and the specific pathophysiology. Posttraumatic stiffness following elbow fractures and dislocations is the most common cause of elbow contracture. Other causes include osteoarthritis or inflammatory arthritis, congenital or developmental deformities, burns, and head injury.

The elbow joint is prone to stiffness for several reasons. Anatomically, the joint is highly congruent. In most joints of the body, the *tendinous portions* of the muscles that act on the joint lie over the joint capsule. In the elbow, however, the brachialis muscle *belly* lies directly over the anterior joint capsule, making adhesion formation between the two structures inevitable following injury. The elbow is often held in 70 to 90 degrees of flexion postinjury because that is the position of greatest intracapsular volume for accommodation of edema. The thin joint capsule responds to trauma by thickening and becoming fibrotic, and quickly accommodating to this flexed position of the elbow. This results in a tethering of joint motion, particularly in the direction of extension. Biomechanically, the strong (and often co-contracting) elbow flexors overpower the weaker elbow extensors, which challenges the ability to regain extension. Last, the elbow joint is prone to heterotopic ossification following trauma and surgery.

Surgical Overview

- Elbow contractures are classified as intrinsic or extrinsic.
    1. *Extrinsic contractures* result from extra-articular pathology, involving the skin, neurovascular structures, joint

capsule, ligaments, muscle tendon units, and hetero-topic bone.

2. *Intrinsic contractures* result from intra-articular pathology, such as joint incongruity, fracture, deformity, and intra-articular heterotopic bone.

- Posttraumatic elbow contractures that are of short duration may respond well to conservative treatment.
- Typically, extrinsic contractures that are 6 to 12 months postinjury have minimal articular incongruity and a soft or firm end feel that will improve with therapy.
- When conservative intervention fails, surgical release is indicated. Surgical options for releasing the joint range from simple arthroscopy to the placement of hinged, external fixation (see Chapter 10).
- Arthroscopic release is generally reserved for patients with minimal joint stiffness, small osteophytes at the coronoid or olecranon, or loose bodies. The anterior joint capsule is well visualized arthroscopically.
- An open release is indicated for more involved cases that may require any one or combination of the following: anterior and posterior capsulectomy, ulnar nerve transposition, removal of large osteophytes, and removal of hardware.
  1. *The open release is performed via a medial, lateral, or posterior incision, or any combination of the three. The approach selected is determined by the type of contracture and location of pathology.*
     - The lateral approach is selected for simple flexion contractures, such as those that result from radial head fractures. The lateral approach is the most simple to perform, yet it provides the least exposure.
     - Situations that present with ulnar nerve involvement require medial exposure. A medial "over-the-top" approach has been advocated by Hotchkiss. This technique allows exposure of the joint, while protecting the ulnar nerve, anterior collateral ligament, and posterolateral ulnohumeral ligament complex. It also allows both anterior and posterior access to the joint.
     - If heterotopic bone is present on the lateral side, a combined medial and lateral approach is used.

- Heterotopic bone that is present on the olecranon warrants a posterior approach.

Rehabilitation Overview

- Rehabilitation following any type of elbow contracture release focuses on regaining functional, pain-free, active range of motion (ROM) of the elbow joint.
- Therapy must be initiated immediately after surgery, and the three members of the patient care team (surgeon, therapist, and patient) must work closely together for an optimal outcome.
- The treatment guidelines for arthroscopic and open contracture releases are similar conceptually, but arthroscopic releases generally require less intervention through all of the phases and progress more quickly.
- Patient compliance is crucial for a successful outcome. Patient selection by the surgeon and patient education by the surgeon and therapist is very essential. The patient must be an active participant in every aspect of his or her rehabilitation program.

Postoperative Phase I: Inflammatory Phase (Days 1 to 7)

GOALS
- Effective edema reduction
- Thorough patient education
- Independence in ROM home program
- Light functional use of the involved elbow and entire upper extremity (UE)

PRECAUTIONS
- Wound

TREATMENT STRATEGIES
- Comprehensive HEP for elbow and forearm active/active assisted ROM
- Shoulder active ROM (AROM)
- Elbow continuous passive motion (CPM) (generally for open releases only)
- Edema reduction: light compression, retrograde massage, elevation, ice

- Creative functional tasks that involve reaching and placing. Tasks should use the entire UE and can include the contralateral UE as well. Pegs, cones, clothespins, and rolling pins are useful tools. Some of these tasks may be too difficult for involved open releases.
- UBE and Nu-Step for endurance (for arthroscopic release)
- Pulleys for increased ROM
- Static progressive splinting for flexion, extension, pronation, and supination, as indicated

CRITERIA FOR ADVANCEMENT
- Wound closure
- Edema reduction
- Pain reduction
- Independence and compliance in comprehensive exercise and splinting program

Postoperative Phase II: Fibroplastic Phase (Weeks 2 to 6)

GOALS
- Full surgical wound closure
- Functional active elbow flexion/extension and forearm pronation/supination
- Pain <1/10
- Full use of involved UE for light functional activities of daily living

PRECAUTIONS
- Exacerbation of pain with overactivity
- Monitor for potential ulnar nerve irritation/compression/entrapment

TREATMENT STRATEGIES
- Active/active assisted/passive ROM (A/AA/PROM) elbow flexion/extension and forearm A/AA/PROM
- Shoulder AROM
- Home CPM (open releases only)
- Continued edema reduction: light compression, retrograde massage, elevation, ice

Continued

Postoperative Phase II: Fibroplastic Phase (Weeks 2 to 6)—Cont'd

- Creative functional tasks that involve reaching and placing. Tasks should use the entire UE and include the contralateral UE as well. Pegs, cones, clothespins, and rolling pins are useful tools.
- Upper body exercise (UBE) and Nu-Step recombent crosstrainer for endurance
- Pulleys for increased ROM
- Static progressive splinting for flexion, extension, pronation, and supination, as indicated
- Surface biofeedback for decreasing biceps co-contraction

CRITERIA FOR ADVANCEMENT
- No pain control issues
- Functional AROM
- Physician clearance

Postoperative Phase III: Scar Maturation Phase (Week 6 and Beyond)

GOALS
- Return to vocational and avocational tasks
- Obtain and maintain intraoperative elbow and forearm ROM
- Independence in comprehensive scapular, shoulder, elbow home exercise program or gym program

PRECAUTIONS
- Heterotopic ossification
- Ulnar nerve irritation/compression/entrapment

TREATMENT STRATEGIES
- Continue A/AA/PROM exercises
- Continue/progress endurance activities: Nu-Step, UBE
- Continue static and static progressive splinting
- Initiate elbow/forearm/shoulder/scapular strengthening with dumbbells and Thera-Band
- Progression to gym program if appropriate for individual

CRITERIA FOR DISCHARGE
- Independence in ROM and strengthening program appropriate for individual's activity level and the functional demands of his or her life
- Achievement and maintenance of intraoperative ROM
- No pain impairments

Bibliography

Griffith, A. Therapist's Management of the Stiff Elbow. In Griffith, A., Mackin, E.J., Skirven, T.M., Schneider, L.H. (Eds). Rehabilitation of the Hand and Upper Extremity, 5th ed. Mosby, St. Louis, 2002, pp. 1245–1262.

Hotchkiss, R. Elbow Contracture. In Hotchkiss, R., Green, D.P., Pederson, W.C. (Eds). Green's Operative Hand Surgery, 4th ed. Churchill Livingstone, New York, 1999, p. 667.

Mansat, P., Morrey, B., Hotchkiss, R.N. Extrinsic Contracture: "The Column Procedure," Lateral and Medial Capsular Release. In Morrey, B. (Ed). The Elbow and Its Disorders, 3rd ed. WB Saunders, Philadelphia, 2000.

CHAPTER 10

Hinged Dynamic External Fixation of the Elbow

Aviva Wolff, OTR/L, CHT

Emily Altman, PT, DPT, CHT

Flexion and extension contractures of the elbow are common complications following injury and trauma to the joint. Open contracture release, closed manipulation, and distraction arthroplasty are three options used to regain functional elbow range of motion (ROM) in the stiff elbow population.

Pain, swelling, and adaptive shortening of the soft tissue and muscle tendon unit can prevent a patient from maintaining the ROM obtained during these procedures. Unfortunately, the skilled use of comprehensive therapy, early active motion, static progressive splinting, and continuous passive motion (CPM) machines does not always guarantee success.

Surgical Overview

- Dynamic hinged external fixation offers a solution for cases that responded poorly to other methods of contracture release. It is defined as a hinged device that separates and distracts the ulna from the humerus while providing varus and valgus stability to the elbow. The hinged fixator allows active and passive motion of the elbow joint and stretches the soft tissue capsule at the end range of both flexion and extension.

- Currently, two dynamic hinged fixators are widely used: the Mayo dynamic joint distractor and the Hotchkiss compass hinge.

- Use of a dynamic fixator may be indicated in several situations, including acute trauma with complex instability, recurrent instability after collateral ligament release, contracted stiff elbow that is mature and has failed conservative therapy, extreme tightness in the muscle tendon unit following a capsular release, and posttraumatic arthritis of the elbow.

- Following a contracture release, the hinged device is applied to maintain the ROM gains achieved intraoperatively and provide elbow stability if it was compromised during the contracture release surgery.

- Application of the hinge allows scar tissue to remodel in an environment that permits joint distraction, joint stability, joint motion, and promotes the healing of the articular surface.

- Through smooth, progressive adjustments of the device while in its locked position, the soft tissue is maintained at its available end range. Motion is performed to condition the muscles with the hinge unlocked.

- Once the underlying pathology has been addressed via contracture release or resurfacing of the joint, the hinge is applied. In most trauma cases, a posterior incision is made and the joint is exposed medially and laterally, depending on the pathology.

- For a stiff elbow both a posterior and an anterior incision may be required for a complete capsular release.

- A temporary axis pin is placed through the distal humerus to align the hinge with the axis of rotation.

- The frame is preassembled so it can freely slide medial to lateral on the axis pin.

- Two humeral pins (medial and lateral) are placed to secure the humerus in two planes. Two pins are placed in the ulna anterior and posterior to the axis of rotation.

- Once all of the pins have been placed and the joint adequately reduced, distraction is applied.

- Both sides of the hinge should be distracted equally.

- Complications of dynamic hinged fixation include compression neuropathy of the ulnar nerve, pin tract infections, heterotopic ossification, pin fractures, and delayed healing.

Rehabilitation Overview

- Dynamic hinged fixators are used following complex elbow dislocation, traumatic elbow fracture, and complex contracture release.

- Despite the various indications for placing a dynamic hinge, the role of the hinge is always the same, that is, to stabilize the joint and permit immediate postoperative movement.
- The therapist must communicate with the surgeon and obtain the details of the original injury and the operative procedure, and confirm an appropriate plan of care.
- Thorough knowledge of exactly what structures were involved and/or repaired is crucial to managing the rehabilitation of these patients.
  1. Examples of common key pieces of information include ligament repair/reconstruction, vascular repair, nerve repair, ulnar nerve transposition, triceps/biceps tendon repair or protection issues, and joint and fracture stability.
  2. The therapist must also be aware of associated injuries of the shoulder and wrist.

Postoperative Phase I:
Inflammatory/Protective (Weeks 0 to 2)

GOALS
- Edema and pain control
- Full ROM of uninvolved joints
- Maximum passive elbow flexion and extension

PRECAUTIONS
- Ulnar nerve compression at elbow
- Pin tract infection

TREATMENT STRATEGIES
- Edema control: ice, elevation, compression
- Wound care, pin care (monitor for infection) draining is common (especially at the medial pin)
- Uninvolved joint ROM: emphasize forearm pronation/supination

SPLINTING
- Wrist support
- Extrinsic flexor/extensor stretcher (resting hand splints) as needed for night
- Sugar tong splint to position forearm in pronation in cases of extreme instability

ELBOW RANGE OF MOTION PROTOCOL
- Continuous axillary block for 24 to 48 hours
- Worm gear is turned in small increments for passive ROM (PROM)
- Postoperative day 1: patient instructed to turn worm gear in direction of extension gradually throughout the day and sleep in maximum tolerated extension
- Postoperative day 2: patient instructed to turn worm gear in direction of flexion gradually throughout the day and sleep in maximum tolerated flexion
- Postoperative day 3: flexion and extension are alternated several times during the day, and nighttime position is alternated between maximum flexion and extension for sleep, or patient is instructed to sleep in the position that is more limiting
- Postoperative day 4: submaximal elbow flexion and extension isometrics with the hinge locked

This program continues for 2 weeks.

Postoperative Phase II: Fibroplastic (Weeks 2 to 8)

GOALS
- Edema reduction
- Wound closure
- Full active ROM (AROM) of uninvolved joint
- Maximum active and passive elbow flexion and extension

PRECAUTIONS
- Ulnar nerve compression at the elbow
- Pin tract infection

TREATMENT STRATEGIES
- Wound care
- AROM elbow flexion and extension, forearm pronation and supination
- Uninvolved joint AROM
- Functional use of upper extremity for light activities of daily living (ADL)

SPLINTING
- As needed for:
  1. Wrist support

Continued

Postoperative Phase II: Fibroplastic (Weeks 2 to 8)—Cont'd

2. Maintenance of extrinsic forearm muscle length
3. Maintenance of elbow stability (forearm pronation)

ELBOW ROM PROTOCOL
- Continue passive ROM (PROM) protocol initiated in phase I
- Initiate AROM elbow flexion and extension (unlock hinge gear), beginning with 10 repetitions, four times a day and progressing to 50% to 70% of the day spent with the hinge unlocked
- Encourage functional use of the upper extremity

Postoperative Phase III: Scar Maturation (Weeks 6 to 8, Post-Hinge Removal)

GOALS
- Regain full functional use of the elbow
- Achieve full wound closure and promote mobile scars
- Achieve independence in comprehensive strengthening and conditioning home exercise program
- Obtain maximum elbow flexion and extension ROM

PRECAUTIONS
- Ulnar nerve compression neuropathy
- Heterotopic ossification
- Persistent joint contracture

TREATMENT STRATEGIES
- AROM, active assisted ROM (AAROM), PROM stretching
- Thermal modalities
- Soft tissue massage/mobilization
- Contract/relax techniques
- Functional use of upper extremity for all ADL
- Progressive resistive exercise
- Comprehensive serial static/static progressive splinting program
- General conditioning

SPLINTING
- Serial static night extension splint
- Static progressive elbow flexion/extension and forearm rotation splints

Bibliography

Griffith, A. Therapist's Management of the Stiff Elbow. In Callahan, A.D., Osterman, A.L., Mackin, E.J., Skirven, T.M., Schneider, L.H. (Eds). Rehabilitation of the Hand and Upper Extremity, 5th ed. Mosby, St. Louis, 2002, pp. 1245–1262.

Hotchkiss, R. Compass Universal Hinge: Surgical Technique. Smith and Nephew, Memphis, 1998.

Hotchkiss, R. Elbow Contracture. In Hotchkiss, R., Green, D.P., Pederson, W.C. (Eds). Green's Operative Hand Surgery, 4th ed. Churchill Livingstone, New York, 1999, p. 667.

Kasparyan, N.G., Hotchkiss, R. Dynamic Skeletal Fixation of the Upper Extremity. *Hand Clin* 1997;13:643.

Mckee, M., Bowden, M.D., King, G.J., Patterson, S.D., Jupiter, J.B., Bamberger, H.B., Paksima, N. Management of Recurrent Complex Instability of the Elbow with Hinged External Fixation. *J Bone Joint Surg Br* 1998;80:1031.

Morrey, B. Post-traumatic Operative Procedures of the Elbow. *J Bone Joint Surg* 1990;72:601.

Morrey, B.F., Hotchkiss, R. External Fixators of the Elbow. In Morrey, B.F. (Ed). The Elbow and Its Disorders, 3rd ed. WB Saunders, Philadelphia, 2000.

CHAPTER 11

Distal Radius Fractures

Coleen T. Gately, PT, DPT, MS

Epidemiologic studies indicate that distal radius fractures are the most common fractures of the forearm. The mechanism of injury usually involves a fall on an outstretched hand (FOOSH). Distal radius fractures resulting from this type of low-energy injury are more common than those sustained secondary to high-energy trauma, such as a motor vehicle accident. The incidence of distal radius fractures in the 35- to 64-year-old population is greater in women than men.

Surgical Overview

- The distal radius articulates with the ulna and proximal row of carpal bones. The radius, ulna, and carpal bones make up the wrist complex.
- The medical management of distal radius fractures varies depending on the extent of the injury.
  1. Common procedures include closed reduction with casting, closed reduction with external fixation (CREF), percutaneous pinning, open reduction with internal fixation (ORIF), or any combination of these techniques.
  2. Reduction may be combined with a graft, depending on the level of comminution or defect. The goal of reduction is to maintain the bone in alignment so that the fracture may heal properly.

Rehabilitation Overview

- As the fracture progresses through the phases of healing, the focus of rehabilitation is to help the patient regain functional use of the hand and upper extremity.

- The stability of the fracture, strength of fixation, and extent of soft tissue trauma will determine the progression of therapy in each phase of healing.
- Direct communication with the doctor is essential to define precautions and set realistic goals.
- Treatment is tailored to the specific needs of the patient and the type of fixation used.

Postoperative Phase I: Protective (Weeks 0 to 6)

GOALS
- Maintain correct protective immobilization
- Minimize edema and pain
- Maintain full range of motion (ROM) of uninvolved joints

PRECAUTIONS
- Obtain physician approval before beginning gentle forearm active ROM (AROM)
- Early motion of the shoulder is critical to prevent adhesive capsulitis
- Report early symptoms of complex regional pain syndrome to physician for early intervention

TREATMENT STRATEGIES
Protection Options
- Custom thermoplastic volar or bivalve wrist splint: 0- to 20-degree wrist extension; thenar crease and distal palmar crease are cleared to prevent thumb web space and metacarpophalangeal joint stiffness
Pin and Wound Care (for CREF, ORIF)
- Pin care regimens may vary: follow physician's specific protocol, for some may not request pin care at all (50% H_2O_2 and sterile water two times per day)
- Standard wound care procedures are followed for ORIF
Edema/Pain Management
- Elevation, rest, ice/cold, compression
- Light, compressive garment or wrap, that is, Isotoner gloves, Coban, Tubigrip stockinette
- Active overhead fisting
Uninvolved Joints ROM
- Tendon gliding exercises
- Hand intrinsic muscle exercises: lumbrical, interossei, thenar, and hypothenar muscles

Continued

Postoperative Phase I: Protective (Weeks 0 to 6)—Cont'd

- Differential tendon gliding exercises to prevent tendon adherence to the fracture site, hardware, or pins, that is, flexor digitorum superficialis, flexor digitorum profundus, extensor pollicis longus, flexor pollicis longus
- Elbow, shoulder ROM is initiated on postoperative day 1
- Gentle forearm rotation in a pain-free range with physician approval

Involved Joint ROM (for Stable/Rigid Fixation)
- Gentle wrist ROM: wrist flexion/extension, radial/ulnar deviation

CRITERIA FOR ADVANCEMENT
- Clinical union at fracture site or stability via surgical fixation

Postoperative Phase II: Stability (Weeks 6 to 8)

Note: Phase II may begin as early as postoperative week 2, if fracture stability is achieved through ORIF

GOALS
- Maximize ROM of the wrist and forearm in a pain-free range
- Restore light, functional use of the involved extremity
- Continue phase I goals as needed

PRECAUTIONS
- Fracture stability must be obtained through bony healing or surgical fixation before initiating wrist ROM or gentle joint mobilization techniques.

TREATMENT STRATEGIES
Protection Options
- Custom thermoplastic volar or bivalve wrist splint: remove for wound and skin care
- Splint is weaned based on fracture stability and bony healing, and following physician's orders.
- External fixator is removed; splinting may be necessary to allow further protection with gradual weaning.

SCAR MANAGEMENT

- Scar massage and silicone gel sheeting may be initiated once the wound is fully healed (to avoid infection).

EDEMA/PAIN MANAGEMENT

- Cold pack
- Retrograde massage
- Gentle heat or contrast baths may be used as edema becomes brawny.
- Light, compressive garment or wrap, that is, Isotoner gloves, Coban, and Tubigrip stockinette

AROM WRIST AND FOREARM

- Initiation of wrist and forearm active ROM (AROM) and gentle active assisted ROM
- Isolated wrist extension exercises are begun early to prevent assistance of the long finger extensors in wrist extension and promote a more functional grip.
- Forearm rotation is performed with the elbow in 90 degrees and the humerus close to the body to prevent substitution with shoulder rotation.
- Gentle distraction and grades I and II joint mobilizations may be initiated in this phase if fracture stability allows.

LIGHT FUNCTIONAL ACTIVITIES

- Fine motor coordination activities, that is, small object manipulation, writing, and typing
- Restoration of normal movement patterns and activities of daily living (ADL), such as eating, dressing, hygiene

CRITERIA FOR ADVANCEMENT

- Evidence of radiographic union or determination by physician of ability of fracture to withstand resistance/stress

Postoperative Phase III: Fracture Consolidation (Weeks 8 to 12)

GOALS

- Restore strength for return to functional activities and work
- Continue phase II goals as needed

Continued

Postoperative Phase III: Fracture Consolidation (Weeks 8 to 12)—Cont'd

PRECAUTIONS
- Progress strengthening exercises gradually, avoiding pain and compensations

TREATMENT STRATEGIES
Passive ROM (PROM) and Splinting
- PROM
  1. Example: prayer stretch
- Stretching
- Joint mobilization to achieve end range potential
- Serial static and static progressive splints to achieve end range potential
  1. Examples: serial static dorsal wrist extension splint, static progressive wrist splint, and static progressive pronation/supination splint

Strengthening
- Isometric and dynamic grip and pinch strengthening
- Examples: putty, hand-helper, Baltimore Therapeutic Equipment (BTE) PRIMUS, Biometrics Ltd., and multi-upper limb exercises (MULE)
- Wrist and forearm progressive resistant exercises
- Examples: gradual progression from weight well to Thera-Band to free weights
- Work conditioning: activity-specific functional activities, BTE
- Return to sport

CRITERIA FOR DISCHARGE
- Restoration of functional AROM and strength, and return to prior ADL, including work
- Independence in home exercise program

Bibliography

Alffram, P.A., Bauer, G.C. Epidemiology of Fracture of the Forearm: A Biomechanical Investigation of Bone Strength. *J Bone Joint Surg Am* 1962;44:105.

Benger, U., Johnell, O. Increasing Incidence of Forearm Fractures: A Comparison of Epidemiologic Patterns 25 Years Apart. *Acta Orthop Scand* 1985;56:158.

Melton, L.J. III, Amadio, P.C., Crowson, C.S., O'Fallon, W.M. Long-term Trends in the Incidence of Distal Forearm Fractures. *Osteoporos Int* 1998;4:341-348.

Owen, R.A., Melton, L.J. III, Johnson, K.A., Ilstrup, D.M., Riggs, B.L. Incidence of Colles' Fracture in North American Community. *Am J Public Health* 1982;72:605-607.

Seitz, W.H. Jr., Froimson, A.I. Reduction of Treatment Related Complications in the External Fixation of Complex Distal Radius Fractures. *Orthop Rev* 1991;2:169-177.

CHAPTER 12

Scaphoid Fractures

Coleen T. Gately, PT, DPT, MS

Of the eight carpal bones, the scaphoid is the most frequently fractured. Seventy-nine percent of all carpal fractures are scaphoid fractures. The mechanism of injury involves a high impact fall on an outstretched hand (FOOSH), with the wrist hyperextended and radially deviated. Scaphoid fractures are more common in young or active individuals and frequently result from contact sports.

Surgical Overview

- The scaphoid is divided anatomically into four parts: the proximal pole, waist, distal pole, and tuberosity.
- The majority of scaphoid fractures occur through the waist (70%), followed by the proximal pole (20%), with the least occurring at the distal pole (10%).
- Although 90% to 95% of scaphoid fractures will heal if treated adequately with immobilization, 5% to 10% result in a nonunion.
- Reduction of scaphoid fractures can be accomplished via several means, depending on the nature of the fracture.
  1. Immobilization in a cast is appropriate for a nondisplaced fracture.
  2. Fractures that are minimally displaced may be treated with closed reduction and percutaneous pinning (CRPP).
  3. Open reduction with internal fixation (ORIF) is performed for displaced fractures. Internal fixation options include Kirschner's wires, cannulated screws, or plating.
- The distal pole of the scaphoid has a rich blood supply in comparison to the proximal pole. Fractures at the scaphoid

waist can disrupt the blood supply to the proximal pole and contribute to avascular necrosis, delayed union, or nonunion.

- Because of the poor blood supply, proximal pole scaphoid fractures take between 12 and 14 weeks to heal and require prolonged immobilization. Therefore, ORIF with a cannulated screw is commonly used to allow for early mobilization even when adequate reduction can be achieved with a closed manipulation.

    1. Surgery may take place through a volar or dorsal approach.
    2. A cannulated screw inserted into a threaded washer provides compression across the fracture site to provide stability as it heals.
    3. A nonvascularized or vascularized bone graft may be used for complex fractures to accelerate bone healing.
    4. Bone healing may also be facilitated by using an electrical bone growth stimulator.
    5. The following rehabilitation guidelines have been developed for scaphoid fractures that have been reduced through ORIF.

Rehabilitation Overview

- The amount of surgical stability achieved, as well as the location of the scaphoid fracture, determine the rate of progression of therapy in each phase of healing.
- Direct communication with the doctor is essential to determine the location and stability of the fracture for appropriate therapeutic progression.

Postoperative Phase I: Protective (Weeks 0 to 4)

GOALS
- Correct protective immobilization
- Edema and pain control
- Full range of motion (ROM) of uninvolved joints

PRECAUTIONS
- Early motion of the shoulder is critical to prevent adhesive capsulitis.

Continued

Postoperative Phase I: Protective (Weeks 0 to 4)—Cont'd

TREATMENT STRATEGIES
Protective Immobilization
- Custom thermoplastic volar or bivalve forearm thumb spica splint: 0- to 20-degree wrist extension and thumb immobilized with interphalangeal joint free

Wound Care
- Standard wound care procedures are followed for ORIF.

Edema/Pain Management
- Elevation, rest, ice/cold
- Light, compressive garment or wrap, that is, Coban, Isotoner gloves, and Tubigrip stockinette

ROM of Uninvolved Joints
- Differential tendon gliding exercises, that is, flexor pollicis longus, extensor digitorum communis, flexor digitorum superficialis, flexor digitorum profundus
- Hand intrinsic muscle exercises, that is, interossei
- Elbow, forearm, and shoulder ROM exercises initiated postoperative day 1

CRITERIA FOR ADVANCEMENT
- Clinical union at fracture site or stability via surgical fixation

Postoperative Phase II: Stability (Weeks 4 to 16)

GOALS
- Maximize ROM of the forearm, wrist, and hand in a pain-free range
- Restore light, functional use of the involved extremity
- Continue phase I goals as needed

PRECAUTIONS
- Fracture stability must be obtained through bony healing or surgical fixation before initiating wrist ROM or gentle joint mobilization techniques.

TREATMENT STRATEGIES
Protection Options
- Thumb spica forearm splint is continued.

Scar Management
- Scar massage and silicone gel sheeting is initiated once the wound is fully healed (to avoid infection).

Edema/Pain Management
- Cold pack
- Retrograde massage
- Gentle heat or contrast baths may be used if edema becomes brawny.

Active ROM (AROM) Wrist
- Initiation of thumb ROM: opposition, MP flexion, abduction
- Initiation of wrist and forearm AROM: wrist flexion/extension, radial/ulnar deviation
- Progression to active assisted ROM and gentle passive ROM (PROM)
- To promote a more functional grip, isolated wrist extension exercises are begun early to prevent assistance of the long finger extensors in wrist extension.

Light, Functional Activities
- Fine motor coordination activities to promote thumb opposition: small object manipulation, writing, typing
- Restoration of normal movement patterns and return to activities of daily living: eating, dressing, hygiene

CRITERIA FOR ADVANCEMENT
- Evidence of radiographic union or determination by physician of ability of fracture to withstand resistance/stress

Postoperative Phase III: Fracture Consolidation (Weeks 8 to 21)

GOALS
- Restore strength for return to functional activities and work
- Continue phase II goals as needed

PRECAUTIONS
- Progress strengthening exercises gradually, avoiding pain and compensatory motion

Continued

Postoperative Phase III: Fracture Consolidation (Weeks 8 to 21)—Cont'd

TREATMENT STRATEGIES

PROM and Splinting

- PROM, stretching, and joint mobilization to achieve end range potential
- Serial static and static progressive splints to achieve end range potential
    1. Examples: static progressive wrist flexion or extension splint

Strengthening

- Isometric and dynamic grip and pinch strengthening: putty, hand-helper, Baltimore Therapeutic Equipment (BTE) PRIMUS, and Biometrics Ltd. upper and lower extremities
- Wrist and forearm progressive resistance exercises: dumbbells, weight well, Thera-Band
- Work conditioning: activity-specific training and BTE PRIMUS

CRITERIA FOR DISCHARGE

- Restoration of functional AROM and strength and return to prior level of function
- Independence in home exercise program

Bibliography

Albert, S.F. Electrical Stimulation of Bone Repair. *Clin Podiatr Med Surg* 1981;8:923-935.

Amadio, P.C. Scaphoid Fractures. *Clin Orthop North Am* 1992;23: 7-17.

Bora, F.W. Jr. Treatment of Nonunion of the Scaphoid by Direct Current. *Orthop Clin North Am* 1984;15:107-112.

dos Reis, F.B., Koeberle, G., Leite, N.M., Katchburian, M.V. Internal Fixation of Scaphoid Injuries Using the Herbert Screw Through a Dorsal Approach. *J Hand Surg* 1993;8A:792-797.

Dunn, A.W. Electrical Stimulation in Treatment of Delayed Union and Nonunion of Fractures and Osteotomies. *South Med J* 1984;77: 1530-1534.

Dunn, A.W. Fractures and Dislocations of the Carpus. *Surg Clin North Am* 1972;52:1513-1538.

Gelberman, R.H., Gross, M.S. The Vascularity of the Wrist. Identification of Arterial Patterns at Risk. *Clin Orthop Relat Res* 1986;202:40-49.

Gelberman, R.H., Menon, J. The Vascularity of the Scaphoid Bone. *J Hand Surg* 1980;5:508-513.

Herbert, T.J. Open Volar Repair of Acute Scaphoid Fractures. *Hand Clin* 2001;17:589-599.

Herbert, T.J., Fisher, W.E. Management of the Fractured Scaphoid Using a New Bone Screw. *J Bone Joint Surg* 1984;66:114-123.

Herndon, J.H. Scaphoid Fractures and Complications. American Academy of Orthopaedic Surgeons, Rosemont, IL, 1994.

Lichtman, D.M., Alexander, C.E. Decision Making in Scaphoid Nonunion. *Orthop Rev* 1982;11:55-67.

Melone, C.P. Scaphoid Fractures: Concepts of Management. *Clin Plast Surg* 1981;8:83-94.

Obletz, B.E., Halbstein, B.M. Non-union of Fractures of the Carpal Navicular. *J Bone Joint Surg* 1938;20:424-428.

O'Brien, L., Herbert, T. Internal Fixation of Acute Scaphoid Fracture: A New Approach to Treatment. *Aust N Z J Surg* 1985;55: 387-389.

Osterman, A.L., Mikulics, M. Scaphoid Nonunion. *Hand Clin* 1988;14:437-455.

Rettig, M.E., Raskin, K.B. Retrograde Compression Screw Fixation of Acute Proximal Pole Scaphoid Fractures. *J Hand Ther* 1999;24A: 1206-1210.

Schaefer, M., Siebert, H.R. Fractures of the Semilunar Bone. *Unfallchirurg* 2002;105:540-552.

Taleisnik, J. Fracture of the Carpal Bones. In Green, D.P. (Ed). Operative Hand Surgery, 2nd ed. Churchill Livingstone, New York, 1988.

Watson, H.K., Pitts, E.C., Ashmead, D. IV, Makhlouf, M.V., Kauer, J. Dorsal Approach to Scaphoid Nonunion. *J Hand Surg* 1993; 18:359-365.

Weber, E.R. Biomechanical Implications of Scaphoid Waist Fractures. *Clin Orthop Relat Res* 1980;149:83-89.

Weber, E.R., Chao, E.Y. An Experimental Approach to the Mechanism of Scaphoid Waist Fractures. *J Hand Surg* 1978;3A:142.

Phalangeal and Metacarpal Phalangeal Fractures

Carol Page, PT, DPT, CHT

Phalangeal and metacarpal fractures are among the most common fractures of the upper extremity. Chung reported that of all hand and forearm fractures reported in the United States in 1998, 23% were phalangeal and 18% were metacarpal. The highest rate of phalangeal fractures was in individuals age 85 and older. The highest rate of metacarpal fractures was found in 15- to 24-year-olds.

Surgical Overview

- The method of fracture management indicated depends on several variables, including fracture location, configuration, stability, whether the fracture is open or closed, and whether there are associated injuries.
- The primary goal of fracture management is proper bony alignment with adequate stability for safe, early motion, and restoration of hand function.
  1. Many phalangeal and metacarpal fractures are stable and can be treated with protective splinting and early mobilization.
  2. Unstable shaft fractures and many articular fractures require fixation to restore stability. Options for surgical fixation of unstable fractures include percutaneous pinning or open reduction with Kirschner's pin fixation, circumferential wiring, intramedullary fixation, compression screws, plate fixation, and external fixation.
- Distal phalanx fractures are the most common fractures in the hand.
  1. Tuft fractures and nondisplaced, stable fractures of the shaft are managed with extension splinting of the distal interphalangeal joint for 3 weeks.

2. Displaced, transverse shaft fractures require fixation with a Kirschner's pin or screw.

3. Injury to the nail matrix often occurs with open, displaced, transverse shaft fractures and with tuft fractures associated with crush injury.

4. Intra-articular fractures of the distal phalanx usually include avulsion of the extensor tendon insertion at the dorsal base (mallet injury), or of the flexor digitorum profundus (FDP) insertion at the volar base.

5. FDP avulsion injuries require surgical fixation, whereas mallet injuries do not, unless there is evidence of volar subluxation of the distal phalanx.

- Metacarpal neck fractures most frequently occur in the ring and small fingers. This common fracture, known as a boxer's fracture, occurs from striking a solid object with a closed fist.

  1. Metacarpal shaft fractures result from direct impact or axial loading through the metacarpal head.

  2. Metacarpal neck and shaft fractures that are stable are treated with closed reduction and immobilization.

  3. Fractures that are unstable, angulated, malrotated, open, or involve multiple metacarpals require surgical fixation.

- Phalangeal fractures of the thumb are treated similarly to those of the fingers.

  1. Surgery to restore stability is indicated for avulsion fractures with disruption of the ulnar collateral ligament (UCL) at the base of the proximal phalanx.

  2. Extra- and intra-articular fractures of the base of the thumb proximal phalanx are more common than metacarpal shaft fractures.

  3. Extra-articular base fractures are treated with closed reduction, with the addition of percutaneous pinning, if required to maintain the reduction.

  4. Fracture subluxation of the thumb metacarpal base, known as a Bennett's fracture, occurs with axial loading of the partially flexed thumb metacarpal. Treatment ranges from nonoperative management to closed or open surgical fixation.

Rehabilitation Overview

- The primary goal of rehabilitation of metacarpal and phalangeal fractures is to restore motion, strength, and functional use of the hand.
- For therapy to be progressed in a safe and timely manner, ongoing communication between the surgeon and therapist regarding the degree of stability and fracture healing is essential.
- Awareness of common complications facilitates early recognition and intervention. Complications of phalangeal and metacarpal fractures include malunion, nonunion, tendon adhesions, capsular contracture, and infection.
- The treatment guidelines that follow specifically address the postoperative management of fractures of the proximal and middle phalangeal shaft, metacarpal neck and shaft, and thumb metacarpal base. These guidelines may be used for fractures managed nonoperatively, with the time frames extended to allow for adequate stability via bony healing.
- Treatment of distal phalanx fractures that involve the disruption of the flexor or extensor tendons follows tendon management guidelines (see Chapters 14 and 15).
- Postoperative management of proximal interphalangeal (PIP) joint injuries, PIP joint arthroplasty, boutonnière reconstruction, and thumb UCL injuries are discussed elsewhere in this book.

Postoperative Phase I: Inflammation/ Protection (Week 1)

GOALS
- Protective immobilization
- Edema control
- Wound healing
- Full motion of uninvolved upper extremity joints

PRECAUTIONS
- Remold splints as edema diminishes for correct fit and positioning
- Accommodate and protect pins

- Avoid compressive gloves that apply uncontrolled forces to fracture during donning and doffing
- No motion of joints adjacent to fracture until stability is achieved through surgical fixation or clinical union

TREATMENT STRATEGIES

Protective Custom Thermoplastic Splint

- Middle and proximal phalanx fractures: hand-based ulnar gutter for middle, long, and small fingers, radial gutter for index finger (metacarpophalangeal [MP] joints flexed 70 to 80 degrees, interphalangeal [IP] joints fully extended); include adjacent finger(s)
- Metacarpal neck and shaft fractures: forearm-based ulnar gutter for middle, long, and small fingers, radial gutter for index metacarpal (wrist extended 20 degrees, MP joints flexed 70 to 80 degrees, IP joints free unless inclusion is specified); include adjacent finger(s)
- Alternative to gutter splints: volar-based splints with or without dorsal protective component
- Thumb metacarpal base fracture: forearm volar-based thumb spica (wrist extended 20 degrees, IP included or free, depending on fracture stability)

Edema Control

- Elevation
- Cold packs, light retrograde massage, and light compressive wraps if fracture is stable
- Active motion of uninvolved joints

Pin and Wound Care

- Pin care as per referring physician's instructions (keep dry, or daily cleaning with solution of 50% hydrogen peroxide and 50% sterile water)
- Sterile dressings to wounds and incisions

A/AAROM of Uninvolved Joints

- Motion of all upper extremity joints, except joints adjacent to the fracture

CRITERIA FOR ADVANCEMENT

- Fracture stability through surgical fixation or clinical union
- Diminished acute, postoperative inflammation

Postoperative Phase II: Stability (Weeks 2 to 6)

GOALS
- Edema control
- Nonadherent scar
- Freely gliding flexor and extensor tendons
- Functional motion of joints adjacent to fracture

PRECAUTIONS
- No resistive exercises or activities
- Avoid excessive passive stress to fracture site
- Avoid strong pinching to protect thumb metacarpal base fractures
- Continue protective splinting, except for hygiene and exercises

TREATMENT STRATEGIES
- Edema control: may add contrast baths and compression glove when wounds have healed and fracture is stable
- Scar management: scar massage, silicone scar pad
- Heat modalities to prepare soft tissue for range of motion (ROM) and scar management
- Active/active assisted ROM (A/AAROM) of joints adjacent to fracture
- Flexor and extensor tendon gliding and blocking exercises
- Light, functional use of hand in splint, progressed to supervised light activities without splint

CRITERIA FOR ADVANCEMENT
- Fracture consolidation as evidenced by radiographic union or physician's clinical examination, indicating ability of fracture to tolerate resistance and stress

Postoperative Phase III: Fracture Consolidation (Weeks 7 to 10)

GOALS
- Full or maximum motion with freely gliding tendons
- Functional strength and endurance
- Independence in activities of daily living (ADL)

PRECAUTIONS
- No resistance, stretching, or static progressive splints until fracture has consolidated
- Avoid overstretching vs gliding of adherent tendons.

TREATMENT STRATEGIES
- Wean from protective custom splint under direction of surgeon.
- Continue edema and scar management.
- Heat modalities, including paraffin and ultrasound, to prepare soft tissues for ROM, joint mobilization, and scar mobilization
- Active ROM (AROM), including flexor and extensor, tendon gliding, and blocking exercises; add blocking splints as needed.
- Passive ROM, stretching, joint mobilization to address joint stiffness
- Serial static or static progressive splinting to address persistent joint stiffness
- Resistive exercises for intrinsic and extrinsic digit musculature and wrist
- Functional activities and conditioning for restoration of independent ADL

CRITERIA FOR DISCHARGE
- Full or maximum digit and wrist AROM with freely gliding tendons
- Functional strength and endurance
- Independence in ADL
- Independence in home program to address any residual impairments

Bibliography

Campbell, P.J., Wilson, R.L. Management of Joint Injuries and Intra-articular Fractures. In Hunter, J.M., Mackin, E.J., Callahan, A.D. (Eds). Rehabilitation of the Hand: Surgery and Therapy, 5th ed. Mosby, St. Louis, 2002, pp. 396-411.

Chung, K.C., Spilson, S.V. The Frequency and Epidemiology of Hand and Forearm Fractures in the United States. *J Hand Surg* 2001;26A:908-915.

Doyle, J.R. Extensor Tendons-Acute Injuries. In Green, D.P., Hotchkiss, R.N., Pederson, W.C. (Eds). Green's Operative Hand Surgery, 4th ed. Churchill Livingstone, New York, 1999, pp. 1950-1987.

Pellegrini, V.D. Fractures at the Base of the Thumb. *Hand Clin* 1988;4:87-102.

Pun, W.K., Chow, S.P., Luk, K.D., Ip, F.K., Chan, K.C., Ngai, W.K., Crosby, C., Ng, C.A. Prospective Study on 284 Digital Fractures of the Hand. *J Hand Surg* 1989;14A:474-481.

Schneider, L.H. Fractures of the Distal Phalanx. *Hand Clin* 1988;4:537-547.

Stern, P.J. Fractures of the Metacarpals and Phalanges. In Green, D.P., Hotchkiss, R.N., Pederson, W.C. (Eds). Green's Operative Hand Surgery, 4th ed. Churchill Livingstone, New York, 1999, pp. 711-771.

CHAPTER 14

Flexor Tendon Repairs

Kara Gallagher, MS, OTR/L, CHT

Flexor tendons are surgically corrected via a primary or secondary repair. Whether a repair is primary or secondary depends on how soon after injury that surgery occurs and the quality of the tendon.

In a *primary repair,* the loose ends of the injured tendon are approximated with sutures. An immediate primary repair is performed within 24 hours of injury, whereas a delayed primary repair is performed between 24 hours and 3 weeks after injury. Primary end-to-end tendon repair performed within the first few days following injury is ideal and guarantees the best outcome. Studies performed on canine and chicken tendons demonstrate that repairs performed within the first few days resulted in improved tendon excursion. It is important to be aware that delayed tendon repair increases the possibility of rupture, tendon elongation, muscle shortening, and joint contractures. A tendon injury that involves bone or neurovascular damage will complicate the rehabilitation process and possibly the outcome but does not contraindicate a primary repair.

A *secondary repair* is considered 3 weeks post-injury, or in situations where the quality of the tendon is beyond surgical correction. After 3 weeks, flexor tendon repair becomes more complicated because of scarring, muscle contracture, and tendon retraction. At this point, available options include a tendon graft, transfer, or two-stage tendon graft. Other situations that require a secondary repair include loss of palmar skin overlying the flexor system, flexor retinacular damage, and pulley destruction.

In a secondary repair, a tendon graft from a noninvolved tendon (often palmaris longus [PL]) is harvested to approximate the free ends of the injured tendon. If scarring or damage to adjacent tissues is severe, a conventional tendon graft is unlikely to resume adequate gliding, and staged tendon grafts are performed. Transformation of the scarred, post-injury flexor tendon and surrounding tissues to a gliding, pliable, effective system is accomplished using a two-stage tendon graft method with a silicone implant. In the first stage, a silicone implant is placed between the free ends, allowing the scar to envelope it and recreate a fibrous sheath to promote healing of the second-stage tendon graft. Tendon injuries may occur in isolation or along with fractures and neurovascular injuries.

This chapter reviews the anatomy, surgery, and rehabilitation related to a flexor tendon injury, specifically an early active mobilization protocol that is appropriate for primary tendon repairs completed with a four-strand core suture and an additional epitendinous suture augmentation crossing the repair site. Flexor tendon injuries in the forearm or hand occur when tendon continuity is disrupted by a laceration, crush, avulsion, or contusion.

Anatomic Overview

- In the distal third of the volar forearm, the flexor tendons arise from the flexor muscles.
    1. The superficial group includes the wrist flexors: flexor carpi radialis, flexor carpi ulnaris, and PL.
    2. The middle group consists of the four tendons of the flexor digitorum superficialis (FDS) that originate from individual muscle bundles. This allows for isolated individual flexion of each digit.
    3. The deep group includes the flexor digitorum profundus (FDP) and flexor pollicis longus. The FDP tendons originate from a common muscle belly and therefore act as a group.
- Several surrounding anatomical structures are significant in flexor tendon injury.
- Flexor tendon injuries are categorized into five zones on the premises of anatomic features to systematically highlight these structures.

Zone V

- Zone V spans the distal third of the forearm to the level of the wrist and contains the musculotendinous junction of the superficial and deep flexors.
- Median and ulnar nerves, as well as the radial and ulnar arteries, course through zone V and are often associated with injury to the tendons.
- The vascular and neural structures must be protected in the early phases of rehabilitation.
- Early repair is especially recommended for tendons in this zone because of the high probability of tendon retraction with muscle contraction.
  1. The tendons lie deep in the skin and subcutaneous tissue and are particularly vulnerable to adhesions.
  2. Contracture and shortening of the tendons in this zone are common. Both adhesions and contracture can be reduced with a strong focus on differential tendon gliding during rehabilitation.

Zone IV

- In zone IV the flexor tendons are enclosed in synovial sheaths as they course through the carpal tunnel.
- Injuries in this zone often include more than one tendon, blood vessels, and nerves because of the close proximity of the structures to one another.
- Adhesions between the tendons are common in the postoperative phase, and differential gliding of the tendons is effective in controlling adhesion formation.

Zone III

- The lumbrical muscles originate from the flexor digitorum profundus tendon at the point where the tendons emerge from the carpal tunnel in zone III.
- Protective positioning in the lumbrical plus position (metacarpophalangeal [MP] flexion with interphalangeal [IP] extension) can lead to adhesions and contracture of the intrinsic muscles in the early weeks. Therefore, gentle, passive MP joint motion and gentle, passive intrinsic minus or hook fist (MP extension with IP flexion)

early in rehabilitation are recommended for injuries in zone II.

Zone II

- Zone II begins at the distal palmar crease and includes the origin of the flexor tendon sheath. Zone II extends to the middle of the middle phalanx, just distal to where the FDP emerges from the two slips of the FDS insertion (Camper's chiasm).
- In zone II the flexor tendons are supported by an intricate pulley system that tethers the tendons to the bones for increased mechanical advantage during flexion.
- Injured and repaired pulleys are potential sites of adhesion formation. Alternatively, unrepaired pulleys may cause "bowstringing" as the tendon pulls away from the bone in the palmar direction under muscle contraction.
- Zone II also includes the viniculae, which provide vascularity and nutrition to the tendons.
- Laceration in zone II often involves both FDS and FDP, in addition to the supporting structures.
- Historically, this region has been referred to as "no man's land" because of the complicated system of synovial sheaths, pulleys, and viniculae supporting the flexor tendons.
- In the past, poor results were expected with tendon injury in zone II because of the combination of intertendinous adhesions as well as the effects of injury to the sheath, viniculae, pulleys, and other surrounding structures.
- During the last 10 years, advances in suture technique, strength, and early postoperative active mobilization protocols have improved the ability to obtain better results.

Zone I

- Zone I, the most distal zone, spans from the insertion of the FDS on the middle phalanx to the insertion of the FDP on the distal phalanx.
- Zone I includes only the FDP tendon as it emerges from the flexor sheath.
- This is a common site for FDP rupture, where the terminal tendon is avulsed with or without a bony component, at its insertion on the distal phalanx.

- Complications following tendon repair in zone I include development of distal interphalangeal (DIP) joint flexion contracture or poor gliding through the A-4 and A-5 pulleys.

Surgical Overview

- Surgical repair of flexor tendons has evolved over the years. For many years, two-strand repairs were performed. In the past decade, four-strand repairs have become more common.
- The strength of a tendon repair is roughly proportional to the number of strands that cross the repair. The number of strands in a repair refers to the number of times the suture material crosses the repair site.
- Today, the most common primary repair is accomplished with a four-strand core suture plus an epitendinous suture crossing the repair site to strengthen the procedure.
- Many core suture designs have been described in the literature, ranging from four to eight strands. These designs include the Bunnell, modified Kessler, Tajima, locking running epitendinous, and double-grasping techniques.
- The surgeons at the Hospital for Special Surgery (HSS) typically use a four-strand modified Kessler core suture with a reinforcing epitendinous suture. Like other early active mobilization programs, this guideline requires a four-strand core repair and an epitendinous suture at the repair site. Therefore, motion can be initiated within the first 3 days post-surgery.
- Early active mobilization requires adequate tensile strength of the suture material and appropriate design of the suture so that the tendon can withstand active muscle pull without rupture or gapping.

Rehabilitation Overview

- There are three approaches to rehabilitating a flexor tendon after surgical repair. They include immobilization, early passive mobilization, and early active mobilization.
    1. Passive mobilization programs, such as those described by Kleinert et al. and Duran and Houser, involve gentle passive flexion and active extension exercises

that are performed in a dorsal block splint, with or without rubber band traction that assists the digits into flexion.

2. Early active mobilization consists of active hold or active place-hold programs.
   - *Active place-hold* indicates that the therapist passively places the digits into flexion and then directs the patient to actively maintain the position with a gentle muscle contraction.
   - This guideline details an active hold/place-hold mobilization program that the authors have found to be most successful. Their version has been modified from protocols designed by Strickland, Cannon, and Silfverskiold and May.
   - The goal of rehabilitation following flexor tendon repair is to promote an opportune environment for a strong repair to support normal forces acting on the tendon in everyday functional use.

3. Research demonstrates that stressing a repaired tendon with early mobilization facilitates healing, tensile strength, excursion, and minimizes adhesion formation.

4. This protocol offers a method to encourage a durable tendon repair that glides freely.

- Passive mobilization techniques based on principles from the Controlled Passive Mobilization Technique by Duran and Houser and the method by Kleinert et al. are also incorporated into this guideline.
  1. The passive mobilization techniques are included to preserve joint motion.
  2. Like most early active mobilization protocols, this guideline was developed for flexor tendon injuries in zone II. However, the principles can be applied to injuries in all zones.

Active Mobilization

- The active mobilization protocol must begin within 1 to 2 days of surgery, when the repair is physiologically strong.
  1. The tensile strength of the immobilized tendon diminishes 3 to 5 days postoperatively because of softening of the tendon ends.

2. A study by Hitchcock et al. determined that the ends of flexor profundus tendons in chickens softened during the inflammatory phase of wound healing. The same study compared the immobilized group to a group that was mobilized 1 to 2 days after repair. The study found that the mobilized group did not encounter a notable inflammatory phase, and rather the repair gained strength, appearing to heal through intrinsic means, with less adhesion formation.

- Active mobilization of the repaired tendon begins with place-hold positions protected by tenodesis (wrist extension with digit flexion/wrist flexion with digit extension).
- Active mobilization progresses toward active flexion along the following ladder: place-hold tenodesis, active tenodesis, differential tendon gliding, blocking, and strengthening.
- Strengthening begins with blocking with resistance, progressing toward isometric grip, and, finally, isotonic strengthening of grip and pinch.

Criteria for Advancement

- Rehabilitation of the repaired flexor tendon progresses through four phases of therapy that can last up to 16 weeks postoperatively.
- The phases of this protocol reflect the three stages of wound healing: inflammation, fibroplasia, and scar maturation.
- Advancement of the patient depends upon the stage of wound healing, excursion of the flexor tendon, and opinions of the surgeon and therapist.
- Ultimately, the surgeon prescribes an early active motion protocol and determines points of advancement based on examination of the patient, tendon excursion, and clinical feedback from the therapist.
- Each phase includes a new set of goals, precautions, splints, treatment strategies, and criteria for advancement.

Stages of Wound Healing

- As the patient is advanced through a regimented rehabilitation program, internal forces applied through the tendon repair site increase.

- Traditionally, therapists have used a timeline based on the stages of wound healing to guide them through the progression of treatment.
  1. The first phase of therapy includes both the inflammatory (0 to 5 days) and fibroplasia stages (5 to 21 days) of wound healing.
  2. The second, third, and fourth phases of therapy occur during the scar maturation or remodeling phase (3 weeks to 2 years) of wound healing. Phase II of therapy typically commences 4 weeks postoperatively, leading into phase III in the sixth postoperative week, and, finally, phase IV in the eighth week after surgery.

Three-Point Adhesion Grading System

- A more clinical approach to the progression of treatment has been described recently.
  1. This approach uses flexor tendon excursion as a guide in selecting the appropriate amount of force to apply across the tendon junction.
  2. Tendon excursion is monitored by determining flexion lag. *Flexion lag* is measured as total passive flexion (sum of passive MP, PIP, and DIP flexion) minus total active flexion (sum of active MP, PIP, and DIP flexion).
- Groth recently developed a model, known as the three-point adhesion grading system, to quantify how adhesions influence flexion lag.
  1. The model is used as an indicator for flexor tendon excursion, providing a clinical method for progressing the patient through the phases of therapy.
  2. *Tendon lag* is defined as absent, responsive, or unresponsive in Groth's three-point adhesion grading system.
  3. Absent tendon lag is indicated by less than or equal to 5 degrees of difference between active and passive flexion.
  4. Responsive and unresponsive tendon lags are determined by measures taken between therapy sessions. A responsive tendon lag improves between sessions. Responsive flexion lag is concluded by greater than or

equal to 10% improvement of lag between therapy sessions. Unresponsive flexion lag indicates less than or equal to 10% improvement of lag between therapy sessions.

5. Change in flexion lag between sessions is determined using the following formula:

$$a = \text{previous session flexion lag}$$
$$b = \text{present session flexion lag}$$
$$c = \text{percent of improvement}$$
$$c = (a - b)/a \times 100\%$$

HSS Criteria for Advancement

- The HSS guideline for progressing patients following flexor tendon repair relies on both wound healing principles and flexor tendon excursion.
- Groth's three-point adhesion grading system can assist in knowing when to progress or delay the therapy program.
  1. In this guideline absent flexion lag indicates excellent tendon glide, and the patient should be progressed slower than the timeline that correlates with wound healing.
  2. Responsive flexion lag suggests that the phase and exercises are appropriate for the strength of the tendon repair and adhesion formation.
  3. Flexion lag must be monitored closely for unresponsiveness.
     - If the lag becomes unresponsive, advancement to the next level occurs sooner than the phase of wound healing indicates.
     - Unresponsive flexion lag reflects adhesion formation.
     - An unresponsive lag indicates advancement through the suggested timeline at a faster pace until the tendon lag resolves.
     - Load application can increase per rehabilitation session until the lag becomes responsive.
     - Once the lag becomes responsive, the patient continues at that level and progresses according to the suggested timeline in accordance with wound healing.

- The rehabilitation overview contains specific guidelines for applying the adhesion grading system to the standard timeline that is based on the principles of wound healing.

Contraindications

- Several factors contraindicate the use of early active motion.
  1. First, a tendon held together with less than a four-strand core repair or lacking the reinforcing epitendinous suture at the repair site cannot withstand such a program. Anything less than the recommended repair parameters may gap or rupture under active forces.
  2. Second, because of the postoperative change in tendon strength, the program should be avoided if the patient is more than 3 days post-surgery.
  3. Third, poor tendon quality or multiple associated injuries may contradict using this program. In such cases, the surgeon should dictate the appropriate postoperative approach.
  4. Last, this program requires active participation, compliance, and commitment from the patient.
     - The patient must have a thorough understanding of the exercises and precautions.
     - Children under age 10 and individuals who lack the ability or desire to commit to this program may not be appropriate candidates. It is worth noting that the authors have used this early active mobilization protocol successfully with a 5-year-old child, who demonstrated the ability and desire to follow through.

**Postoperative Phase I
(24 Hours to 3–4 Weeks)**

GOALS
- Fabrication of custom immobilization splint
- Instruction in passive range of motion (PROM) and protected active range of motion (AROM)
- Increased tendon excursion
- Edema control and scar management
- Independence in home exercise program (HEP)

PRECAUTIONS
- Wear splint at all times—remove for hygiene and specific exercises
- No simultaneous wrist and digital extension
- Digital nerve injuries: IP position as per surgeon (slight flexion)

TREATMENT STRATEGIES
- *Splint: Static, dorsal, forearm based*
  1. Dorsal block splint (DBS)
  2. Wrist 15- to 30-degree flexion
  3. Metacarpophalangeal joints 60- to 70-degree flexion
  4. IP joints strapped into extension against DBS, unless digital nerves were repaired
  5. PIP extension splint if needed to achieve full PIP extension
- *PROM*
  1. Passive PIP/DIP flexion in splint followed by active extension to roof of splint
  2. Composite passive flexion followed by active extension to roof of splint
  3. 10 times each, every 2 hours
- *AROM (protected, supervised in therapy)*
  1. Tenodesis: Place and hold composite and straight fist
  2. 10 times each, every 2 hours
  3. AROM
     - Active digital extension with wrist flexed
     - FDS blocking to uninvolved digits and tendons
     - FDP blocking to uninvolved digits, if FDP is not involved
     - 10 times each, every 2 hours
- *Scar management: to prevent tendon adhesions*
  1. Silicone scar pads
  2. Cross-frictional massage
- *Edema control*
  1. Coban-light, pinch method; remove for AROM exercises
  2. Retrograde massage
- *HEP*
  1. PROM exercises every 2 hours
  2. Tenodesis and AROM added when 100% competent in therapy

Continued

**Postoperative Phase I
(24 Hours to 3–4 Weeks)—Cont'd**

- Scar management as previous, 2 times a day
- Edema management as previous, as
  needed

CRITERIA FOR ADVANCEMENT
- Per surgeon
- Based on stage of wound healing
- Contingent upon tendon excursion measured 3 weeks
  postoperative and weekly thereafter
  1. Determine flexion lag
     - Absent: Prolong phase I until 6 weeks postoperative
     - Responsive: Progress to phase II at 4 weeks
       postoperative
     - Unresponsive: Progress to phase II at 3 weeks
       postoperative, continuing to increase load to tendon
       until lag becomes responsive

Postoperative Phase II (3 to 6 Weeks)

GOALS
- Increased tendon excursion
- Decreased adhesion formation
- Increased active flexion of the involved digit

PRECAUTIONS
- Continue DBS, unless patient shows unresponsive flexion
  lag
- Watch for PIP flexion contracture; initiate extension
  splinting if needed
- No active or passive simultaneous wrist and digital
  extension

TREATMENT STRATEGIES
- *Splint*
  1. Continue with DBS, if absent flexor lag
  2. Modify DBS, if responsive flexor lag
     - Wrist extension to neutral and MP extension to 30 to
       45 degrees
  3. Discontinue DBS, if unresponsive flexor lag at 4 weeks
     postoperative

- *PROM*
  1. Continue as in phase I
  2. Begin joint mobilization for joint stiffness
- *AROM*
  1. Begin place and hold hook fist tenodesis
  2. Progress to active tenodesis for composite, straight, and hook fists
  3. Increase repetition of exercises
- *HEP*
  1. Add active tenodesis for tabletop, composite, straight, and hook fists
  2. Increase repetition of each exercise
  3. Reduce frequency of sessions at home to three times per day

CRITERIA FOR ADVANCEMENT
- Tendon integrity determined by surgeon
- Based on stage of wound healing
- Contingent upon tendon excursion
  1. Determine flexion lag
     - Absent: Prolong phase II until 8 weeks postoperative
     - Responsive: Progress to phase III at 6 weeks postoperative
     - Unresponsive: Progress to phase III as early as 4 weeks postoperative, continuing to increase load to tendon until lag becomes responsive

Postoperative Phase III (6 to 8 Weeks)

GOALS
- Full passive motion by 8 weeks
- Increased tendon excursion and controlled adhesion formation
- Independence with activities of daily living (ADL)

PRECAUTIONS
- No strengthening with good tendon excursion (absent tendon lag)
- No grip and strength testing because this requires maximal effort

Continued

Postoperative Phase III (6 to 8 Weeks)—Cont'd

TREATMENT STRATEGIES

- *Splints*
  1. Discontinue DBS
  2. Continue PIP and/or DIP extension splint
  3. Consider flexor stretcher for night
     - Wrist neutral, digits at comfortable end range
     - Wear at night
     - Continue to modify flexor stretcher to position flexor tendons at end of available range
- *Passive Motion*
  1. Upgrade PROM as needed
  2. In therapy *only:*
     - Passive digit extension, with wrist in flexion advancing to neutral
  3. Joint mobilization for stiff joints
- *Active Motion*
  1. Active tenodesis for composite, straight, and hook fists
  2. Progression toward active tendon glides
  3. Isolated FDS and FDP glide of repaired tendon
  4. Neuromuscular electric stimulation (NMES) for muscle reeducation may be necessary
  5. Gentle blocking FDS and FDP at 6 weeks, if unresponsive flexion lag
- *Functional Activities*
  1. Resistive exercises with isometric pinch and grip
  2. NMES with functional activities
- *HEP*
  1. Tendon gliding
  2. Education for light activity-use of newly splint-free hand

CRITERIA FOR ADVANCEMENT

- Absent flexor lag: Prolong phase III until 10 to 12 weeks postoperatively
- Responsive flexor lag: Progress to phase IV by week 8
- Unresponsive flexor lag: Progress to phase IV by week 6

Postoperative Phase IV (8 to 16 Weeks)

GOALS
- Full active motion (absent flexor lag)
- Functional grip strength (75% of noninjured hand)
- Independence with self-care, homemaking, work, school, leisure
- Independent knowledge of precautions

PRECAUTIONS
- Do not measure grip and pinch with excellent tendon excursion
- Extreme uncontrolled force against the tendon may cause tendon rupture up to 12 weeks
- No lifting until 12 weeks with good tendon glide
- No sports or heavy labor until 16 weeks

TREATMENT STRATEGIES
- Splints
  1. Continue flexor stretcher as needed
  2. Continue PIP extension splinting as needed
  3. Blocking splints
     - MP block for hook fisting
     - PIP block for DIP flexion
- Passive Motion
  1. Full PROM
- Joint Mobilization Active Motion
  1. Tendon gliding
  2. Blocking with resistance
  3. NMES
- Functional Activity
  1. Full participation in ADL by 12 weeks
  2. Grip and pinch strengthening
     - Progress from isometrics to sponge to putty to hand helper
     - Avoid specific strengthening if excellent tendon excursion
- HEP
  1. Blocking exercises
  2. Progress to full use of involved hand in all ADL

CRITERIA FOR DISCHARGE
- Functional active motion (less than 5 degree flexor lag)

Continued

Postoperative Phase IV (8 to 16 Weeks)—Cont'd

- Functional strength (involved 75% of noninjured hand)
- Able to return to full duty work, homemaking, sports by 16 weeks postoperatively

Bibliography

Allen, B.N., Frykman, G.K., Unsell, R.S., Wood, V.E. Ruptured Flexor Tendon Tenorrhaphies in Zone II: Repair and Rehabilitation. *J Hand Surg* 1987;12A:18.

Bainbridge, L.C., Robertson, C., Gillies, D., Elliot, D. A Comparison of Post-operative Mobilization of Flexor Tendon Repairs with "Passive Flexion-active Extension" and "Controlled Active Motion" Techniques. *J Hand Surg* 1994;19B:517.

Cannon, N. Post Flexor Tendon Repair Motion Protocol. *Indiana Hand Cent Newsl* 1993;1:13.

Cullen, K.W., Tolhurst, P., Lang, D., Page, R.E. Flexor Tendon Repair Zone 2 Followed by Controlled Active Mobilisation. *J Hand Surg* 1989;14B:392.

Culp, R.W., Taras, J.S. Primary Care of Flexor Tendon Injuries. In Mackin, E.J., Callahan, A.D., Skirven, T.M., Schneider, L.H., Osterman, A.L., Hunter, J.M. (Eds). Rehabilitation of the Hand and Upper Extremity. Mosby, St. Louis, 2002, pp. 415-430.

Duran, R., Houser, R. Controlled Passive Motion Following Flexor Tendon Repair in Zones 2 and 3. In AAOS Symposium on Tendon Surgery in the Hand. Mosby, St. Louis, 1975, pp. 105-144.

Duran, R., Houser, R. Management of Flexor Tendon Lacerations in Zone 2 Using Controlled Passive Motion Post-operatively. In Hunter, J., Schneider, L., Mackin, E., Bell, J. (Eds). Rehabilitation of the Hand. Mosby, St. Louis, 1978, pp. 217-224.

Elliot, D., Moiemen, N.S., Flemming, A.F., Harris, S.B., Foster, A.J. The Rupture Rate of Acute Flexor Tendon Repairs Mobilized by the Controlled Active Motion Regimen. *J Hand Surg* 1994;19B:607.

Gelberman, R.H., Amifl, D., Gonsalves, M., Page, R.E. The Influence of Protected Passive Mobilization on the Healing Flexor Tendons: A Biomechanical and Microangiographic Study. *Hand Clin* 1981;13:120.

Gelberman, R.H., Botte, M.J., Spiegelman, J.J., Akeson, W.H. The Excursion and Deformation of Repaired Flexor Tendons Treated with Protected Early Motion. *J Hand Surg* 1986;11A:106.

Gelberman, R.H., Manske, P.R., Akeson, W.H., Woo, S.L., Lundborg, G., Amiel, D. Flexor Tendon Repair. *J Orthop Res* 1986;4:119.

Gelberman, R.H., Nunley, J.A. II, Osterman, A.L., Breen, T.F., Dimick, M.P., Woo, S.L. Influences of the Protected Passive Mobilization Interval on Flexor Tendon Healing. *Clin Orthop* 1991;264:189.

Gelberman, R.H., Woo, S.L., Lothringer, K., Akeson, W.H., Amiel, D. Effects of Early Intermittent Passive Mobilization on Healing Canine Flexor Tendons. *J Hand Surg* 1982;7:170.

Gratton, P. Early Active Mobilization after Flexor Tendon Repairs. *J Hand Ther* 1993;6:285.

Groth, G.N. Pyramid of Progressive Force Exercises to the Injured Flexor Tendon. *J Hand Ther* 2004;17:31.

Hitchcock, T.F., Light, T.R., Bunch, W.H., Knight, G.W., Sartori, M.J., Patwardhan, A.G., Hollyfield, R.L. The Effect of Immediate Constrained Digital Motion on the Strength of Flexor Tendon Repairs in Chickens. *J Hand Surg* 1987;12A:590.

Kleinert, H.E., Kutz, J.E., Cohen, M.J. Primary Repair of Lacerated Flexor Tendons in No-man's-land. *J Bone Joint Surg* 1967;49A:577.

Kleinert, H.E., Kutz, J.E., Cohen, M.J. Primary Repair of Zone 2 Flexor Tendon Lacerations. In AAOS Symposium on Tendon Surgery in the Hand. Mosby, St. Louis, 1975, pp. 91–104.

Lee, H. Double Locking Suture: A Technique of Tendon Repair for Early Active Mobilization Part I. *J Hand Surg* 1990;15A:945.

Lee, H. Double Loop Locking Suture: A Technique of Tendon Repair for Early Active Mobilization Part II. *J Hand Surg* 1990;15A:953.

Mackin, E., Callahan, A.D., Skirven, T.M., Schneider, L.H., Osterman, A.L., Hunter, J.M. Staged Flexor Tendon Reconstruction. In Mackin, E.J. (Eds). Rehabilitation of the Hand and Upper Extremity. Mosby, St. Louis, 2002, pp. 469–497.

Mason, J., Allen, H. The Rate of Healing Tendons: An Experimental Study of Tensile Strength. *Ann Surg* 1941;113:424.

Matthews, J.P. Early Mobilisation after Flexor Tendon Repair. *J Hand Surg* 1993;14B:363.

Pettengill, K.M., Van Strien, G. Postoperative Management of Flexor Tendon Injuries. In Mackin, E.J., Callahan, A.D., Skirven, T.M., Schneider, L.H., Osterman, A.L., Hunter, J.M. (Eds). Rehabilitation of the Hand and Upper Extremity. Mosby, St. Louis, 2002, pp. 431–456.

Pruitt, D.L. Cyclic Stress Analysis of Flexor Tendon Repair. *J Hand Surg* 1991;16A:701.

Riaz, M. Long Term Outcome of Early Active Mobilization Following Flexor Tendon Repair in Zone II. *J Hand Surg* 1999;24B:157.

Robertson, G.A., Al-Qattan, N.M. A Biomechanical Analysis of a New Interlock Suture Technique for Flexor Tendon Repair. *J Hand Surg* 1992;17B:92.

Savage, R. Flexor Tendon Repair Using a "Six-strand" Method of Repair and Early Active Mobilization. *J Hand Surg* 1989;14B:396.

Savage, R. The Influence of Wrist Position on the Minimum Force Required for Active Movement of the Interphalangeal Joints. *J Hand Surg* 1988;13B:262.

Silfverskiold, K.L., May, E.J. Flexor Tendon Repair in Zone II with a New Suture Technique and an Early Mobilization Program Combining Passive and Active Flexion. *J Hand Surg* 1994;18A:654.

Small, J.O., Brennen, M.D., Colville, J. Early Active Mobilisation Following Flexor Tendon Repair Zone 2. *J Hand Surg* 1989;14B:383.

Stewart, K.M. Tendon Injuries. In Stanley, B.J., Tribuzzi, S.M. (Eds). Concepts in Hand Rehabilitation. FA Davis Company, Philadelphia, 1992, pp. 353–392.

Stewart Pettengill, K. Postoperative Therapy Concepts in Management of Tendon Injuries: Early Mobilization. In Hunter, J., Schneider, L., Mackin, E. (Eds). Tendon and Nerve Surgery in the Hand: A Third Decade. Mosby, St. Louis, 1997, pp. 332–341.

Strickland, J.W. Flexor Tendons-Acute Injuries. In Green, D.P., Hotchkiss, R.N., Pederson, W.C. (Eds). Green's Operative Hand Surgery, 4th ed. Churchill Livingstone, New York, 1999, pp. 1851–1897.

Strickland, J.W. Flexor Tendon Injuries: Foundations of Treatment. *J Am Acad Orthop Surg* 1995;3:44.

Strickland, J.W. Flexor Tendon Injuries II: Operative Technique. *J Acad Orthop Surg* 1995;3:55.

Thurman, R.T., Trumble, T.E., Hanel, D.P., Tencer, A.F., Kiser, P.K. Two-, Four-, and Six-strand Zone II Flexor Tendon Repairs: An In Situ Biomechanical Comparison Using a Cadaver Model. *J Hand Surg* 1998;23A:261.

Trail, I.A., Powell, E.S., Noble, J. The Mechanical Strength of Various Suture Techniques. *J Hand Surg* 1992;17B:89.

Woo, S.L., Gelberman, R.H., Cobb, N.G., Amiel, D., Lothringer, K., Akeson, W.H. The Importance of Controlled Passive Mobilization on Flexor Tendon Healing. *Acta Orthop Scand* 1981;52:615.

Yii, N., Urban, M., Elliot, D. A Prospective Study of Flexor Tendon Repair in Zone 5. *J Hand Surg* 1998;23B:642.

CHAPTER 15

Extensor Tendon Repairs

Kara Gallagher, MS, OTR/L, CHT

The extensor tendons in the hand are particularly susceptible to injury because of their unique anatomy and superficial location as the tendons course distally beyond the wrist. The extensor system is divided into eight zones that extend from the fingertips to the forearm. The thumb is divided into five zones (T-1 through T-5). Research in human cadavers indicates that the thickness of the extensor tendons ranges from 1.7 mm in the forearm to 0.65 mm in the distal fingertip. Limited subcutaneous tissue and elastic skin cover the extensor tendons on the dorsal wrist, hand, and digits, leaving the extensor tendons vulnerable to injury. Laceration, deep abrasion, crush, forceful rupture, and avulsion fracture are the major causes of extensor tendon injuries. Systemic disease, such as rheumatoid arthritis, also affects the integrity of the extensor tendons, predisposing them to attenuation and rupture.

Extensor tendon injuries are treated conservatively via immobilization or with surgical repair. Immobilization is used to treat closed terminal tendon disruption in the digits and thumb, because injury to the terminal tendon does not result in retraction of the tendon ends because of soft tissue attachments and interconnections at multiple levels. All other extensor tendon injuries are treated surgically. This allows for early mobilization to begin as early as 24 hours postoperatively. Suture techniques that have been used successfully for flexor tendon repair have been modified to accommodate the thinner extensor tendons in the fingers. Extensor tendons exhibit approximately 50% of the strength of repaired flexor tendons because of reduced tendon dimension and collagen cross linking. Postoperative extensor tendons require protective splinting and carefully controlled mobilization following surgery.

Rehabilitation Overview

- Historically, extensor tendon repairs have been immobilized in a splint, whether conservatively or surgically managed, for a minimum of 3 weeks. Studies over the last 20 years indicate that immobilization of tendons following surgical repair leads to a high percentage of fair to poor results because of adhesion formation that limits tendon excursion and joint motion.

- In the past several years, early mobilization, supported by evidence related to flexor tendon management, has been advocated in the care extensor tendon injuries. Studies on postoperative flexor and extensor management demonstrate that repaired tendons tolerate early active motion and have better outcomes.

- Evans has described the following principles for the therapeutic management of extensor tendons.
  1. Extensor tendons in all zones (with the exception of zones I and II) tolerate early controlled active motion.
  2. Wrist position affects tendon excursion by decreasing the resistive forces from the flexor system.
  3. Early therapeutic intervention, within 24 hours to 3 days postoperatively, is critical.
  4. Accurate splint design and diligent postoperative control of force, excursion, and design prevent gapping and rupture.

- The decision to use an immobilization or early mobilization protocol depends on several factors.
  1. To withstand the force of early mobilization, a strong surgical repair and good tendon quality are required.
  2. Conservatively managed tendons, not surgically managed, require a period of immobilization to allow the gap between the interrupted tendons to heal sufficiently.
  3. In addition, the physiology of the tendons over the distal phalanges of the fingers and thumb prevents these tendons from being able to tolerate the stress of early mobilization.
  4. Therefore, tendons in zones I, II, and T-I, whether treated conservatively or surgically, benefit from an immobilization period.

5. Tendons in zones III through VIII and T-II through V tolerate and benefit from early mobilization protocols.
- At the Hospital for Special Surgery (HSS), the authors use an early mobilization program for postoperative care of extensor tendons in all zones, except zones I, II, and T-I, where active force is not tolerated by the flat, thin, and broad extensor tendon.
  1. *Early mobilization* refers to either controlled passive motion or early active motion.
  2. Early mobilization programs require a strong surgical repair, good tendon integrity, patient compliance, and referral to therapy within 24 hours to 3 days after surgery.
  3. The early active motion program is based on the scientific studies describing an immediate active short arc motion protocol by Evans and studies regarding positive effects of active mobilization for flexor tendons.
  4. The early mobilization guidelines for thumb zones T-II and T-IV are also based on Evans' suggestions.
  5. Early active motion requires a strong repair to withstand active tension of the involved extensor tendon.
  6. In addition, early active motion must begin when the repaired tendon quality is at its best 24 hours to 3 days after surgery.
  7. Studies indicate that the projected tensile strength of an unstressed tendon repair may decrease as much as 25% to 50% at 5 to 51 days after surgery because of softening of the tendon ends.
  8. The following guideline describes extensor tendon anatomy, injury, surgery, and rehabilitation by zone, expected outcome, and criteria for discharge from therapy.
- Early active motion for zones III through VIII and zones T-IV and T-V in the thumb begins with passive wrist tenodesis exercises, followed by active placehold extension, and protected active extension.
- A *safe arc of motion* is described for each zone to protect the repair site and promote healing. The arc of motion has been determined by calculations of tendon excursion measured in radians.

- *Protected joint motion* allowing for 3 to 5 mm of tendon excursion has been defined as safe and effective in preventing rupture or gapping while promoting functional glide and cellular healing.

Calculating Extensor Tendon Excursion

- To theoretically determine how much joint motion provides 3 to 5 mm of tendon excursion, Evans synthesized information from excursion studies in the literature, mathematical calculations by radians, and intraoperative measurements.
- In zones III and IV, 30 degrees of proximal interphalangeal (PIP) flexion creates 4mm of extensor digitorum communis (EDC) excursion.
- In zones V through VIII, 30 to 40 degrees of metacarpophalangeal (MP) flexion offers 4 to 5 mm of EDC excursion.
- In zones T-III through T-V, 60 degrees of interphalangeal (IP) flexion allows 5mm of extensor pollicis longus (EPL) excursion.

Contraindications for Early Active Motion

- As described previously, closed zone I and II tendon injuries in the digits and zone I in the thumb are treated via immobilization.
- Children under age 10 and noncompliant or incompetent adult patients are better managed with immobilization protocols.
- Patients referred to therapy more than 3 days postoperatively cannot begin early mobilization because of decreased tensile strength of the repair. In this case, immobilization for 3 weeks is indicated to allow for healing to occur.

Splinting

- Splint design varies by zone of injury and associated structures involved in the injury.
- The basic splints included in this guideline are static finger or forearm-based splints that include only the joints crossed by the affected tendon.

- Static progressive and dynamic splints to affect tendon extensibility or joint stiffness may or may not be incorporated into the rehabilitation process, depending on progress and functional gains. These splints will be mentioned in considerations for each zone.

Edema Control

- Postoperative edema relates directly to the fibroblastic response and collagen production at the injury site. Edema control is mandatory in treating the postoperative extensor tendon.
- Digital edema is minimized with a single layer of Coban (3M Health Care, St. Paul, MN) for as long as any excessive volume is present around the PIP joint (up to 8 to 12 weeks postoperatively).
- Dorsal hand edema is controlled with bulky, compressive dressing between exercises and therapy sessions.
- Elevation, motion of the uninvolved joints, and controlled motion of the involved joints assist in decreasing edema.

Scar Management

- Superficial finger digital scars are managed with a silicone gel pad.
- Dorsal hand and forearm scars often require custom silicone scar pads for improved fit and effectiveness.
- Cross-friction scar massage helps soften adhesions and increase the pliability of the skin and underlying structures.

Home Exercise Program

- The patient is instructed in a specific home exercise program (HEP) that is appropriate for the repaired zone.
- The HEP also includes education for safe splint donning/doffing techniques.
- Exercises are performed in the confines of the splint until the patient demonstrates competence.
- The therapist determines the frequency of exercise based on the quality of tendon glide.
- Each zone in this guideline recommends a specific HEP with suggested frequency.

Criteria for Advancement

- The criterion for advancement in all zones is the presence of an extensor lag.
- *Extensor lag* is defined as passive extension that exceeds active extension. When full active extension is present, there is no lag, and treatment is progressed according to the phases in the guideline.
- When an extension lag of 10 degrees or more is present, active flexion is curtailed and the focus is aimed at obtaining full active extension before advancement to the next phase.
- It is important to concentrate on the extension exercises and avoid emphasizing flexion at the expense of extension.
- Increases in passive and active flexion are avoided unless full active extension has been achieved.

Zones I and II: Immobilization

GOALS
- 0 to 6 weeks
  1. Splint to prevent DIP extensor lag and educate patient for proper donning/doffing of splint to protect healing extensor tendon
  2. Weekly check splint fit to ensure DIP joint is held in full to slight hyperextension
- 6 to 12 weeks
  1. Maintain 0 degrees of active DIP extension
  2. Attain 70 degrees of active DIP flexion

PRECAUTIONS
- Do not splint DIP joint in so much hyperextension that beginning signs of ischemia develop (volar distal phalange blanches)
- No active or passive DIP motion until week 6 (if no surgery)
- No active or passive DIP motion until week 5 (if surgery)
- Avoid moderate to heavy ADL until week 12.

TREATMENT STRATEGIES
Splints
- Static DIP extension splint with two points of counterpressure
  1. Include volar and dorsal distal phalanx
  2. Cross the dorsal DIP joint, covering the dorsal middle phalanx distal to the PIP joint

   3. 0 to 10 degrees of DIP joint hyperextension
   4. Continuous splinting for at least 6 weeks (if no surgery)
   5. Continuous splinting for at least 5 weeks (if surgery)
   6. Possibly continue splinting between exercise sessions and at night if extensor lag present
- Static DIP extension and PIP flexion (figure-eight design)
   1. If patient develops PIP hyperextension in addition to mallet finger
   2. DIP 0 to 10 degrees extension, PIP 30 to 45 degrees of flexion
- Blocking splints: 6 weeks+
   1. Static palm-based MP extension blocker for hook fisting
   2. Static palm-based MP and PIP extension blockers for isolated DIP flexion

Motion
- 0 to 6 weeks
   1. No active or passive DIP joint motion
   2. Active motion of uninvolved joints
- 6+ weeks
   1. 6 to 7 weeks
      – Active DIP flexion/extension 0 to 25 degrees
   2. 7 to 8 weeks
      – Active/passive DIP flexion/extension 0 to 35 degrees
      – Gentle tendon gliding-tabletop, straight, hook, full fists
      – ORL stretch
   3. 8 to 12 weeks
      – Gradually increase DIP extension/flexion to 0 to 70 degrees
      – Add composite fist to tendon gliding

Functional Activity
- 0 to 6 weeks
   1. Light ADL with splint donned at all times, including bathing/showering
- 6 to 12 weeks
   1. Incorporate prehension and fine motor coordination activities into therapy session
   2. Light ADL without splint (if no extensor lag)
   3. Light ADL with splint until extensor lag resolves
- 12 weeks
   1. Resume all ADL without splint
- 16 weeks
   1. Return to heavy labor and sports

Continued

Zones I and II: Immobilization—Cont'd

HOME EXERCISE PROGRAM
- 0 to 6 weeks: patient educated for safe donning/doffing of splint
- 6+ weeks: incorporate exercises from therapy (10 times each, 3 times/day)

CRITERIA FOR DISCONTINUING SPLINT
- No extensor lag at 6 weeks indicates initiation of active DIP motion
- Extensor lag at 6 weeks indicates 2 additional weeks of splinting full-time

Zones III and IV: Early Active Motion (Short Arc Motion)

GOALS
- Full active DIP and PIP extension and flexion
- Incorporate injured digit into ADL
- Independence with premorbid ADL

PRECAUTIONS
- Do not use this protocol unless involved tendons were surgically repaired
- Avoid emphasizing flexion gains over extension
- Position wrist in 30 degrees flexion/MP joints in 0 degrees during active IP motion during first 6 weeks

TREATMENT STRATEGIES
Splints
- Immobilization splint
  1. Static volar gutter extension splint with DIP and PIP in 0 degrees extension
  2. Immobilization straps placed over joints to ensure full extension
  3. Continue 5 to 6 weeks postoperatively
- Exercise splints
  1. Splint A: DIP allowed 25 degrees of flexion; PIP allowed 30 degrees of flexion
  2. Splint B: PIP extension blocking splint for active DIP flexion

- Static progressive or dynamic PIP flexion splint
  1. Not until week 4
  2. Intermittent use to decrease joint stiffness

Motion
- Early active short arc motion
  1. 0 to 1 week
     - Splint A: active flexion to splint limits followed by active extension to 0 degrees
     - Splint B: full active DIP flexion, if lateral bands are not involved
     - Splint B: limit active DIP flexion to 30 to 35 degrees, if lateral bands are repaired
     - Repeat each exercise 20 times, with a hold for three counts
  2. 2 to 3 weeks
     - Splint A: increase flexion angle to allow 40 degrees of active flexion/extension
     - Splint B: continue with unlimited active DIP flexion; if lateral bands were repaired, increase angle to 45 degrees
  3. 4 to 5 weeks
     - Splint A: increase flexion angle to 50 degrees in beginning of week 4; continue to increase angle up to 80 degrees by end of week 5
     - Splint B: allow full DIP flexion
     - Gentle passive ROM of all joints on individual basis with others held in protected position
  4. 5+ weeks
     - Discontinue exercise splints
     - Unrestricted isolated and composite DIP and PIP active motion (hold MP joints in 0 degrees extension)
     - Initiate tendon glides (hook, tabletop at 5 weeks; straight, composite at 6 weeks)
     - Manual mobilization to increase PIP flexion
     - Isometric, then isotonic grip strengthening
- MP joint and wrist AROM
  1. Begin immediately with static extension splint in place.

Functional Activity
- 0 to 6 weeks: light ADL with immobilization splint donned
- 6 to 8 weeks:
  1. Light ADL without splint (unless extensor lag)

Continued

Zones III and IV: Early Active Motion (Short Arc Motion)—Cont'd

   2. Incorporate static prehension and coordination activities into therapy sessions (dowel putty stamping, BTE Work Simulator, MULE)
- 8 to 12 weeks
   1. Moderate ADL without splint (unless extensor lag)
   2. Incorporate dynamic prehension and grip activities into therapy sessions
- 12 weeks: resume full participation in all ADL
- 16 weeks: heavy labor and sports permitted

HOME EXERCISE PROGRAM
- 0 to 6 weeks: add template splint exercises when patient becomes competent (10 times each, 3 times/day)
- 6+ weeks: tendon gliding, fine motor coordination activities, static grip strengthening

Zones V and VI: Early Active Mobilization

GOALS
- Full active DIP and PIP extension and flexion
- Incorporate injured digit into ADL
- Independence with premorbid ADL

PRECAUTIONS
- Do not use this protocol unless involved tendons were surgically repaired
- Avoid emphasizing flexion gains over extension
- Progress slowly if MP joint extension lag develops at any point

TREATMENT STRATEGIES
Splints
- Static volar forearm-based splint with wrist and MP joints included
   1. Wrist in 40 to 45 degrees of extension; MP joints in 15 to 20 degrees of flexion; IP joints and thumb free
   2. Full time 0 to 6 weeks; nighttime 6 to 8 weeks; discontinue at 8 weeks

- Nighttime removable volar IP extension splint with IP joints in 0 degrees of extension
- Static progressive MP flexion splints
  1. 4 weeks postoperative if active MP and/or PIP flexion is limited at 30 to 40 degrees with hard end-feel
     Note: separate splints for MP and PIP flexion; no composite flexion at this point
  2. 6 weeks postoperative if active MP and /or PIP flexion is limited at 50 to 60 degrees with hard end-feel
     Note: can treat MP and PIP flexion tightness with one splint; composite flexion permitted

Motion
- Phase I: 0 to 21 days postoperatively
  1. Passive wrist tenodesis by therapist
     - Passive full wrist extension with passive MP flexion to 40 degrees
     - Passive wrist flexion to 20 degrees with passive MP extension to 0 degrees
  2. Active place-hold MP and IP extension at 0 degrees with wrist in 20 degrees of flexion
  3. Protected active MP extension
     - Wrist placed in 20 degrees of flexion
     - MP joints placed in 30 degrees of flexion
     - Active MP extension to 0 degrees from start position
  4. Active hook fisting with MP and wrist supported in splint
- Phase II: 3 weeks postoperatively
  1. Discontinue place-hold if patient extends to 0 degrees from a position of 60 degrees of flexion
  2. Continue passive wrist tenodesis
  3. Continue protected active extension, but increase the arc of motion 10 to 20 degrees
- 4 weeks
  1. Transition to active tenodesis
  2. Add graded composite MP and IP flexion with neutral wrist
  3. Add tendon gliding with the wrist extended
  4. Add EDC glides and digital abduction/adduction with neutral wrist
- 5 weeks
  1. Add passive flexion of individual finger joints and wrist
- Phase III: 6+ weeks postoperatively

Continued

Zones V and VI: Early Active Mobilization—Cont'd

1. Add graded composite MP, IP, and wrist flexion
2. Add graded strengthening for wrist extension/flexion and forearm supination/pronation

Functional Activity
- 0 to 6 weeks postoperatively
  1. Light ADL with splint protection
- 6 to 8 weeks postoperatively
  1. Static grip and prehension activities in therapy
  2. Light ADL without splint protection unless MP joint extensor lag; if lag use splint until 8 weeks
- 8 to 12 weeks postoperatively
  1. Dynamic grip and prehension activities in therapy
  2. Moderate ADL without splint
- 12 weeks postoperatively: Resume full participation in ADL without restriction
- 16 weeks postoperatively: Heavy labor and sports permitted

HOME EXERCISE PROGRAM
- 0 to 4 weeks
  1. Active hook fisting in the splint
  2. Active place-hold MP extension
- 4 weeks: Add active tenodesis, tendon gliding with wrist extended, and EDC gliding with wrist neutral
- 8 weeks: Add strengthening for digital extension, wrist extension/flexion, forearm supination/pronation

Zones VII and VIII: Early Active Mobilization

GOALS
- Full active DIP and PIP extension and flexion
- Incorporate injured digit into ADL
- Independence with premorbid ADL

PRECAUTIONS
- *Do not* use this protocol unless involved tendons were surgically repaired
- *Do not* flex the wrist past neutral until 3 to 4 weeks after wrist extensor tendon repair

- Avoid emphasizing flexion gains over extension
- Progress more slowly if MP joint or wrist extension lag develops at any point
- Wrist position with active MP motion from 0 to 21 days postoperatively depends on whether digital extensor tendons or wrist extensor tendons were repaired

TREATMENT STRATEGIES
Splint
- Static volar forearm-based splint with MP joints included
  1. Wrist extended 40 degrees
  2. MP joints flexed 30 degrees
  3. Continuous wear except for exercises
     - Digital extensor tendon repair: 5 to 6 weeks
     - Wrist extensor repair: 8 weeks

Motion
- 0 to 21 days
  1. Passive wrist tenodesis:
     - Passive full wrist extension with passive MP flexion to 40 degrees
     - Passive wrist flexion to 20 degrees with passive MP extension to 0 degrees
  2. Active place-hold MP extension with digital extensor tendon repair
     - Wrist placed in 20 degrees of flexion
     - MP and IP joints placed in 0 degrees of extension for active hold
  3. Active place-hold MP extension with wrist extensor tendon repair
     - Wrist placed and supported in 0 to 20 degrees of extension
     - MP and IP joints placed in 0 degrees of extension for active hold
  4. Protected active MP extension with digital extensor tendon repair
     - Wrist placed and supported in 20 degrees of flexion
     - MP joints placed in 30 degrees of flexion
     - Active extension to 0 degrees from start position
  5. Protected active MP extension with wrist extensor tendon repair
     - Wrist placed and supported in 20 degrees of extension
     - MP joints placed in 30 degrees of flexion
     - Active extension to 0 degrees from start position

Continued

Zones VII and VIII: Early Active Mobilization— Cont'd

- 3 weeks
  1. Add placed MP flexion to 40 to 60 degrees, followed by active-assisted MP extension to 0 degrees (all with wrist held in full extension)
  2. Add active wrist extension and ulnar deviation with gravity eliminated (0 degrees to end range)
  3. Add extensor digitorum communis gliding and digital abduction/adduction
  4. Discontinue active place-hold
- 5 to 8+ weeks
  1. Begin active wrist flexion to 15 degrees maximum
  2. Increase wrist flexion arc by 10 to 15 degrees/week
  3. Begin active wrist extension and ulnar/radial deviation against gravity

Functional Activity

See recommendations for zones V and VI

HOME EXERCISE PROGRAM

See recommendations for zones V and VI

Note: Position of wrist with active place-hold MP extension depends upon whether the digital or wrist extensor tendons were repaired.

Thumb Zones T-I and T-II: Immobilization

GOALS

- Full active thumb IP extension and flexion
- Incorporate injured digit into ADL
- Independence with premorbid ADL

PRECAUTIONS

- No early active motion
- Avoid emphasizing flexion gains over extension
- Progress more slowly, if thumb IP joint extension lag develops at any point

TREATMENT STRATEGIES

Splint

- Thumb in 0 degrees
- Continuous splint for 6 weeks
- At 6 weeks, discharge splint if no lag

Motion
- 0 to 6 weeks
  1. AROM: MP extension/flexion 0 to 70 degrees
  2. AROM: Wrist extension/flexion
- 6 weeks
  1. AROM: IP flexion/extension
  2. AROM: Composite IP and MP flexion
- 8 weeks
  1. PROM: for each thumb joint and composite thumb flexion
  2. Graded grip and prehension activities

Functional Activity
- 0 to 6 weeks
  1. Light ADL with splint donned
- 6 to 8 weeks
  1. Light prehension activities without splint in therapy
  2. Light ADL with splint donned
- 8 to 12 weeks
  1. Light to moderate ADL without splint
- 12 weeks
  1. Resume full participation in all ADL without splint; sports/heavy labor at 16 weeks

HOME EXERCISE PROGRAM
- 0 to 6 weeks: Patient is educated for safe donning/doffing of splint and incorporates exercises from therapy
- 6+ weeks: Incorporate exercises from therapy, 10 times each, 3 times/day

Thumb Zones T-III and T-IV: Controlled Passive Motion

GOALS
- Full active thumb IP and MP extension and flexion
- Incorporate injured digit into ADL
- Independence with premorbid ADL

PRECAUTIONS
- Avoid emphasizing flexion gains over extension
- Progress more slowly if thumb MP joint extension lag develops at any point

Continued

Thumb Zones T-III and T-IV: Controlled Passive Motion—Cont'd

TREATMENT STRATEGIES
Splint
- Thumb IP and MP extension to 0 degrees, CMC midway between palmar and radial abduction, wrist 30 to 45 degrees of extension
  1. 0 to 6 weeks: At all times except exercises
  2. 3 weeks: Modify to allow active IP extension/flexion
  3. 6 weeks: Discontinue splint as long as no extensor lag
- Static progressive MP flexion splint
  1. Begin at week 7 if MP flexion proves difficult to recover
  2. Wear intermittently throughout the day

Motion
- 0 to 4 weeks
  1. Passive wrist tenodesis in therapy (20 times)
     - Wrist passively moved to full extension with relaxed thumb
     - Wrist passively flexed to neutral with the thumb held in full extension
  2. Controlled passive thumb MP extension/flexion during therapy only
     - Passive MP extension/flexion in a 30-degree arc (20 times)
     - Thumb IP and wrist held in maximum extension during passive motion
- 4 weeks
  1. Begin active MP extension and flexion
  2. Okay to use joint mobilization to increase extension/flexion
- 6 weeks
  1. PROM: Individual and composite joint flexion
  2. Grip and prehension activities
- 8 weeks
  1. Strengthening: Grip, pinch, wrist

Functional Activity
- 0 to 4 weeks: Light ADL within the splint
- 4 to 8 weeks: Light ADL without splint
- 8 to 12 weeks: Moderate ADL without splint
- 12 weeks: Resume full participation in ADL
- 16 weeks: Heavy labor and sports permitted

HOME EXERCISE PROGRAM
- Integrate previous functional activity and exercises into daily home program 3 times/day, 10 repetitions each

Thumb Zone T-V: Early Active Motion

GOALS
- Full active thumb IP and MP extension and flexion
- Incorporate injured digit into ADL
- Independence with premorbid ADL

PRECAUTIONS
- Avoid emphasizing flexion gains over extension
- Progress more slowly if thumb MP joint extension lag develops at any point

TREATMENT STRATEGIES
Splints
- Thumb IP and MP extension to 0 degrees, CMC midway between palmar and radial abduction, wrist 30 to 45 degrees of extension
  1. 0 to 6 weeks: At all times except exercises
  2. 3 weeks: Modify to allow active IP extension/flexion
  3. 6 weeks: Discontinue splint as long as no extensor lag
- Static progressive MP flexion splint
  1. Begin at week 7 if MP flexion proves difficult to recover
  2. Wear intermittently throughout the day

Motion
- 0 to 3 weeks
  1. Passive wrist tenodesis (20 times)
  2. Controlled passive thumb MP extension/flexion (20 times)
  3. Active place-hold thumb MP extension (20 times)
  4. Active thumb IP flexion/extension in dynamic IP extension splint (10 times/hr)
- 3 weeks
  1. Graded active flexion of thumb IP and MP joints
  2. Graded active motion of thumb CMC joint (palmar abduction, radial abduction, extension)
  3. Graded active wrist flexion/extension

Continued

Thumb Zone T-V: Early Active Motion—Cont'd

- 5 weeks (AROM only)
  1. Graded opposition
  2. Composite thumb flexion across the palm
  3. Radial and palmar abduction
- 6 weeks
  1. PROM: Individual and composite joint flexion

Functional Activity
- 0 to 3 weeks: Light ADL within splint
- 3 to 6 weeks: Shower/bathe without splint, exercise without splint; otherwise, wear splint
- 6 to 12 weeks: Wean from splint, light ADL without splint
- 12 weeks: Resume full participation in ADL

HOME EXERCISE PROGRAM
- Integrate above functional activity and exercises into daily home program 3 times/day, 10 repetitions each

Note: Perform all above exercises with remaining joints in the kinetic chain of the thumb held in full extension

Bibliography

Brand, P.W. Biomechanics of the Hand. Mosby, St. Louis, 1985.

Brand, P.W., Hollister, A. Clinical Mechanics of the Hand, 2nd ed. Mosby, St. Louis, 1993.

Chang, J. Molecular Studies in Flexor Tendon Wound Healing: The Role of Basic Fibroblastic Growth Factor Gene Expression. *J Hand Surg* 1998;23A(6):1052-1058.

Crosby, C.A., Wehbe, M.A. Early Protected Motion after Extensor Tendon Repair. *J Hand Surg* 1999;24A(5):1061-1070.

Doyle, J. Extensor Tendons-Acute Injuries. In Green, D.P., Hotchkiss, R.N., Pederson, W.C. (Eds). Green's Operative Hand Surgery, 4th ed. Churchill Livingstone, New York, 1999, pp. 1950-1986.

Evans, R. Clinical Management of Extensor Tendon Injuries. In Callahan, A., Mackin, E.J., Skirven, T.M., Schneider, L.H., Osterman, A.L., Hunter, J.M. (Eds). Rehabilitation of the Hand and Upper Extremity, 5th ed. Mosby, Philadelphia, 2002, pp. 542-579.

Evans, R. Early Active Short Arc Motion for the Repaired Central Slip. *J Hand Surg* 1994;19A(6):991-997.

Evans, R.B. Immediate Short Arc Motion Following Extensor Tendon Repair. *Hand Clin* 1995;11(3):483-512.

Evans, R.B. Rehabilitation Techniques for Applying Immediate Active Tension to the Repaired Extensor System. *Tech Hand Up Extrem Surg* 1999;3:139.

Evans, R.B., Buckhalter, W.E. A Study of the Dynamic Anatomy of Extensor Tendons and Implications for Treatment. *J Hand Surg* 1986;11A(5):774-779.

Evans, R.B., Thompson, D.E. An Analysis of Factors that Support Early Active Short Arc Motion of the Repaired Central Slip. *J Hand Ther* 1992;5:187-201.

Evans, R.B., Thompson, D.E. The Application of Stress to the Healing Tendon. *J Hand Ther* 1993;6(4):262-284.

Gelberman, R.H., Botte, M.J., Spiegelman, J.J., Akeson, W.H. The Excursion and Deformation of Repaired Flexor Tendons Treated with Protected Early Motion. *J Hand Surg* 1986;11A:106-110.

Gelberman, R.H., Gonsawes, M., Woo, S., Akeson, W.H. The Influence of Protected Passive Mobilization on the Healing Flexor Tendons: A Biomechanical and Microangiographic Study. *Hand* 1981; 13(2):120.

Gelberman, R.H., Nunley, J.A. II, Osterman, A.L., Breen, T.F., Dimick, M.P., Woo, S.L. Influences of the Protected Passive Mobilization Interval on Flexor Tendon Healing. *Clin Orthop* 1991;264:189-196.

Gelberman, R.H., Woo, S.L., Lothringer, K., Akeson, W.H., Amiel, D. Effects of Early Intermittent Passive Mobilization on Healing Canine Flexor Tendons. *J Hand Surg* 1982;7(2):170.

Gratton, P. Early Active Mobilization after Flexor Tendon Repairs. *J Hand Ther* 1993;6(4):285-289.

Hitchcock, T.F., Light, T.R., Bunch, W.H., Knight, G.W., Sartori, M.J., Patwardhan, A.G., Hollyfield, R.L. The Effect of Immediate Constrained Digital Motion on the Strength of Flexor Tendon Repairs in Chickens. *J Hand Surg* 1987;12A(4):590-595.

Kaplan, E. Anatomy, Injuries, and Treatment of the Extensor Apparatus of the Hand and Fingers. *Clin Orthop* 1959;13:24-41.

Khan, U., Occleston, N.L., Khaw, P.T., McGrouther, D.A. Differences in Proliferative Rate and Collagen Lattice Contraction Between Endotenon and Synovial Fibroblasts. *J Hand Surg* 1998;23A:266.

Mason, M.L., Allen, H.S. The Rate of Healing Tendons: An Experimental Study of Tensile Strength. *Ann Surg* 1941;113:424.

McFarlane, R.M., Hampole, M.K. Treatment of Extensor Tendon Injuries of the Hand. *Can J Surg* 1973;16:366-375.

Rosenthal, E. The Extensor Tendons: Anatomy and Management. In Callahan, A., Mackin, E.J., Skirven, T.M., Shcneider, L.H.,

Osterman, A.L., Hunter, J.M. (Eds). Rehabilitation of the Hand and Upper Extremity, 5th ed. Mosby, Philadelphia, 2002, pp. 498-540.

Saldana, M.J., Choban, S., Westerbeck, P., Schacherer, T.G. Results of Acute Zone III Extensor Tendon Injuries Treated with Dynamic Extension Splinting. *J Hand Surg* 1991;16A(6):1145-1150.

CHAPTER 16

Flexor Tenolysis

Amy Barenholtz-Marshall, OTR, CHT

Tenolysis is a surgical release of nongliding adhesions that form along the surface of a tendon after injury or repair. It is an elective surgical procedure that is performed in an effort to salvage tendon function after all therapy techniques have failed. If the patient has been compliant with a continuous therapy program for a minimum of 3 to 6 months with no significant improvement in active range of motion (AROM), a tenolysis is considered. Prerequisites for this procedure include full fracture and wound healing and resolution of joint contractures with normal or nearly normal passive range of motion (PROM).

To improve the likelihood of successful results, the patient must be motivated, committed, and able to follow through with a postoperative therapy program. In addition, close communication among the therapist, surgeon, and patient is essential. A preoperative visit for patient education is strongly recommended to reinforce the commitment and expectations during the postoperative phase. Poor compliance with therapy following tenolysis leads to poor results.

Surgical Overview

- The tenolysis procedure is performed under local anesthesia that is supplemented with an intravenous sedative drug. This allows for a thorough evaluation of AROM in which the patient is participatory.
- The involved flexor system is approached via a zigzag incision, long enough to expose the adhered tendon.
- The adhesions are excised with all efforts made to preserve the pulley systems, specifically the A2 and A4 pulleys.

- These pulleys are critical in maintaining the correct moment arm for the tendons to function most efficiently and prevent tendon bowstringing. Without the pulleys, more force is required to generate tension to produce full digital flexion.
- When it is not possible to preserve the pulleys, they are reconstructed at this time.
- Joint contractures, if present, are released through a capsulectomy. During this procedure, the active motion is reevaluated frequently to confirm adequate tissue release.
- The tendon is assessed for gapping at the repair site. A tendon with a large gap that has filled in with scar tissue will be too long, inefficient, and prone to rupture.
- Staged flexor tendon reconstruction may be necessary, if an adequate pulley system cannot be preserved and/or the flexor mechanism cannot be salvaged.

Rehabilitation Overview

- Immediate initiation of a hand therapy program is crucial to the success of a tenolysis.
- Early and frequent therapy will reduce the opportunity for rescarring.
- Referral information should include the integrity of the lysed tendon, intraoperative AROM and PROM measures, digit vascularity, prognosis for motion, and any concomitant procedures performed, such as a capsulectomy or pulley reconstruction.
- Additional corrective procedures complicate the patient's recovery.
- A tendon of good quality, with intact pulleys, requires a more vigorous postoperative therapy program.
- When the quality is poor (also known as *frayed tendon*) and/or there is pulley reconstruction, a less aggressive approach is used to decrease the demands of the involved structures and reduce the risk of tendon rupture.
- General rehabilitation goals are to achieve and maintain intraoperative AROM/PROM, prevent adhesion formation, maximize tendon glide/excursion, and maximize strength for restoration of normal hand function.
- The protocol that follows is similar to that following a tendon repair (see Chapter 14).

Postoperative Phase I: Inflammation (Week 1)

GOALS
- Control edema
- Achieve or maintain AROM/PROM obtained in surgery
- Decrease pain
- Promote wound healing
- Patient education
- Maintain ROM of uninvolved joints

PRECAUTIONS
- Avoid exacerbation of pain and inflammation
- Prevent flexion contractures
- Avoid neurovascular compromise

TREATMENT STRATEGIES
- Initiate therapy on the day of surgery
- Nighttime extension splinting
- Wound care: nonbulky, sterile protective dressing, as not to impede motion
- Elevated positioning at all times
- Compression wraps: Coban wrap, Ace wrap, or Isotoner glove applied with little to no tension
- Gentle PROM (all planes) to involved joints
- Active tendon gliding exercises
  1. Tenodesis place-hold may be the only appropriate exercise if the tendon quality is poor
- Active isolated/composite extension exercises
- Cryotherapy
- Daily therapy with strong emphasis on home exercise program (HEP)

CRITERIA FOR ADVANCEMENT
- Evidence of wound healing
- Reduction in edema
- Minimal inflammatory responsiveness

Postoperative Phase II: Fibroplasia (Weeks 2 to 3)

GOALS
- Facilitate wound healing
- Promote scar mobility and minimize adhesions

Continued

**Postoperative Phase II: Fibroplasia
(Weeks 2 to 3)—Cont'd**

- Reduce edema
- Maximize AROM
- Maintain full PROM
- Encourage functional hand use in light activities of daily living (ADL)

PRECAUTIONS
- Same as phase I
- Monitor soft tissue responses to treatment and upgrade techniques accordingly
- Watch for signs of adhesions (i.e., discrepancy in ROM where PROM is significantly greater than AROM); if adhesions are significant, upgrade AROM/blocking exercises

TREATMENT STRATEGIES
- Discharge splint during the day, continue at night
  1. May need to adjust splint to achieve greater extension if it has not already been achieved
- Retrograde massage
- Initiate scar management after sutures are removed and incision is fully closed
  1. Scar massage
  2. Silicone sheets
  3. Compression wraps during day, at night if tolerated
- Tendon gliding exercises
- Blocking exercises to isolate flexor digitorum superficialis and flexor digitorum profundus
  1. Assistive blocking splints if needed
- PROM
- Light soft tissue stretching
- Day splinting (static-progressive) for joint stiffness or soft tissue tightness
- Dexterity exercises
- Functional activities
- Sensibility testing if indicated
- HEP

CRITERIA FOR ADVANCEMENT
- Evidence of soft tissue healing
- Complete wound closure
- AROM is close or equal to PROM
- *AROM is WNL*

Postoperative Phase III: Scar Maturation (Weeks 4 to 10)

GOALS
- Maximize AROM to achieve intraoperative range
- Eliminate any residual edema
- Scar management
- Improve endurance
- Increase grip-and-pinch strength
- Return to full hand use

PRECAUTIONS
- Graded introduction of progressive resistive exercises

TREATMENT STRATEGIES
- Continue night splinting for 6 to 8 weeks (10 to 12 weeks for the frayed tendon)
- Continue with edema reduction as needed
- Scar management
  1. Scar mobilization techniques
  2. Deep friction massage
- Upgrade AROM exercises
- Tendon gliding
- Passive stretching
- Joint mobilizations if joint stiffness is present
- Continue with day splinting (static or static-progressive) as needed
- Dexterity exercises
- Functional activities
- If tendon integrity is good, sustained gripping exercises may be initiated at 3 to 4 weeks postoperatively
  1. Isometrics
  2. Rubber dowel squeezes
  3. Dowel stamping in firm putty
- Heavy resistance activities can begin at 8 weeks postoperatively (12 weeks for frayed tendon). If noted to have significant adhesions, patient can add resistive exercises sooner

CRITERIA FOR DISCHARGE
- Elimination of edema
- AROM/PROM has plateaued for 4 weeks
- Patient has resumed full use of hand in all ADL/vocational and recreational tasks

Bibliography

Feldshcer, S.B., Schneider, L.H. Flexor Tenolysis. *Hand Surg* 2002;
7(1):61–74.

Schneider, L.H. Flexor Tendons-Late Reconstruction. In Green, D.P.,
Hotchkiss, R.N., Pederson, W.C. (Eds). Green's Operative Hand
Surgery, 4th ed. Churchill Livingstone, New York, 1999,
pp. 1921–1925.

Schneider, L.H., Feldscher, S.B. Tenolysis: Dynamic Approach to
Surgery and Therapy. In Mackin, E.J., Callahan, A.D., Skirven, T.M.,
Schneider, L.H., Hunter, J.M. (Eds). Rehabilitation of the Hand,
5th ed. Mosby, St. Louis, 2002, pp. 457–467.

Strickland, J.W. (Ed). Flexor Tenolysis. In Hand Clinics, vol 1, no 1.
WB Saunders, Philadelphia, 1985.

Wehbe, M.A. Flexor Tendon Injury-Late Solution. *Hand Clin*
1986;1:133–137.

CHAPTER *17*

Upper Extremity Surgical Intervention in Patients with Cerebral Palsy: Musculotendinous Procedures

Kara Gallagher, MS, OTR/L, CHT

Jennifer P. Lewin, OTR/L

Cerebral palsy is a general term used to describe a condition characterized by irreversible brain damage and associated neuromotor dysfunction in the developing child. Cerebral palsy results from an injury to the brain before birth, during birth, or during the first 2 to 3 years of childhood. The extent of involvement of motor function, sensibility, and intelligence is highly variable. Cerebral palsy occurs in an estimated 0.6 to 2.5 of 1000 live births. It occurs in an estimated 5.2 of 1000 live births in the United States and in approximately 1 of 7 children worldwide. The number of cases is difficult to determine, because there is no system for monitoring the occurrence of cerebral palsy in the United States.

Several systems are used to classify cerebral palsy. The most common systems use the number of involved extremities and type of muscle tone. The main terms used to describe the extent of involved extremities include monoplegia (one limb), hemiplegia (one arm, one leg), quadriplegia (all limbs), and diplegia (quadriplegia with upper limb involvement milder than lower limbs). Terms used to describe muscle tone are spasticity (high tone), flaccidity (markedly low tone), athetosis (mixed tone), and ataxia. Ataxia is associated with primitive movement patterns and decreased coordination, such as dysmetria, dysdiadochokinesia, tremors at rest, and balance. Spastic involvement of a muscle (i.e., agonist) often pairs with a weak antagonistic muscle, which leads to deformity in the direction of the agonist.

Cerebral palsy is a static, nonprogressive condition, although abnormal movement patterns and imbalanced muscle tone, combined with the effects of gravity and normal growth, may cause the child to develop contractures and deformities. As a result, function becomes increasingly impaired. Upper extremity reconstructive surgery in the patient with cerebral palsy improves function and prevents further deformity. The goals of surgery are to correct deformity, rebalance the muscles to increase functional use, and improve hygiene and appearance. Rehabilitation following surgery is essential to facilitate active use of the muscles and integrate the upper extremity into functional activity. The following guideline describes common surgical reconstructive procedures and the preoperative and postoperative therapeutic interventions.

Surgical Overview

- The typical pattern of deformity in the spastic upper extremity is shoulder adduction and internal rotation, elbow flexion, forearm pronation, wrist flexion, finger flexion, and thumb flexion. The pattern of deformity is evident by the time the child reaches the age of 3.
- The goals of upper extremity reconstructive surgery are to correct these patterns and prevent further impairment.
- It is imperative that therapists, patients, and caregivers appreciate that surgery can augment function, yet rarely provides restoration of a normal arm.
- The surgeon establishes a realistic operative plan, based on a thorough physical examination, videotaped motion analysis, and, occasionally, a dynamic electromyography (EMG) test, to meet the patient's functional goals.
- To rebalance agonist and antagonistic muscles, the agonist is released and the antagonist is augmented through muscle transfers.
- Muscular release can take several forms, including release of the origin of the muscle, release of the insertion of the muscle, and lengthening of the muscle.
- A spastic muscle often provides a good choice for transfer to a weak muscle.
- Box 17-1 is a summary of the common procedures performed to correct upper extremity deformities in the patient with cerebral palsy.

BOX 17-1

Summary of Upper Extremity Surgical Reconstruction in the Patient with Cerebral Palsy

- Shoulder internal rotation
  1. Release of subscapularis
- Shoulder external rotation
  1. Release of supraspinatus, infraspinatus, and teres minor
- Elbow flexion
  1. Release of biceps, brachialis, and brachioradialis
  2. Flexor-pronator slide
- Forearm pronation
  1. Release of PQ and flexor aponeurosis
  2. PT rerouting
  3. Flexor-pronator slide
- Wrist flexion
  1. Wrist arthrodesis
  2. Muscle transfers for wrist and digital extension
     - ECU to ECRB
     - FCU to ECRB
     - PT to ECRB
     - BR to ECRB
     - FCU to EDC
  3. Wrist flexor tendon tightness
     - Tendon lengthening of FCR
     - Tendon lengthening of FCU
  4. Volar wrist capsule contracture
     - Proximal row carpectomy
     - Wedge resection arthrodesis
- Digital flexion tightness
  1. Flexor-pronator slide
  2. Fractional lengthening of FDS and/or FDP
  3. Z-lengthening of FDS and FDP
  4. Transfer of FDS to FDP (superficialis to profundus or STP)
- Intrinsic muscle spasticity
  1. Interosseous muscle origin slide
  2. Ulnar motor neurectomy
  3. Central slip tenotomy (for swan-neck deformity)

Continued

BOX 17-1

Summary of Upper Extremity Surgical Reconstruction in the Patient with Cerebral Palsy—cont'd

    4. FDS tenodesis (for swan-neck deformity)
- Thumb-in-palm deformity
    1. Web space release
    2. Release or lengthening of first dorsal interosseous, AP, FPB, and/or FPL
    3. EPL rerouting
    4. Transfer of BR to EPB
    5. Thumb MP joint capsulodesis

AP, adductor pollicis; BR, brachioradialis; ECRB, extensor carpi radialis brevis; ECU, extensor carpi ulnaris; EDC, extensor digitorum communis; EPB, extensor pollicis brevis; EPL, extensor pollicis longus; FCR, flexor carpi radialis; FCU, flexor carpi ulnaris; FDP, flexor digitorum profundus; FDS, flexor digitorum superficialis; FPB, flexor pollicis brevis; FPL, flexor pollicis longus; MP, metacarpophalangeal; PQ, pronator quadratus; PT, pronator teres.

Shoulder

- The shoulder postures in adduction and internal rotation. This position is caused by spasm or contracture of the subscapularis and pectoralis major.
  1. An adducted and internally rotated shoulder prevents the patient from reaching overhead and out to the side.
  2. With the arm in this position, tasks such as bathing and dressing are difficult to perform.
  3. Hygiene within the axilla may also be a problem in more severe cases.
  4. A lengthening or release of the subscapularis is performed to correct the adduction and internal rotation deformity.
- Occasionally, a patient postures in external rotation and abduction of the shoulder.
  1. This position makes it difficult to perform activities in midline.
  2. A release of the supraspinatus, infraspinatus, and teres minor can place the shoulder joint in a more functional position, permitting midline activities.

- Glenohumeral dislocation can occur in athetoid cerebral palsy and is treated surgically with a glenohumeral arthrodesis.

Elbow

- The elbow typically postures at rest in some degree of flexion. The degree of flexion increases with associated reactions caused by spastic contracture of any or all of the muscles of the elbow (biceps, brachialis, and brachioradialis [BR]).
- Long-standing deformities may result in soft tissue contractures and skin breakdown in the antecubital fossa.
- Elbow flexion contractures inhibit the patient's ability to reach forward for objects and effectively perform bimanual activities, such as placing an object on a table with two hands.
- Elbow flexion deformities, in a functional upper extremity, that are greater than 45 degrees at rest, with activity, or during ambulation benefit from surgical correction.
- Elbow flexion deformities, in the nonfunctional upper extremity, that are greater than 100 degrees benefit from surgery to improve functional transfers and hygiene.
- Elbow flexion deformities between 45 and 100 degrees in the nonfunctional elbow may be surgically addressed only if cosmesis is a concern.
- Surgery to correct an elbow flexion deformity includes a musculocutaneous neurectomy, a flexor-pronator slide, or lengthening of the elbow flexor muscles.
- The most direct method to address an elbow flexion deformity is via fractional lengthening of the biceps, brachialis, and brachioradialis (BR). The patient can anticipate a gain of 40 degrees of elbow extension with minimal loss of flexion or functional power.
- Musculocutaneous neurectomy is contraindicated for a functional upper extremity because active control of the biceps and brachialis is required for elbow flexion. It is also contraindicated in situations where muscle contracture exists.

Forearm

- Spasticity in the pronator teres (PT) and pronator quadratus (PQ) creates a pronation deformity.
  1. This prevents the patient from being able to bring the palms together for tasks requiring bimanual manipulation of objects.
  2. Furthermore, the pronated forearm cannot be used effectively to carry large objects because of the palm-down position of the hand.
- Procedures to correct pronation deformity include a flexor pronator slide, release of the pronator quadratus, pronator teres (PT) and flexor aponeurosis, and a pronator rerouting.
  1. A flexor-pronator slide involves the release of the PT at its origin, whereas a pronator tenotomy, or rerouting, involves the release of the PT at its insertion.
  2. When active pronation is present in the absence of active supination, a PT rerouting provides active supination.
  3. When both active supination and pronation are lacking, a pronator teres rerouting suspends the forearm in a neutral position, using a tenodesis effect.

Wrist and Digits: Extrinsic Musculature

- The wrist often postures in flexion with fisted digits, which is a result of weak wrist and digital extensors, contracted or spastic wrist and digital flexor tendons, or a volar wrist capsular contracture.
  1. The flexed position interferes with the normal tenodesis balance between the wrist and digital flexor and extensor muscles, thereby impairing grasp and release of everyday objects.
  2. The poor mechanical advantage of the digital flexors in wrist flexion impairs grip strength.
  3. Weak extensors and/or contracted flexors inhibit the release of objects.
- Ulnar deviation is another common posture of the wrist, which is caused by spasticity or contracture of the flexor carpi ulnaris (FCU) or extensor carpi ulnaris (ECU).
  1. The FCU causes ulnar deviation with wrist flexion, whereas the ECU causes ulnar deviation with wrist extension.

2. The flexor muscle causing the deformity often serves as the transfer muscle to the weak extensor group. For example, if the FCU pulls the wrist into ulnar deviation with wrist flexion, then the FCU may be transferred to the extensor carpi radialis brevis (ECRB) to augment extension.

3. An FCU to ECRB transfer improves wrist extension while eliminating the ulnar deviating force with wrist flexion.

- Impaired wrist/digital extension caused by contracture or spasticity of the flexors requires release or lengthening of the involved flexor muscles.
- When wrist and digital extension is impaired without flexor contracture or spasticity, surgery involves muscle transfers to augment extension.
- A combination of flexor contractures (or spasticity) with extensor weakness requires both release and lengthening of the flexors, as well as a transfer to the extensors for increased power.

Wrist and Digital Extensor Weakness

- One or more of the following procedures may be performed to improve wrist and digital extension, depending on the strength of donor muscles ECU to ECRB, FCU to ECRB, PT to ECRB, BR to ECRB, or FCU to extensor digitorum communis (EDC).
- When the flexion deformity at the wrist is severe, and a joint contracture has developed, a proximal row carpectomy may be the only option to position the wrist in neutral.

Wrist and Digital Flexor Tightness

- Spasticity or contracture of the FCU tendon is the dominant cause of a wrist flexion deformity in patients with cerebral palsy.
- Spasticity or contracture of flexor carpi radialis (FCR), palmaris longus, flexor digitorum superficialis (FDS), flexor digitorum profundus (FDP), and flexor pollicis longus (FPL) can also contribute to the deformity.

- Procedures to lengthen the flexor tendons include flexor-pronator slide, fractional lengthening, Z-lengthening, superficialis to profundus transfer, and bony shortening at the wrist.
- Digital flexor lengthening decreases the strength of the flexors, yet provides improved wrist extension, which enhances force.

Hand: Intrinsic Musculature

- Spasticity or contracture of the intrinsic muscles of the hand (lumbricals and interossei) leads to flexion at the metacarpophalangeal (MP) joints and extension at the proximal interphalangeal (PIP) joints.
- The EDC can usually overpower intrinsic spasticity to extend the MP joints and open the hand. A functional problem arises when the EDC cannot overcome the intrinsic spasticity to open the hand, thereby preventing effective grasp and release.
- The imbalance created by spastic intrinsic muscles and weak flexor muscles can lead to a swan-neck deformity over time. In a swan-neck deformity, the PIP joint can lock in hyperextension, making flexion of this joint very difficult.
- Surgical correction for intrinsic muscle spasticity includes interosseous muscle origin slide or ulnar motor neurectomy.
  1. The muscle origin slide adjusts the spasticity of the muscle, decreases the contracture, and permits some intrinsic function.
  2. Ulnar motor neurectomy releases the spasticity of the intrinsic muscles but does not address the joint contracture.
- A swan-neck deformity can be corrected with a central slip tenotomy or FDS tenodesis.

Thumb

- Flexion of the thumb into the palm greatly impairs hand function by preventing opposition and prehension grasp. This deformity is caused by web space contracture; spasticity or contracture of the adductor pollicis (AP), flexor pollicis brevis (FPB), and first dorsal interosseous; spasticity of the FPL with the wrist extended and flexed; or a weak abductor pollicis longus (APL), extensor pollicis longus (EPL), or extensor pollicis brevis (EPB).

- Hyperextension of greater than 20 degrees in the thumb MP joint is also a concern and may need to be addressed.
- Surgery is determined according to the cause of the deformity.
- Common reconstructive thumb procedures include release of the spastic muscles, augmentation of the impaired extensor and abductor muscles, stabilization of the thumb MP joint, and release of the web space contracture.
- Thumb abduction and extension can be improved by various tendon transfers, including BR, palmaris longus, FCR, FCU, ECRB, extensor carpi radialis longus (ECRL), and FDS.
- FPL rerouting and abductorplasty also improve extension and abduction.
- If the thumb MP joint actively extends more than 20 degrees past zero, MP joint arthrodesis or capsulodesis is performed to prevent hyperextension.

Rehabilitation Overview
Preoperative Care

- The preoperative phase is critical in providing the surgeon with the information required to formulate and finalize the surgical plan.
- This phase focuses on completing a thorough upper extremity evaluation that includes a videotaped motion analysis, functional performance tests, and, occasionally, a dynamic EMG study.
- The preoperative evaluation is completed by an occupational or hand therapist and reviewed with the treating hand surgeon.
- The therapist, surgeon, and patient determine preoperative therapy goals once the evaluation has been reviewed.
- Preoperative therapy is not always necessary, depending on the needs of the patient. It is indicated to maximize range of motion (ROM) before surgery. For example, botulinum toxin A (BTX-A) injection is used preoperatively to

temporarily relax a spastic muscle. A serial cast or splint is then applied to elongate this spastic muscle in preparation for surgery.

* BTX-A may also be used to determine whether a particular surgical procedure will enhance function in the hand.
    1. The surgeon injects BTX-A into a specific muscle to determine whether its release will enhance function.
    2. The therapist then instructs the patient in exercises to test the effects of the BTX-A and the function of the antagonistic muscles.

Preoperative Therapy

GOALS
* Complete upper extremity evaluation, motion analysis video, and functional performance testing
* Refer patient for EMG study, when necessary
* Maximize AROM/PROM

PRECAUTIONS
* None

TREATMENT STRATEGIES
* BTX-A injection into spastic muscle
* Apply serial cast or splint within 3 days of injection and continue until PROM stabilizes (6 weeks)
* Home exercise program for AROM/PROM of spastic and/ or contracted muscle

CRITERIA FOR ADVANCEMENT
* PROM is stabilized
* BTX-A demonstrates a positive effect on upper extremity function
* Consider surgery to permanently recreate effects of BTX-A

Postoperative Care Overview

* Rehabilitation focuses on the following goals: protection of the rebalanced length-tension relationship of the postoperative structures; neuromuscular reeducation of the transferred muscles; and integration of the arm into functional use.

- The postoperative upper extremity in a patient with cerebral palsy is subject to muscle spasms and spasticity following surgery.
  1. Therefore, despite the trend in rehabilitation toward early mobility, this patient is immobilized for 4 weeks following surgery during phase I.
  2. Immobilization is necessary to protect the rebalanced muscles at their resting lengths, despite postoperative, unpredictable spasms and increased tone.
- Phase II begins 4 weeks after surgery, once the immobilization period has ended.
  1. This phase consists of protective splinting and intensive therapy to assist the patient in developing increased control over the rebalanced limb.
  2. During phase II the patient is splinted according to the surgical procedures and surgeon's orders. The splint remains in place at all times, except during therapy, the home exercise program (HEP), and bathing.
  3. Clinicians should use traditional therapeutic methods to improve ROM and strength, as well as neurorehabilitative techniques to facilitate movement out of the preoperative synergistic patterns.
- Phase III begins 8 weeks after surgery.
  1. The clinician assists the patient in integrating the arm into functional use through activity practice.
  2. Therapeutic activities include both unilateral and bilateral tasks to integrate the upper extremity into function.
  3. The splint is removed during the day to complete activities of daily living (ADL).
  4. The splint continues to be worn at night, sometimes up to 16 weeks postoperatively, to prevent recurrence of the preoperative deformities.
- This guideline delineates desired goals, precautions, and treatment strategies to facilitate motion, strength, motor control, and function in the upper extremity after reconstructive surgery in the patient with cerebral palsy.
- Criteria for advancement are included for each phase. In addition, the guideline includes splint designs applicable for phases II and III.

Postoperative Phase I (Weeks 0 to 4)

GOALS
- Immobilization of surgical areas
- Independence with HEP
- Independence with edema control techniques
- Preparation for phase II therapy

PRECAUTIONS
- Bulky postoperative dressing may not be removed
- Loose dressing must be secured and the surgeon contacted
- No heavy grasping or pinching; light self-care acceptable

TREATMENT STRATEGIES
- HEP
  1. AROM/PROM of uninvolved joints
  2. 3 times/day, 10 repetitions each, with 5-second hold
- Edema control
  1. Ice, compression, elevation
  2. Sleep with arm elevated

CRITERIA FOR ADVANCEMENT
- Immobilization period ends at 4 weeks with cast removal by surgeon
- Surgeon's approval to proceed to phase II

SPECIAL CONSIDERATIONS
- If problems arise with the cast, surgeon may remove it and initiate splint earlier than 4 weeks postoperatively

Postoperative Phase II (Weeks 4 to 8)

GOALS
- Protective immobilization with custom splint
- Active firing of transferred and lengthened muscles
- Patient education

PRECAUTIONS
- Wear splint at all times, except during bath, exercise, and scar management
- Protective splint must be worn during physical education classes and recess

- No passive forearm pronation, wrist flexion, or heavy grasp/pinch

TREATMENT STRATEGIES
- Custom splint, as ordered by surgeon
- Isolated motion: AA/AROM/PROM progressing from a gravity-eliminated position to against-gravity position
  1. Elbow extension/flexion: supine then standing
  2. Forearm supination/pronation: seated, elbow by side
  3. Wrist extension/flexion: seated, forearm supported
  4. Digital extension/flexion: open/close fist
  5. Thumb abduction and extension: hand on table, palm down, bring thumb out to side
- Neuromuscular reeducation
  1. Facilitation of transferred muscle
  2. Tapping, cold, or vibration to stimulate the transferred muscle
  3. NDT and PNF techniques to facilitate movement out of synergy
- Functional activities (Week 6)
  1. Grasping objects to encourage spherical or cylindrical patterns
  2. Pinching light objects to promote tip-to-tip or 3-jaw chuck prehension
  3. School, art, athletic, self-care activities of low demand on muscles
  4. Examples: turning pages in book, finger painting, catching/rolling lightweight ball, finger foods
- Scar management
  1. Scar massage (cross-frictional) 5 minutes each scar
  2. Scar pressure: silicone pads at night only
- HEP
  1. Place-hold and AROM/PROM of involved joints
  2. Keep simple: one exercise per joint

CRITERIA FOR ADVANCEMENT
- Active control of muscle transfers
- Beginning to use hand for light activities
- Clearance from surgeon

SPECIAL CONSIDERATIONS
- Consider electric stimulation for transferred muscle in case of poor active initiation of movement

Continued

Postoperative Phase II (Weeks 4 to 8)—Cont'd

- Focus therapy on new muscle patterns via neuromuscular reeducation and functional activities
- Preference for adduction of thumb and initiation of movement from the tip may persist; splint thumb IP in 10 to 15 degrees of flexion to encourage radial abduction

Postoperative Phase III (Week 8 to 6 Months)

GOALS

- Reinforce HEP and scar management
- Initiate strengthening
- Resume full participation in ADL and functional tasks in school/work
- Use splint for nighttime only

PRECAUTIONS

- Begin strengthening, only per surgeon's orders
- Do not strengthen forearm pronation
- Needs surgeon's approval to participate in gym and recess without splint protection

TREATMENT STRATEGIES

- Motion: AROM against gravity progressing toward resistance of the following:
  1. Elbow extension, forearm supination, wrist extension/flexion, digital extension, thumb extension and abduction, grasp, and prehension
- Neuromuscular reeducation
  1. Use NDT or PNF patterns with functional activities to encourage new movement patterns
- Functional activities
  1. Grasping objects that encourage spherical or cylindrical patterns
  2. Pinching light objects that promote tip-to-tip or 3-jaw chuck prehension
  3. School, art, athletic, self-care activities of low demand on muscles
  4. Examples: carrying textbook, molding clay, wall push-ups, donning socks and shoes

- HEP
  1. Modify program so that all exercises are performed against gravity
  2. Continue scar management until week 12
  3. Add grip-and-pinch strengthening as needed

CRITERIA FOR ADVANCEMENT
- Maintains good form as resistance increases
- Able to perform graded activities with minimal to no assistance
- Progress under guidance from surgeon

SPECIAL CONSIDERATIONS
- Integrate upper extremity into both unilateral and bilateral activities
- Forearm procedure may result as a suspension in neutral rather than an active supinator; active supination may not evolve
- Ulnar deviation preference may persist with active wrist extension; block this preference as patient strengthens wrist extension

Bibliography

Autti-Ramo, I., Larsen, A., Taimo, A., von Wendt, L. Management of the Upper Limb with Botulinum Toxin Type A in Children with Spastic Type Cerebral Palsy and Acquired Brain Injury: Clinical Implications. *Eur J Neurol* 2001;8(Suppl 5):136–144.

Bobath, K. A Neurophysiological Basis for the Treatment of Cerebral Palsy. Lippincott, Philadelphia, 1980.

Boyd, R.N., Morris, M.E., Graham, H.K. Management of Upper Limb Dysfunction in Children with Cerebral Palsy: A Systematic View. *Eur J Neurol* 2001;8(Suppl 5):150–166.

Carlson, M.G. Cerebral Palsy. In Hotchkiss, R. (Ed). Green's Operative Hand Surgery. Elsevier, New York, 1999.

Chin, T.Y., Graham, H.K. Botulinum Toxin A in the Management of Upper Limb Spasticity in Cerebral Palsy. *Hand Clin* 2003; 19(4):591–600.

Cooper, W. Surgery of Upper Extremity in Spastic Paralysis. *Q Rev Pediatr* 1952;7:139–144.

Goldner, J.L. Surgical Reconstruction of the Upper Extremity in Cerebral Palsy. *Hand Clin* 1988;4(2):223–265.

Goldner, J.L. Upper Extremity Tendon Transfers in Cerebral Palsy. *Orthop Clin North Am* 1974;5(2):389-414.

Gordon, K.Y., Schanzenbacher, K.E., Case-Smith, J., Carrasco, R.C. Diagnostic Problems in Pediatrics. In Case-Smith (Ed). Occupational Therapy for Children. Mosby, St. Louis, 1996.

Koman, L.A., Smith, B.P., Goodman, A. Botulinum Toxin Type A in the Management of Cerebral Palsy. Wake Forest University Press, Winston-Salem, NC, 2002.

Leclercq, C. General Assessment of the Upper Limb. *Hand Clin* 2003;19:557-564.

Mowery, C.A., Gelberman, R.H., Rhoades, C.E. Upper Extremity Tendon Transfers in Cerebral Palsy: Electromyographic and Functional Analysis. *J Pediatr Orthop* 1985;5:69-72.

Renshaw, T.S. Cerebral Palsy. In Morrissy, R.T., Weinstein, S.L. (Eds). Lovell and Winter's Pediatric Orthopedics, 5th ed., vol. 1. Lippincott Williams & Wilkins, New York, 2001, pp. 563-599.

Samilson, R.L., Morris, J.M. Surgical Improvement of the Cerebral-palsied Upper Limb: Electromyographic Studies and Results of 128 Operations. *J Bone Joint Surg* 1964;46A:1203-1216.

Skoff, H., Woodbury, D.F. Management of the Upper Extremity in Cerebral Palsy. *J Bone Joint Surg* 1985;67A(3):500-503.

Statistic from "How common is cerebral palsy?" Centers for Disease Control and Prevention (CDC). Available online at http://www.cdc.gov.

Stranger, M. Orthopedic Management. In Tecklin, J.S. (Ed). Pediatric Physical Therapy, 3rd ed. Lippincott Williams & Wilkins, New York, 1999, pp. 394-396.

Tachdjian, M.O., Minear, A.L. Sensory Disturbances in the Hands of Children with Cerebral Palsy. *J Bone Joint Surg* 1958;40A:85-90.

Van Heest, A.E., House, J.H., Cariello, C. Upper Extremity Surgical Treatment of Cerebral Palsy. *J Hand Surg* 1999;24A(2):323-330.

Wall, S.A., Chait, L.A., Temlett, J.A., Perkins, B., Hillen, G., Becker, P. Botulinum A Chemodenervation: A New Modality in Cerebral Palsied Hands. *Br J Plast Surg* 1993;46:703-706.

Waters, P.M., Zurakowski, D., Patterson, P., Bae, D.S., Nimec, D. Interobserver and Intraobserver Reliability of Therapist-assisted Videotaped Evaluations of Upper-limb Hemiplegia. *J Hand Surg* 2004;29A:328-334.

Wong, D.L. Whaley and Wongs Essentials of Pediatric Nursing, 4th ed. Mosby, St. Louis, 1993.

CHAPTER 18

Ulnar Nerve Transposition

Amy Barenholtz-Marshall, OTR, CHT

At the elbow, the ulnar nerve passes posterior to the medial epicondyle through a narrow space known as the cubital tunnel. Because of the anatomical configuration and the superficial course of the nerve, this is a common entrapment site and is referred to as cubital tunnel syndrome. At this level the nerve is responsible for motor activity of the fourth and fifth flexor digitorum profundus (FDP) tendons, flexor carpi ulnaris (FCU) muscle, intrinsic hand muscles, and sensation of the fifth and ulnar one-half of fourth fingers.

Injury to the nerve can be caused by a blunt trauma to the elbow (such as a fracture or fracture dislocation), compression, traction, friction, or subluxation. Compression to the nerve can originate from external or internal sources. Externally sustained, prolonged pressure on the medial side of the elbow, or repetitive motion, results in compression of the nerve. Internal sources of compression include tight fascial bands, arthritic spurs, rheumatoid synovitis, and soft tissue tumors. Other conditions that contribute to compression by lowering the nerve threshold include diabetes, chronic alcoholism, and renal disease.

Ulnar nerve compression symptoms can mimic other conditions. A differential diagnoses must be made to exclude thoracic outlet syndrome (TOS), cervical disc lesion with nerve root compression, and ulnar nerve entrapment at Guyon's canal. Early symptoms of ulnar nerve compression include sharp or aching pain on the medial side of the proximal forearm, that radiates proximally or distally. This is accompanied by intermittent paresthesias in the fourth and fifth fingers. Symptoms are aggravated by elbow flexion and frequently awaken the patient at night. Later symptoms include muscle atrophy of the intrinsics, slight clawing of the fourth and fifth digits accompanied by sensory changes, hand weakness, and impaired dexterity. The last changes to appear are FDP and FCU weakness.

Nerve compression that is detected early, with the compression attributed to external sources, is treated conservatively by anti-inflammatory medication, nighttime splinting (to avoid prolonged elbow flexion), postural education, and activity modification. If a 4- to 6-week trial of conservative treatment fails, surgery is considered. Electromyography (EMG) testing before surgery confirms compression of the nerve.

Surgical procedures to decompress the nerve range from a simple ligament release (in situ decompression) to an anterior transposition of the nerve to a medial epicondylectomy. Functional results vary depending on the severity and duration of nerve compression, clinical symptoms, and surgical procedure. Symptoms that have been present for less than 6 months and limited to paresthesias can expect complete recovery.

Anatomic Overview

- The ulnar nerve arises from the medial cord of the brachial plexus.
- As the ulnar nerve courses medially toward the elbow, it pierces the medial intermuscular septum through the arcade of Struthers. This is a fascial band that lies 8 cm proximally to the medial epicondyle and traverses the medial head of the triceps to the medial intramuscular septum.
- The nerve descends subfascially on the medial aspect of the triceps muscle and changes to a more posterior course.
- Before the nerve enters the forearm, it passes posteriorly to the medial epicondyle through the cubital tunnel.
  1. The tunnel begins at the condylar groove between the medial epicondyle of the humerus and the olecranon of the ulna.
  2. The floor of the tunnel is composed of the medial collateral ligament of the elbow joint, and the two heads of the FCU form the sides.

3. The roof is formed by the triangular arcuate ligament, which bridges the medial epicondyle of the humerus and the medial tip of the olecranon.
4. The capacity of the cubital tunnel is greatest when the elbow is extended, because this puts the arcuate ligament on slack.

- The nerve then passes into the forearm between the ulnar and humeral heads of the FCU muscle.
- Compression at the elbow can occur at various sites along the course of the nerve, including the arcade of Struthers, the medial intermuscular septum, the medial epicondyle, the cubital tunnel, or between the two heads of the FCU origin.

Surgical Overview

- The purpose of surgical intervention is to decompress the nerve while retaining adequate blood supply.
- If in situ decompression cannot adequately relieve compression, the nerve is removed from the tunnel and transposed anteriorly either subcutaneously or submuscularly. The nerve is moved to lie anteriorly to the elbow flexion/extension axis of motion to avoid compression and traction with elbow flexion.
- The approach is a posteromedial longitudinal incision approximately 8 to 10 cm long, with proximal exposure of the medial intermuscular septum and the arcade of Struthers and distal exposure of the nerve between the two heads of the FCU.
- The arcade of Struthers is released, and the intermuscular septum is removed.
- The nerve is then identified and freed in the proximal forearm at the level deep to the FCU origin.
- It is elevated from its bed and placed anteriorly to the medial epicondyle.
- At this point the nerve is placed in an intermuscular, subfascial, subcutaneous, or submuscular position.

Subcutaneous Transposition

- The ulnar nerve and its neurovascular bundle are transposed anteriorly beneath the elevated skin flap.

- A loose fasciodermal sling, created from the flexor muscle mass or the intermuscular septum, is created to support the nerve in the new position.
- This approach is appropriate for mild cases of compression.
- Clinical symptoms are present, but EMG tests are normal.

Submuscular Transposition (Learmonth Procedure)

- This procedure places the nerve in a protected position and is indicated in moderate to severe neuropathies, thin-skinned individuals, or high demand elbows, such as throwing athletes.
- It is also performed as a second procedure in people who had a failed anterior subcutaneous transposition.
- The muscles of the flexor-pronator group are detached 1 cm distally to the medial epicondyle.
- The ulnar nerve is moved beneath the flexor muscle group and aligned adjacently to the median nerve.
- The flexor-pronator origin is repaired and reattached to the epicondyle, with the forearm positioned in pronation.

Rehabilitation Overview

- Rehabilitation goals are to reduce pain, reduce paresthesias, optimize nerve glide, increase elbow range of motion (ROM), prevent deformity, increase muscle strength, restore full functional hand use, and educate the patient in sensory precautions, if necessary.
- Protected ROM begins early to prevent nerve adhesions and joint stiffness.
- Full active elbow motion is expected by 3 weeks post-surgery.
- Resistive exercises are initiated in accordance with the stages of soft tissue healing and are aimed at restoring normal upper extremity function to perform all relevant activities of daily living (ADL), vocational, and leisure activities.

Postoperative Phase I: Inflammation (Weeks 0 to 2)

GOALS
- Edema and pain control
- Maximum elbow and forearm AROM within safe parameters
- Promote wound healing
- Awareness of precautions
- Full ROM of uninvolved joints
- Independence in HEP

PRECAUTIONS
- Avoid exacerbation of pain and inflammation
- Avoid neurovascular compromise
- No elbow extension beyond 90 degrees
- If the flexor-pronator group is reattached, no active wrist flexion or extension or forearm pronation
- Sensory precautions

TREATMENT STRATEGIES
Splinting
- Elbow positioned either in sling or splint (posterior elbow shell: elbow at 90 degrees with forearm and wrist in neutral) full-time, remove three to four times a day for Therex
- Splinting to prevent deformity
- Figure-eight splint for motor weakness and muscle imbalance (clawing of digits IV and V)

Wound care
- Wound care: maintain sterile protective dressing as thin as possible as not to impede motion

Edema control
- Elevated positioning at all times
- Compression wraps: coban or Ace wrapping
- Cryotherapy

Therapeutic exercises
- AROM elbow flexion and graded extension to pain tolerance
- AROM forearm pronation and supination to pain tolerance
- Gentle PROM elbow flexion
- AROM to uninvolved joints: shoulder, wrist and hand, tendon gliding exercises

Continued

Postoperative Phase I: Inflammation (Weeks 0 to 2)—Cont'd

  1. If there is motor involvement in hand; intrinsic muscle exercises
- HEP

CRITERIA FOR ADVANCEMENT
- Evidence of wound healing
- Reduction in edema
- Minimal inflammatory responsiveness

Postoperative Phase II: Fibroplasia (Weeks 3 to 7)

GOALS
- Scar management
- Promote scar mobility and minimize adhesions
- Promote nerve glide
- Reduce edema
- Maximize AROM/PROM
- Task modification
- Encourage functional hand use in light ADL

PRECAUTIONS
- Same as phase I
- Monitor soft tissue responses to treatment and upgrade techniques accordingly
- Watch for signs of nerve adhesions
- Sensory precautions
- Avoid provocative positioning
- Avoid repetitive elbow flexion/extension tasks

TREATMENT STRATEGIES
Splinting
- Wean splint/sling during day; use only for protection and sleep
- Splinting to prevent deformity

Edema reduction
- Elevation
- Retrograde massage
- Compression wrapping

Scar management (initiate after sutures are removed and incision is fully closed)
- Scar massage
- Silicone sheets
- Compression wraps during day and at night if tolerated

Therapeutic exercises
- Heat modalities pretreatment
- Elbow/forearm AROM and progress to PROM
- Graded progression of active elbow extension
- Upgrade forearm ROM
- Light soft tissue stretching
- Ulnar nerve gliding exercises
- Pain relief via appropriate modalities
- Hand strengthening with putty or bands
  1. Lumbricals
  2. Thumb adductor
  3. Dorsal/volar interossei
- Pinch strengthening
  1. Lateral pinch
  2. Three- and two-point pinch
- Isometric elbow exercises in midrange at 4 weeks
- Weeks 6 to 8: PREs to wrist begin at week 4 for subcutaneous transposition

Function
- Functional activities
- Sensibility retraining/reeducation if necessary

CRITERIA FOR ADVANCEMENT
- Evidence of soft tissue healing without an inflammatory response
- Achieve full elbow AROM/PROM

Postoperative Phase III: Scar Maturation (Weeks 8 to 12)

GOALS
- Maximize AROM/PROM
- Improve upper extremity endurance
- Increase elbow/forearm strength
- Increase grip/pincher strength
- Return to full functional activity

Continued

Postoperative Phase III: Scar Maturation (Weeks 8 to 12)—Cont'd

PRECAUTIONS
- Grade introduction of PREs

TREATMENT STRATEGIES
Scar management
- Scar mobilization techniques

Therapeutic exercises
- Ulnar nerve gliding exercises
- Passive stretching
- Joint mobilizations if joint stiffness is present
- Continue with grip-and-pinch strengthening
- PREs to elbow
- Forearm and wrist strengthening
  1. Free weights
  2. Thera-Band
  3. Putty
  4. UBE
  5. BTE

Function
- Functional activities
- Dexterity exercises

CRITERIA FOR DISCHARGE
- Minimal to no pain
- AROM/PROM has plateaued for 4 weeks
- Patient has resumed full use of extremity in all ADL, vocational, and recreational tasks

Bibliography

Aeillo, B. Ulnar Nerve Compression. In Clark, G.L., Wilgis, E.F., Aiello, B., Eckhaus, D., Eddington, L.V. (Eds). Hand Rehab, A Practical Guide, 2nd ed. Churchill Livingstone, New York, 1998, pp. 213-220.

Omer, G. Diagnosis and Management of Cubital Tunnel Syndrome. In Mackin, E.J., Callahan, A.D., Skirven, T.M., Schneider, L.H., Hunter, J.M. (Eds). Rehabilitation of the Hand, 5th ed. Mosby, St. Louis, 2002, pp. 672-677.

Osterman, A.L., Davies, C.A. Subcutaneous Transposition of the Ulnar Nerve for Treatment of Cubital Tunnel Syndrome. In Plancher, K.D. (Ed). Hand Clinics, WB Saunders, Philadelphia, 1996, pp. 421-433.

Spinner, R.J., Spinner, M. Nerve Entrapment Syndromes. In Morrey, B.F. (Ed). The Elbow and Its Disorders, 3rd ed. WB Saunders, Philadelphia, 2000, pp. 847-859.

Szabo, R.M. Entrapment and Compression Neuropathies. In Green, D.P., Hotchkiss, R.N., Pederson, W.C. (Eds). Green's Operative Hand Surgery, 4th ed. Churchill Livingstone, New York, 1999, pp. 1422-1429.

CHAPTER 19

Thumb Carpometacarpal Joint Arthroplasty

Carol Page, PT, DPT, CHT

Osteoarthritis, the most common type of arthritis, frequently affects the hands. The thumb carpometacarpal (CMC) joint is the second most frequently affected joint of the hand, following the distal interphalangeal (IP) joint. Thumb CMC joint osteoarthritis is more common in women than in men and is associated with aging. Thumb CMC joint osteoarthritis may be degenerative or posttraumatic in origin. The chief complaint is thumb pain, with joint stiffness being a later finding. The severity of symptoms may not correspond radiographically to the degree of change in the joint.

Initial treatment consists of nonoperative measures, such as splinting, education in joint protection principles, oral anti-inflammatory medications, and corticosteroid injections. Surgery is indicated when pain is no longer controlled by these nonoperative measures and when pain impairs sleep and functional use of the hand.

Surgical Overview

- The thumb CMC joint comprises the articulation of the trapezium and the first metacarpal. The scaphotrapezial joint may demonstrate degenerative changes as well.
- The most commonly performed surgery for thumb CMC osteoarthritis is resection arthroplasty of a portion of or the entire trapezium, with ligament reconstruction and use of filler for the excised bone.
- At the Hospital for Special Surgery (HSS), the two most commonly performed basal joint arthroplasties are ligament reconstruction tendon interposition (LRTI) arthroplasty and hematoma and distraction arthroplasty (HDA).

- LRTI arthroplasty involves excision of the distal portion of the trapezium, if the scaphotrapezial joint is in satisfactory condition. If not, the entire trapezium is excised.
  1. The base of the thumb metacarpal is excised and a hole is made in the radial base.
  2. Half of the flexor carpi radialis tendon is harvested, passed through the trapezial fossa into the medullary canal of the thumb metacarpal, and advanced through the hole in the metacarpal radial base.
  3. The tendon slip is pulled tightly and sutured to the periosteum of the metacarpal, resurfacing the metacarpal base.
  4. The remainder of the tendon slip is folded into the trapezial space to act as a spacer.
  5. Some surgeons use one or more longitudinal Kirschner's wires to stabilize the metacarpal in an abducted, distracted position.
  6. LRTI arthroplasty has been shown to provide pain relief and thumb stability and restore grip-and-pinch strength for as long as 11 years after surgery.
- HDA involves excision of the entire trapezium without ligament reconstruction or tendon interposition.
  1. A Kirschner's wire is passed through the first metacarpal base into the trapezoid or second metacarpal with the thumb in palmar abduction, slight opposition, and distraction.
  2. The Kirschner's wire is left in place for approximately 5 weeks.
  3. The hematoma filling the trapezial void becomes fibrotic, thus supporting the base of the second metacarpal.

Rehabilitation Overview

- The treatment guidelines that follow are designed for postoperative management of LRTI arthroplasty. However, they can be easily modified, as will be specified, for use following HDA.
- The goals of therapy after thumb CMC arthroplasty are to provide correct protective splinting; manage edema, pain, and the postoperative wound and resulting scar; and, ultimately, facilitate restoration of stable thumb and wrist

motion and strength adequate to the functional demands of the individual.

- Individuals who underwent postoperative therapy following thumb CMC arthroplasty should be well versed in joint protection principles and able to consistently apply them during their daily activities.
- Overaggressive motion and strengthening exercises, as well as too rapid a return to full hand use, may increase pain and inflammation, delaying recovery.

Postoperative Phase I: Inflammation/ Protection (Weeks 0 to 3)

GOALS
- Protect the arthroplasty through splinting and activity modification/joint protection
- Reduce edema and pain
- Maintain full AROM of uninvolved joints

PRECAUTIONS
- No ROM of thumb MP or CMC joints
- No ROM of wrist unless specifically prescribed by MD
- No strong pinching or other resistive activities

TREATMENT STRATEGIES
- Splinting: thumb spica splint when postoperative splint is discharged by MD
- Joint protection: avoid strong pinch and any aggravating activities; use hand for light ADL to tolerance only
- Edema and pain reduction: elevation, cold modalities, retrograde massage (avoiding surgical incision until fully closed)
- ROM exercises for uninvolved joints: fingers, thumb IP joint, elbow, forearm, and shoulder

CRITERIA FOR ADVANCEMENT
- Edema and pain controlled (minimal)
- Patient cleared by MD for thumb and wrist AROM, typically at 3 to 4 weeks postoperatively, depending on MD preference; some MDs may allow wrist AROM earlier.

Note: If a Kirschner's wire is used, phase II does not begin until its removal, at 4 weeks following LRTI arthroplasty and at 5 weeks following HDA.

**Postoperative Phase II: Fibroplasia
(Weeks 4 to 8)**

GOALS
- Protect arthroplasty through continued splinting and activity modification
- Reduce residual edema and pain
- Minimize scarring
- Restore stable AROM of thumb CMC and MP joints and wrist within tolerance
- Restore independence in light ADL while maintaining joint protection

PRECAUTIONS
- No resistive activities or exercises

TREATMENT STRATEGIES
- Splinting: thumb spica splint is removed for therapeutic exercises and hygiene, until discharged by surgeon
- Phase I edema treatments continue; contrast baths and light compression wrapping, avoiding overly tight application
- Scar management when incision has healed: scar massage, silicone pad
- A/AAROM of thumb MP and CMC joints and wrist; PROM to regain functional motion (see section on troubleshooting phase II)
- Light, functional activities to encourage use of hand to tolerance, avoiding forceful pinch and any aggravating activities

CRITERIA FOR ADVANCEMENT
- Minimal pain with light activities and motion exercises
- Patient cleared by MD for strengthening exercises and discharge of splint

**Postoperative Phase III: Scar Maturation
(Weeks 8 to 12)**

GOALS
- Restore functional, pain-free ROM in thumb and wrist
- Achieve functional strength for pinch, grip, and wrist

Continued

Postoperative Phase III: Scar Maturation (Weeks 8 to 12)—Cont'd

- Restore independent activities of daily living (ADL) while maintaining joint protection

PRECAUTIONS
- Avoid pain-provoking activities and overaggressive, resistive exercises

TREATMENT STRATEGIES
- Gradual weaning from splint
- Scar management until scar is pale and flat
- Thumb and wrist ROM exercises continue, with emphasis on functional motion vs extreme end range motion
- Light resistance for wrist and grip strengthening for return to independent ADL
- Light resistance for pinch strength for return to independent ADL

CRITERIA FOR DISCHARGE
- Independence in home program
- Understanding and use of joint protection principles
- Functional thumb and wrist ROM
- Functional hand and wrist strength
- Independence in ADL with minimal discomfort

Bibliography

Berger, R.A., Beckenbaugh, R.D., Linscheid, R.L. Arthroplasty in the Hand and Wrist. In Green, D.P., Hotchkiss, R.N., Pederson, W.C. (Eds). Green's Operative Hand Surgery, 4th ed. Churchill Livingstone, New York, 1999, pp. 166–168.

Burton, R.I., Pellegrini, V.D. Surgical Management of Basal Joint Arthritis of the Thumb. Part II: Ligament Reconstruction with Tendon Interposition Arthroplasty. *J Hand Surg* 1986;11A:324–332.

Chaisson, C.E., Zhang, Y., McAlindon, T.E., Hannan, M.T., Aliabadi, P., Naimark, A., Levy, D., Felson, D.T. Radiographic Hand Osteoarthritis: Incidence, Patterns, and Influence of Pre-existing Disease in a Population Based Sample. *J Rheumatol* 1997;24:1337–1343.

Kuhns, C.A., Emerson, E.T., Meals, R.A. Hematoma and Distraction Arthroplasty for Thumb Basal Joint Osteoarthritis: A Prospective,

Single Surgeon Study Including Outcome Measures. *J Hand Surg* 2003;28A:381–389.

Tomaino, M.M. Ligament Reconstruction Tendon Interposition Arthroplasty for Basal Joint Arthritis. *Hand Clin* 2001;17(2): 207–221.

Tomaino, M.M., Pellegrini, V.D., Burton, R.I. Arthroplasty of the Basal Joint of the Thumb. *J Bone Joint Surg* 1995;77A(3):346–355.

CHAPTER 20

Ulnar Collateral Ligament Repair

Coleen T. Gately, PT, DPT, MS

The ulnar collateral ligament (UCL) is the primary valgus stabilizer of the thumb metacarpophalangeal (MP) joint. The UCL is more frequently injured than the radial collateral ligament. A 10 to 1 ratio of injury is reported in the literature.

Historically, UCL laxity was observed in gamekeepers as a result of repetitive valgus stress placed on the thumb while pinning game between the thumb and index finger, and was subsequently referred to as "gamekeeper's thumb." Acute injury to the UCL results from a fall on an extended thumb forced into hyperabduction. This is a common skiing injury and is frequently referred to as "skier's thumb." The UCL can be ruptured or avulsed at the origin, with or without a bony fragment of the proximal phalanx. Symptoms following a UCL tear include pain, swelling, and instability of the MP during pinch activities. Many patients do not seek immediate medical attention. If left untreated, this injury can lead to long-term weakness, joint deformity (subluxation), and arthritis.

Surgical Overview

- UCL ruptures may be treated conservatively with immobilization splinting for 6 to 8 weeks in a hand-based thumb immobilization splint with the interphalangeal (IP) joint free. Surgical indications for a UCL injury include failure of conservative management, clinical joint instability, fracture or displacement, and a Stener lesion.
- A Stener lesion prevents the UCL from healing without surgery because of interposition of the adductor aponeurosis between the ligament's torn edges.
- Several surgical techniques are used to repair a UCL tear.

1. They include a simple ligament repair and tendon reconstruction.
2. Suture anchors are used for the repair, and a Kirschner's wire is used to stabilize larger avulsion fractures.
3. In certain cases, a temporary transarticular pin is used to control stress across the repair site.
4. The surgical technique is based on the extent of joint involvement and the time elapsed since injury. An acute injury is often treated with a simple repair, whereas a chronic injury may require a complex procedure.

Rehabilitation Overview

- The amount of surgical stability achieved will determine the rate of progression of therapeutic techniques in each phase of healing.
- Direct communication with the doctor is essential to determine the stability of the joint for appropriate therapeutic progression.

Postoperative Phase I: Protection (Weeks 0 to 4)

GOALS
- Correct protective immobilization
- Edema and pain control
- Full ROM of uninvolved joints

PRECAUTIONS
- No thumb MP motion
- Valgus forces

PIN AND WOUND CARE
- Pin care regimens vary: commonly, 50% peroxide and sterile water two times per day
- Standard wound care procedures followed for ORIF

TREATMENT STRATEGIES
Protection options
- Hand-based thumb immobilization splint, IP free
  1. Accommodate any pins
  2. Remold to accommodate changes in edema
Edema/pain management
- Elevation, rest, ice/cold

Continued

Postoperative Phase I: Protection (Weeks 0 to 4)—Cont'd

- Light, compressive garment or wrap (i.e., Coban™, compression sleeve, stockinette)

Uninvolved joints ROM
- Tendon gliding exercises
- Thumb IP motion
- Shoulder, elbow, wrist, and forearm motion

Light, functional activities
- Restoration of normal movement patterns and light, functional activities with splint on

CRITERIA FOR ADVANCEMENT
- Determination by MD of ability of repair site to withstand stress and motion

Postoperative Phase II: Stability (Weeks 4 to 8)

GOALS
- Maximize ROM of the thumb MP and IP joints
- Restore functional use of the involved extremity
- Continue phase I goals as needed

PRECAUTIONS
- Avoid excessive PROM/stretching

TREATMENT STRATEGIES

Splinting
- Splint is weaned during the day and continued for sleep and travel

Scar management
- Scar massage and silicone gel sheeting are initiated once the wound is fully healed (to avoid infection)

Edema/pain management
- Cold pack
- Retrograde massage

MP joint ROM
- Thumb MP motion: flexion, abduction, and opposition

PROM and splinting
- PROM, stretching
- Serial static and static progressive splints to achieve end range potential
  1. Example: serial static thumb web spacer

Functional activities
- Restoration of normal movement patterns/activities of daily living (ADL)
- May require hand-based thumb immobilization splint, IP free for heavy activity

CRITERIA FOR ADVANCEMENT
- Determination by MD of ability of injury site to withstand stress

Postoperative Phase III: Repair Consolidation (Weeks 8 to 12)

GOALS
- Restore strength for return to functional activities and work
- Continue phase II goals as needed

PRECAUTIONS
- Progress strengthening exercises gradually, avoiding pain and compensations

STRENGTHENING
- Isometric and dynamic grip-and-pinch strengthening: putty, hand-helper, BTE PRIMUS (Baltimore Therapeutic Equipment Co., Hanover, MD), and Upper Limb Exerciser (ULE) (Biometrics LTD., UK)
- Wrist and forearm progressive resistive exercises (PREs): dumbbells, weight well, Thera-Band
- Work and sport conditioning: activity-specific activities

CRITERIA FOR DISCHARGE
- Restoration of functional AROM and strength, and return to prior ADL and work
- Independence in home exercise program

Bibliography

Alldred, A.J. Rupture of the Collateral Ligament of the Metacarpophalangeal Joint of the Thumb. *J Bone Joint Surg* 1955;37B:443-445.

Bowers, W.H., Hurst, L.C. Gamekeeper's Thumb. Evaluations by Arthrography and Stress Roentgenography. *J Bone Joint Surg* 1977;59A(4):519-524.

Campbell, C.S. Gamekeeper's Thumb. *J Bone Joint Surg* 1955;
  37A:148.

Frank, W.E., Dobyns, J.H. Surgical Pathology of Collateral Ligamentous
  Injury of the Thumb. *Clin Orthop* 1972;83:102-114.

Frykman, G., Johansson, O. Surgical Repair of Rupture of the Ulnar
  Collateral Ligament of the Metacarpophalangeal Joint of the Thumb.
  Acta Chir Scand 1956;112:58-64.

Green, D. Dislocations and Ligamentous Injuries of the Hand. Churchill
  Livingstone, New York, 1990, pp. 385-448.

Heyman, P., Gelberman, R.H., Duncan, K., Hipp, J.A. Injuries of the
  Ulnar Collateral Ligament of the Thumb Metacarpophalangeal Joint.
  Clin Orthop Relat Res 1993;292:165-171.

Kaplan, E.B. The Pathology and Treatment of Radial Subluxation of the
  Thumb with Ulnar Displacement of the Head of the First
  Metacarpal. *J Bone Joint Surg* 1961;43A:541-546.

Louis, D.S., Huebner, J.J., Hankin, F.M. Rupture and Displacement of
  the Ulnar Collateral Ligament of the Metacarpophalangeal Joint of
  the Thumb. Preoperative Diagnosis. *J Bone Joint Surg* 1986;
  6A(9):1320-1325.

Moberg, E. Fractures and Ligamentous Injuries of the Thumb and
  Fingers. *Surg Clin North Am* 1960;40:297-309.

Moberg, E., Stener, B. Injuries to the Ligaments of the Thumb and
  Fingers. *Acta Chir Scand* 1953;106:166-186.

Moutet, F. Les entorse de la metacarpo-phalangienne due pouce a une
  experience de plus de 1000 cas. *Ann Chir Main Memb Super*
  1989;8:99.

Osterman, A.L., Hayken, G.D., Bora, W.M. A Quantitative Evaluation of
  the Thumb Function after Ulnar Collateral Repair and
  Reconstruction. *J Trauma* 1981;21:854-860.

Posner, M.A. Metacarpophalangeal Joint Injuries of the Thumb. *Hand
  Clin* 1992;8:713.

Sennwald, G., Segmuller, G., Egli, A. The Late Reconstruction of the
  Ligament of the Metacarpophalangeal Joint of the Thumb. *Ann Chir
  Main* 1987;6:15-24.

Smith, R.J. Post-traumatic Instability of the Metacarpophalangeal Joint
  of the Thumb. *J Bone Joint Surg* 1977;59A:14-21.

Stener, B. Displacement of the Ruptured Ulnar Collateral Ligament of
  the Metacarpophalangeal Joint of the Thumb. A Clinical and
  Anatomical Study. *J Bone Joint Surg* 1962;44B:869-879.

Strandell, G. Total Rupture of the Ulnar Collateral Ligament of the
  Metacarpophalangeal Joint of the Thumb. Results of Surgery in 35
  Cases. *Acta Chir Scand* 1959;118:72-80.

CHAPTER 21

Volar Plate Arthroplasty

Aviva Wolff, OTR/L, CHT

Dislocations of the proximal interphalangeal (PIP) joint may be dorsal, lateral, or volar, depending on the position of the middle phalanx at the moment of joint deformation. The mechanism of injury in dorsal dislocations is usually hyperextension with longitudinal compression. In a more severe injury, rupture of the volar plate occurs proximally.

Surgical Overview

- Volar plate arthroplasty is a surgical technique used to treat unstable dorsal fracture dislocations of the PIP with disruption of the volar plate complex, the collateral ligaments, and greater than 40% of the volar articular surface of the middle phalanx.
- Surgical exposure is through a volar incision on the PIP joint surface.
- The flexor sheath is excised between the A2 and A4 pulleys and the tendons are retracted.
- The PIP joint is hyperextended, and the collateral ligaments are excised.
- Large fragments are reduced by K-wires, and loose bone fragments are debrided.
- The volar plate is mobilized to advance 4 to 6 mm into the middle phalanx defect.
  1. The plate is advanced by means of a pullout wire along the lateral margins of the volar plate and then exits the dorsal middle phalanx through the triangular ligament of the extensor mechanism.
  2. The pullout suture is then tied over a button.
- The lateral margins of the volar plate are sutured to the adjacent collateral ligament remnants.

173

- A longitudinal K-wire or PIP compass hinge may be used to maintain the reduced joint in 30-degree flexion in severely unstable fractures (see chapter on PIP compass hinge).
- Complications of volar plate arthroplasty include redisplacement, angulation, flexion contracture, distal interphalangealk (DIP) joint stiffness, oblique retinacular ligament (ORL) tightness, and flexor and extensor tendon adherence.

Rehabilitation Overview

- Because this is a complex injury that requires postoperative protection, it is often difficult to achieve adequate PIP range of motion (ROM).
- It is essential that postoperative management by the hand therapist begins in the early phases of wound healing.
- To avoid complications, such as contraction of the scarred volar plate and flexor tendons, protected motion must be initiated as early as possible.
- The PIP joint is particularly prone to adhesions and contractures because multiple structures cross the joint. The structures include collateral ligaments, volar plate, central slip, lateral bands, transverse retinacular ligaments, oblique retinacular ligament, and flexor tendons.
- Even loose adhesions have been found to significantly limit motion.

Postoperative Phase I: Inflammation/ Protection (Weeks 0 to 3)

GOALS
- Provide correct splinting to maintain stability and protect repaired structures
- Control inflammation and reduce edema
- Maintain stability and protect repaired structures
- Maintain ROM in uninvolved joints
- Begin gentle protective active motion within the confines of the splint

PRECAUTIONS
- No active or passive PIP extension beyond prescribed position

TREATMENT STRATEGIES

Protective Immobilization
- Dorsal block splint in 35- to 40-degree PIP flexion

Edema Control
- Standard principles of edema control
- Gentle compressive wraps, such as Coban
- Avoid compression garments (such as Isotoner gloves) that place the digit in too much extension during donning

Protect Repaired Structures
- PIP joint not to be extended beyond prescribed limit
- Splint is not to be removed at home

ROM Exercises of Uninvolved Joints
- Active DIP flexion exercises
- Active metacarpophalangeal flexion and ROM of all uninvolved joints

Early Protective Mobilization
- Active PIP flexion when the K-wire is removed (3 weeks), or at 1 week (no K-wire)
- Gentle active composite flexion
- Active extension to the limit of the splint
- Active flexor digitorum profundus (FDP) and flexor digitorum superficialis (FDS) glides

Criteria for Advancement
- Removal of K-wire
- Joint stability determined by surgeon

Postoperative Phase II: Fibroplasia/Early Remodeling (Weeks 3 to 6)

GOALS
- Achieve maximum PIP flexion
- Begin to progress PIP extension
- Encourage scar remodeling
- Encourage functional and protected use of hand

PRECAUTIONS
- No active or passive PIP extension beyond prescribed limits

Continued

Postoperative Phase II: Fibroplasia/Early Remodeling (Weeks 3 to 6)—Cont'd

TREATMENT STRATEGIES
PIP Flexion Exercises
- Gentle passive stretch into flexion at 3 to 4 weeks after surgery
- Gentle hook and composite fisting

PIP Extension
- Progression of dorsal block splint into extension
- Active PIP extension following button removal
- The dorsal splint is worn between exercises and at night up to 6 weeks

Scar Remodeling
- Begin gentle scar massage
- Use Otoform mold or silicone gel with Coban for night use
- Massage over the dorsal hood and lateral bands at 3 weeks

CRITERIA FOR ADVANCEMENT
- Removal of dorsal button
- Clinical union at fracture site
- Joint stability determined by surgeon

Postoperative Phase III: Scar Maturation (Weeks 6 to 12)

GOALS
- To achieve full ROM (active and passive) at the PIP and DIP joints
- To prevent a PIP extension lag
- To prevent a PIP flexion contracture

TREATMENT PLAN
Achieve Maximum Range of Motion
- Splint to be discharged (6 to 8 weeks)
- Intensive ROM and blocking exercises initiated
- Blocking splints
- Joint mobilization in both directions with physician authorization
- Static progressive flexion splinting for end range flexion (6 to 8 weeks)

- Neuromuscular electrostimulation to encourage flexor tendon pull-through

Prevent PIP Extension Lag
- Finger gutter extension splint for night to prevent joint contracture
- Intrinsic exercises and progressive strengthening to the extensor mechanism
- Resistive exercises to decrease extensor mechanism adherence and cross adhesions of the FDS/FDP at Camper's chiasm

Prevent and Treat PIP Flexion Contractures
- Ultrasound to the PIP joint, followed by vigorous massage, exercise, and splinting
- Extension splinting/serial casting to the PIP

CRITERIA FOR DISCHARGE
- Maximum PIP flexion and extension
- Functional grip strength
- Return to premorbid level of function

Bibliography

Glickel, S.Z., Baron, O.A., Eaton, R. Dislocations and Injuries in the Digits. In Green, D.P. (Ed). Operative Hand Surgery, 4th ed., vol. 1. Churchill Livingstone, Philadelphia, 1999, pp. 772–800.

Kiefhaber, T.R., Stern, P. Fracture Dislocations of the Proximal Interphalangeal Joint. *J Hand Surg* 1998;23A:368–380.

Lanz, U., H.P. Tendon Adhesions. In G.A. Bruser, P. (Eds). Finger, Bone and Joint Injuries. Dunitz, UK, 1999.

CHAPTER 22

Proximal Interphalangeal (PIP) Joint Replacement

Emily Altman, PT, DPT, CHT

The proximal interphalangeal (PIP) joint can be affected by posttraumatic arthritis and osteoarthritis. Impairments typically include pain, weakness, joint stiffness, and deformity. Even though patients often present with only one affected digit, the impact on the function of the entire hand is significantly impacted secondary to the quadriga effect. Because the four tendons of the flexor digitorum profundus (FDP) share a common muscle belly, a surgical procedure results in limited proximal tendon excursion (in this case, because of limited PIP flexion range of motion [ROM]). When the ulnar digits are involved, grip is impaired. When the index is involved, pinch strength and dexterity are affected. Surgical options for this condition include joint fusion, joint replacement (arthroplasty), and amputation.

Joint replacement is the only option that preserves joint motion. To date, options for joint replacement include fibrous interposition, volar plate advancement, metallic or metallo-plastic hinges, or one-piece polymeric plastic hinge devices. Surgical placement of early prostheses requires extensive resection of the joint, including the collateral ligaments. This compromises the postoperative stability of the PIP joint.

At the Hospital for Special Surgery (HSS), the Avanta PIP finger prosthesis (Avanta Orthopaedics, San Diego, CA) is the option most often used. It is a *semiconstrained* prosthesis that more closely mimics the anatomy and kinematics of the PIP joint than other, earlier prostheses. The proximal phalanx component is a metallic cobalt chromium (CoCr) alloy, and the middle phalanx component is titanium with an ultra high molecular weight polyethylene surface. Minimal bony excision is required for placement of the Avanta prosthesis, permitting preservation of the collateral ligaments and enhanced joint stability.

Surgical Overview

- The Avanta prosthesis replaces the articular surfaces of the head of the proximal phalanx and the base of the middle phalanx.
- The surgery can be done via a dorsal, lateral, or volar approach.
    1. The dorsal approach is preferred because there is better exposure of the joint and easier placement of the prosthesis.
    2. Flexor tendon adherence can be a complication of the volar approach.
- With the dorsal approach, the author recommends that the central slip *not* be dissected from its insertion on the middle phalanx. Instead, the central slip is isolated proximal to the dorsal rim of the middle phalanx for 1 to 2 cm (via parallel incisions on either side of the central slip) then cut transversely and reflected distally, exposing the PIP joint.
    1. This technique permits a larger (and therefore stronger) area of repair of the central slip/extensor apparatus once the prosthesis has been placed.
    2. The distal end of the proximal phalanx and the proximal end of the middle phalanx are excised, and the implant is fitted and placed.
    3. The extensor apparatus is repaired with multiple fine sutures, the skin is closed, and the finger is immobilized in full extension.
- If a volar approach is used, the flexor tendons are released and retracted, and the volar plate is released to obtain access to the volar aspect of the PIP joint.
    1. The distal end of the proximal phalanx and the proximal end of the middle phalanx are excised, and the implant is fitted and placed.
    2. The volar plate and the tendon sheath complex (annular pulleys) are repaired.
    3. Immediately postoperatively the finger is immobilized in 15- to 20-degree PIP flexion for 1 to 3 days to protect the repaired volar plate.

Rehabilitation Overview

- The goal of rehabilitation following PIP joint arthroplasty is to regain a pain-free functional arc of PIP joint motion.
- With both dorsal and volar approaches, certain structures must be protected following surgery.
- Appropriate postoperative splinting is essential.
- Once the protection phase is over, gradually regaining ROM of the joint is the goal of therapy. Strengthening is not a priority.

Postoperative Phase I (Days 1 to 14)

GOALS
- Edema reduction
- Patient education
  1. Wound care
  2. Signs of infection
- Independence in home exercise program
- Independence in splint regimen

PRECAUTIONS
- No hyperextension force at the PIP joint
- Passive range of motion (PROM) of the PIP joint is contraindicated
- No strengthening

TREATMENT STRATEGIES
- Splint fabrication-static and dynamic splints
- Instruction in specific home exercise program
- Instruction in precautions
- Instruction in edema reduction techniques

CRITERIA FOR ADVANCEMENT
- Wound closure
- PIP joint stability (determined by surgeon)

Postoperative Phase II (Weeks 2 to 6)

GOALS
- Independence in scar management
- AROM PIP joint 0 to 70 degrees

PRECAUTIONS
- No PROM of PIP joint
- No strengthening
- Careful monitoring for PIP joint extension lag
- Prevent scar adherence to dorsal apparatus

TREATMENT STRATEGIES
- Precise progression of PIP AROM
- Template exercise splinting for PIP AROM
- Scar mobilization

CRITERIA FOR ADVANCEMENT
- Acceptable arc of motion at PIP joint

Postoperative Phase III (Weeks 6 to 14)

GOALS
- To regain full functional use of hand for grasping, holding, lifting, and manipulating objects
- Greater than 1/10 pain

PRECAUTIONS
- No strengthening
- No aggressive PROM of PIP joint

TREATMENT STRATEGIES
- Replace tendon gliding and AROM exercises with functional activities

CRITERIA FOR DISCHARGE
- Able to perform ADL without assistance

Bibliography

Kobayashi, K.Y., Terrono, A. Proximal Interphalangeal Joint Arthroplasty of the Hand. *J Am Soc Surg Hand* 2003;3(4):219-226.

Proximal Interphalangeal (PIP) Finger Prosthesis-Surgical Technique. Available online at http://www.avanta.org.

Sauerbier, M., Cooney, W.P., Linscheid, R.L. Operative Technique of Surface Replacement Arthroplasty of the Proximal Interphalangeal Joint. *Tech Hand Up Extrem Surg* 2001;5(3):141-147.

CHAPTER 23

Dynamic External Fixation of the Proximal Interphalangeal (PIP) Joint

Emily Altman, PT, DPT, CHT

Injury to the proximal interphalangeal (PIP) joint is frequently the result of a fall or participation in sports. Many injuries are managed with closed reduction, open reduction and internal fixation (ORIF), or splinting. However, complex, unstable fracture dislocations are very difficult to successfully treat. Poor results include severely limited joint range of motion (ROM), chronic joint pain, posttraumatic arthritis, and chronic joint instability. ROM impairments affect the patient's ability to grasp objects. Severe PIP joint flexion contractures make it very difficult to open the hand enough to get around objects, don a glove, slip a hand in a garment pocket, or shake another person's hand.

Use of the Compass PIP joint hinge (Smith & Nephew, Orthopedic Division, Memphis, TN) can be an effective way to treat complex PIP joint injuries. The Compass PIP joint hinge (hereafter referred to as "hinge") is an external fixation device composed of a unilateral external hinge that attaches with skeletal fixation to either side of the joint. The design permits controlled passive motion of the joint when the gear is engaged and protected active motion when the gear is not engaged. Indications for use of the hinge include acute fracture dislocations with comminution, volar plate arthroplasty, contracture release of the PIP joint, and chronic boutonnière reconstruction.

Surgical Overview

- The PIP joint is a ginglymus, or hinge joint, whose instant center of rotation moves only slightly as the joint moves through its arc of motion. This kinematic fact permits the use of this hinged external fixator whose axis of rotation is fixed.

- For the hinged external fixator to work effectively, its axis of rotation must be aligned perfectly with the joint's axis of rotation.
  1. The hinge is attached to the skeleton by two pins in the proximal phalanx and two pins in the middle phalanx.
  2. Exactly four pins are necessary to handle the mechanical requirements of maintaining joint stability (two pins), applying distraction, if needed (one pin), and controlling joint rotation (one pin).
  3. Distraction creates tension in the ligaments and capsule, which maintains reduction (the principle of ligamentotaxis).
- The hinge is often used in conjunction with other surgical procedures, such as volar plate arthroplasty, internal fracture fixation, extensor tendon reconstruction, or tenolysis.
- The hinge is usually removed after 5 to 6 weeks. It can be removed as early as 3 weeks, depending on the specifics of the injury and surgery.

Rehabilitation Overview

- Because the hinged external fixator can be used in the surgical management of several different diagnoses (e.g., fracture dislocations, volar plate arthroplasties, contracture releases), postoperative rehabilitation guidelines will vary widely.
- Variables include the duration of immediate postoperative immobilization, the preferred resting position for the hinge, the rate of progression of ROM, the initiation of active range of motion (AROM), and specific precautions.
- The therapist must communicate with the surgeon and obtain the details of the original injury and the operative procedure and confirm an appropriate plan of care.

Postoperative Phase I (Days 1 to 14)

GOALS
- Effective edema reduction
- Thorough patient education
  1. Hinge use
  2. Signs of infection
  3. Pin and wound care

Continued

Postoperative Phase I (Days 1 to 14)—Cont'd

- Independence in HEP targeting uninvolved joints
- Independence in appropriate hinge program for PROM of PIP joint

PRECAUTIONS
- Close monitoring for pin tract infection
- Close monitoring for pin loosening

TREATMENT STRATEGIES
- Instruction in very specific HEP
- Cryotherapy instruction
- Instruction in edema reduction techniques
- Marks on hinge itself (with permanent ink marker) to monitor progress and/or delineate boundaries of "safe" PIP ROM

CRITERIA FOR ADVANCEMENT
- Wound closure
- Suture removal
- Independence in hinge management, independence in HEP
- Bone and soft tissue able to tolerate initiation of PIP AROM

Postoperative Phase II (Weeks 2 to 6)

GOALS
- Independence in scar management
- Independence in progressed HEP
- AROM PIP joint 15 to 70 degrees

PRECAUTIONS
- Persistent edema
- Poor progression of ROM
- Pin site infection
- Pin loosening
- Strengthening is contraindicated

TREATMENT STRATEGIES
- Precise instruction in AROM program to normalize digit flexion
- Instruction in scar management

CRITERIA FOR ADVANCEMENT
- Joint is ready for hinge removal = fracture has healed sufficiently and joint is stable
- Maximum PROM/AROM of involved PIP joint has been achieved

Postoperative Phase III: Hinge Removal (Weeks 6 to 14)

GOALS
- Increased use of hand and digit in performance of ADL
- Continued increase in PIP AROM/PROM

PRECAUTIONS
- Inability to maintain PIP extension that was obtained in surgery (return to flexion contracture)
- Poor progression of ROM

TREATMENT STRATEGIES
- Therapeutic putty activities/exercises
- Exercise splints (MP blocking splint, PIP blocking splint)
- Dynamic PIP extension splinting

CRITERIA FOR DISCHARGE
- Functional composite fist
- Acceptable PIP active extension (25 degrees)
- Independent in advanced HEP
- Full use of hand in performance of ADL

Bibliography

Bain, G.I., Mehta, J.A., Heptinstall, R.J., Bria, M. Dynamic External Fixation for Injuries of the Proximal Interphalangeal Joint. *J Bone Joint Surg Br* 1998;80B:1014-1019.

Hotchkiss, R. Surgical Technique: Compass Proximal Interphalangeal (PIP) Joint Hinge. Available online at http://www.ortho.smith-nephew.com.

Meals, R.A., Foulkes, G.D. Hinged Device for Fractures Involving the Proximal Interphalangeal Joint. *Clin Orthop* 1996;327:29-37.

CHAPTER *24*

Dupuytren's Fasciectomy

Carol Page, PT, DPT, CHT

Dupuytren's disease is a condition of increased fibrous tissue growth in the hand, characterized by nodule and cord formation. The changes in the palmar and digital fascia result in flexion contractures of the proximal interphalangeal (PIP) and metacarpophalangeal (MP) joints. The distal interphalangeal (DIP) joints may also become contracted. Although any of the digits can be involved, the fourth and fifth fingers are most commonly affected. As the flexion contractures progress, hand function becomes increasingly impaired.

Although Dupuytren's disease is considered to be idiopathic, there is evidence of a genetic component. The disorder occurs more commonly in Northern European populations, particularly in men and with advancing age. Additional links have been made with diabetes, epilepsy, alcohol use, and cigarette smoking.

Surgical Overview

- Dupuytren's disease typically presents with a nodule in the palm of the hand.
- The disease progresses more quickly in some individuals than others.
  1. The normal fibrous tissue changes into fibrous cords that form longitudinally along the lines of tension placed on the tissue with hand motion and use.
  2. Formation of the cords causes joint contractures of the MP and PIP joints.
- Indications for surgical intervention include impairment of hand function as a result of digital flexion contractures and demonstrated disease progression.

- Impairment of digital extension may interfere with the ability to perform various functions, such as reaching into pockets, purses, and briefcases, and opening the hand for face washing and hand shaking.
- The purpose of surgery is to restore the ability to straighten the digits to promote hand function.
- The surgical approach to treating contractures resulting from Dupuytren's disease ranges from the less frequently performed simple fasciotomy, the division of contracted tissue, to various types of fasciectomy.
- In a limited fasciectomy, the diseased tissue in the digits is excised.
- In a radical fasciectomy, the diseased palmar fascia is excised in addition.
- A dermofasciectomy, in which the skin as well as the diseased fascia are excised, may be performed in the attempt to minimize the rate of recurrence.
- Closure of surgical incisions is handled in several ways. The incisions made on the digits are usually primarily closed, and the surgical wounds on the palm are either left open to heal by secondary intention or primarily closed, with or without skin grafting.

Rehabilitation Overview

- Preoperative rehabilitation for Dupuytren's contracture has not been demonstrated to be effective and is therefore not indicated. However, rehabilitation is widely recognized to be a critical component in a successful postoperative outcome.
- The purpose of postoperative therapy is to use interventions, such as scar and edema management techniques, splinting, and therapeutic exercise, to promote motion, strength, and function.
- Scar management is particularly important to prevent loss of digit extension gained in surgery and flexor tendon adherence.
  1. Extension splinting, which is used throughout the course of therapy, continues at night until scar tissue is mature to prevent recurrence of flexion contractures resulting from scar contraction.

2. Although passive motion is helpful for regaining motion, it should never substitute for the active gliding of the tendons that can adhere in the scarred region, causing impairment of hand function.

3. Continuous passive motion machines have not been found to be useful for this diagnosis and are therefore not recommended.

- Therapists treating patients following Dupuytren's fasciectomy need to be on the alert for the onset of complications and communicate with the referring surgeon if signs are present.

  1. The most common complications are hematoma, skin loss, loss of digital flexion, and complex regional pain syndrome (formerly known as *reflex sympathetic dystrophy*).

  2. Additional complications include infection, excessive edema, and persistent or recurrent proximal phalangeal joint flexion contractures.

  3. Complications are best caught and addressed early. They will be discussed in further detail in the following sections.

Postoperative Phase I: Inflammation/ Protection (Weeks 0 to 2)

GOALS
- Provide correct positioning in splint for reduction of inflammation and maintenance of tissue length
- Facilitate wound healing
- Reduce edema and pain
- Prevent tendon adherence and joint stiffness in involved joints
- Maintain full AROM of uninvolved joints

PRECAUTIONS
- Positioning in excessive digit extension can compromise circulation and prolong the inflammatory phase
- In cases of skin grafting, delay ROM exercises until graft is well vascularized and protect from shearing forces
- Alert physician to signs of hematoma or infection

TREATMENT STRATEGIES

- Splinting: volar-based extension splint for involved digits and wrist
- Wound care: dressing changes and patient education, monitoring of wound status
- Edema and pain reduction: elevation, cold modalities, retrograde massage on dorsum of hand and wrist (avoid surgical wounds)
- ROM exercises for uninvolved joints: uninvolved digits, wrist, elbow, forearm, shoulder
- AROM/AAROM/PROM to involved digits when acute postoperative edema has diminished (and skin graft, if present, is well vascularized): tendon gliding, blocking, and extension exercises

CRITERIA FOR ADVANCEMENT

- Sutures removed and well-vascularized skin graft, if present
- Controlled (minimal) edema and pain

Postoperative Phase II: Fibroplasia (Weeks 2 to 6)

GOALS

- Reduce residual edema and pain
- Minimize scar adherence
- Maximize AROM and PROM of involved digits
- Restore independence in light activities of daily living (ADL)

PRECAUTIONS

- Overzealous stretching and resistive exercises may increase inflammation
- Compression wraps that are too tight may increase rather than decrease edema

TREATMENT STRATEGIES

- Splinting: remold extension splint if needed to maximize MP and IP joint extension or to accommodate silicone insert; splint worn at night only
- Edema control: continue treatments from phase I, adding (if needed) light compression, contrast baths (when wounds are fully healed)

Continued

Postoperative Phase II: Fibroplasia (Weeks 2 to 6)—Cont'd

- Scar management when wounds have healed: scar massage, silicone scar pad or mold
- Heat modalities to prepare soft tissues for ROM
- AROM, AAROM to promote tendon gliding, balancing focus on flexors and extensors
- PROM, gentle stretching
- Light, functional activities to encourage use of hand to tolerance

CRITERIA FOR ADVANCEMENT
- Complete wound closure
- Minimal edema and pain with light activities and motion exercises

Postoperative Phase III: Scar Maturation (Weeks 6 to 12)

GOALS
- Achieve flat, nonadherent scars
- Achieve maximum AROM/PROM in involved digits, without flexion contractures
- Achieve functional strength
- Restore independence in ADL

PRECAUTIONS
- Night extension splinting with silicone insert should continue until scar maturity (up to a year postoperatively) to avoid digital flexion contractures

TREATMENT STRATEGIES
- Continue night extension splinting and scar management until scar is mature.
- Heat modalities, including ultrasound, as needed, to prepare soft tissues for ROM and scar techniques
- Edema control measures as needed
- AROM, PROM, and stretching with emphasis on end range flexion and extension
- Resistance exercises to promote tendon gliding and strengthening of digits (flexors and extensors) and wrist

- Functional activities to promote restoration of independent ADL

CRITERIA FOR DISCHARGE
- Independence in home program of night splinting, scar management, and therapeutic exercise
- Full or maximum digit AROM with freely gliding tendons
- Functional hand strength
- Independence in ADL

Bibliography

Abbott, K., Denney, J., Burke, F.D., McGrouther, D.A. A Review of Attitudes to Splintage in Dupuytren's Contracture. *J Hand Surg Br* 1987;12:326-328.

Boyer, M.I., Gelberman, R.H. Complications of the Operative Treatment of Dupuytren's Disease. *Hand Clin* 1999;15:161-166.

Fietti, V.G.Jr., Mackin, E.J. Open-palm Technique in Dupuytren's Disease. In Hunter, J.M., Mackin, E.J., Callahan, A.D. (Eds). Rehabilitation of the Hand: Surgery and Therapy, 4th ed. Mosby, St. Louis, 1995, pp. 995-1006.

Gosset, J. Dupuytren's Disease and the Anatomy of the Palmodigital Aponeuroses. In Hueston, J., Tubiana, R. (Eds). Dupuytren's Disease, 2nd ed. Churchill Livingstone, London, 1985, pp. 13-26.

McFarlane, R.M., MacDermid, J.C. Dupuytren's Disease. In Hunter, J.M., Mackin, E.J., Callahan, A.D. (Eds). Rehabilitation of the Hand: Surgery and Therapy, 5th ed. Mosby, St. Louis, 2002, pp. 971-988.

McFarlane, R.M., McGrouther, D.A. Complications and Their Management. In McFarlane, R.M., McGrouther, D.A., Flint, M.H. (Eds). Dupuytren's Disease: Biology and Treatment. Churchill Livingstone, Edinburgh, Scotland, 1990, pp. 377-382.

McGrouther, D.A. Dupuytren's Contracture. In Green, D.P., Hotchkiss, R.N., Pederson, W.C. (Eds). Green's Operative Hand Surgery, 4th ed. Churchill Livingstone, New York, 1999, pp. 563-591.

Mullins, P.A. Postsurgical Rehabilitation of Dupuytren's Disease. *Hand Clin* 1999;15(1):167-174.

Prosser, R., Conolly, W.B. Complications Following Surgical Treatment for Dupuytren's Contracture. *J Hand Ther* 1996;9:344-348.

Ross, D.C. Epidemiology of Dupuytren's Disease. *Hand Clin* 1999; 15(1):53-62.

Sampson, S.P., Badalamente, M.A., Hurst, L.C., Dowd, A., Sewell, C.S., Lehmann-Torres, J., Ferraro, M., Semon, B. The Use of a Passive

Motion Machine in the Postoperative Rehabilitation of Dupuytren's Disease. *J Hand Surg Am* 1992;17:333-338.

Watson, H.K., Fong, D. Dystrophy, Recurrence, and Salvage Procedures in Dupuytren's Contracture. *Hand Clin* 1991;7:745-755.

C H A P T E R *25*

Lower Extremity Surgical Intervention in Patients with Cerebral Palsy: Bone and Musculotendinous Procedures

Deborah Corradi-Scalise, PT, DPT, MA
Cathi Wagner, PT, MBA
Amanda R. Sparrow, PT

Cerebral palsy (CP) is defined as a condition characterized by a chronic, nonprogressive disorder of movement or posture of early onset. It presents as abnormal control of motor function/coordination as a result of damage to one or more specific areas of the brain. The damage to the brain can occur during the prenatal, perinatal, postnatal, as well as the infancy period. The primary lesion is static; however, the manifestations can change, especially in the musculoskeletal system, because of muscle imbalances, growth, development, and the effects of gravity.

Rehabilitation Overview
Preoperative Considerations

- Orthopedic management of a child with CP is best accomplished via a team approach.
- The medical and rehabilitation team must consider the "total" child when evaluating a patient with CP for surgical intervention.
- An understanding of **atypical development and movement compensations** is imperative to determine how surgery will likely impact the child's future function.

193

1. Muscular tightness and joint limitations at any one joint impact the alignment and function of adjacent muscles and joints.
2. Surgically treating one problem, without consideration of the rest of the body in CP, may have a poor outcome.
3. Additionally, one must also remember that lengthening a muscle also weakens it. This is very important to remember when considering any surgical procedure in the ambulatory patient.
4. The current trend in orthopedic surgery is to develop a strategy and prepare an operative plan that addresses all of the patient's impairments at one time.

- Additionally, a differentiation must be made between **primary impairments and secondary compensations** to adequately address CP.
- A comprehensive physical therapy examination for each presurgical candidate should be performed and the findings discussed with the team.
- Another tool that may be used in the preoperative evaluation process is quantitative gait analysis.
   1. Gait analysis, using a three-dimensional (3-D) motion analysis laboratory, provides the clinician with important objective data.
   2. Kinematic, kinetic, and electromyographic (EMG) data collected in this fashion help identify, simultaneously, the presence of multiple abnormalities (bone and soft tissue) at multiple levels, in three anatomical planes.
   3. Gait analysis provides the team with data to assist in the differentiation of primary gait deviations and secondary coping strategies.

Postoperative Considerations

- Immediate postoperative concerns for any surgical procedure in the patient with CP include pain and spasm management and decreasing the anxiety level of both the child and caregiver/family.
- It is important to overcome the early weakness, stiffness, and discomfort postoperatively.
   1. Rapid mobilization following surgery is essential in overcoming early postoperative stiffness and weakness;

however, traumatized muscles should be given enough time to recover, and the child should be as comfortable as possible when beginning therapy.
2. Analgesic medication and muscle relaxants are used immediately postoperatively.
3. A compassionate and supportive staff is also essential to help the patient and family during the postoperative rehabilitation phase.
- Postoperative rehabilitation focuses on:
  1. The restoration of range of motion (ROM)
  2. Regaining preoperative muscle strength
  3. Optimizing mobility/gait and functional ability.
- All goals will be directly related to and dependent upon the overall functional ability of the patient.
  1. During the initial rehabilitative period, it may be beneficial to use splints for comfort and prevent joint positioning that could contribute to recurrent contractures.
  2. If only soft tissue procedures have been performed, ambulation typically begins on postoperative day one (POD 1). If bone procedures are performed, radiographic evidence of bone healing and physician clearance are necessary before initiating weight-bearing activities.
  3. When multiple surgical procedures are performed on the lower extremity, it may take a long time for the patient to regain preoperative level of strength and function.
- A home exercise program (HEP) will greatly assist the patient in the recovery and rehabilitative process.
  1. The patient's HEP is continually updated based on evaluative findings.
  2. Compliance to the HEP is very important and should be reinforced with the patient and family.
  3. In the rehabilitation process of a patient with a primary neurological impairment, it is important to incorporate principles of motor learning into the treatment program.
  4. Direct hands-on therapeutic input, in addition to providing the patient with feedback through all of the sensory systems, is important.

5. Repetition is necessary for learning a movement skill, and a focus on functional tasks will provide meaning to the activity for the patient.

- It is very important that the medical team **identify and address the patient/family goals** when making decisions regarding surgical interventions.

1. Typically, there is an increase in frequency of physical therapy intervention postoperatively for a period of time to address the immediate weakness and functional limitations/disability associated with surgical lengthening, bone procedures, and immobilization.

2. Once the acute and subacute phase of rehabilitation is complete, the patient typically returns to his or her pre-existing, preoperative therapeutic program.

The following pages provide postoperative guidelines following bone and joint tissue surgical procedures commonly performed at HSS for the management of CP. For the sake of clarity, only one anatomical deformity/surgery is presented at a time. The reader must realize that, characteristically, many of the deformities coexist in patients with CP and therefore multiple surgical procedures are typically performed simultaneously. The total rehabilitation course must reflect this and be coordinated/modified according to the surgical procedures performed on each individual patient. As always, the physical therapist should maintain open communication with the treating surgeon on how to progress each individual patient.

Varus Rotational Osteotomy

- Children with CP commonly present with coxa valga and excessive femoral anteversion, as reported on radiograph.

1. Both of these findings can contribute to hip subluxation and dislocation.

2. Functionally, increased femoral anteversion presents as an in-toeing gait pattern.

3. Excessive hip internal rotation during gait carries with it an associated cosmetic and functional disability.

4. Increased femoral anteversion can result in hip flexion and adduction contractures with shortening of the psoas muscles. This can lead to hip instability and subsequent hip subluxation or dislocation.

- The *varus rotational osteotomy* (VRO) is a surgical intervention performed to correct femoral anteversion, coxa valga, and hip subluxation.
    1. The goal of this procedure in individuals with CP is to improve cosmetic and functional gait parameters as well as stabilize the hip joint.
    2. In individuals with CP, VRO outcomes have reportedly included an increase in hip external rotation and extension, a decrease in anterior pelvic tilt, and an increase in knee extension strength.
    3. Surgical indications are based on clinical examination, gait analysis, and radiographic findings.
- Indications for a VRO are:
    1. In-toeing gait with excessive femoral anteversion greater than 40 to 45 degrees.
    2. Clinically, passive internal rotation greater than 45 degrees with less than 30 degrees of external rotation on physical exam.
    3. Hip subluxation.

Surgical Overview

- The VRO procedure is performed prone, as described by Dr. Leon Root.
- An osteotomy is performed at the upper level of the lesser trochanter in the intertrochanteric aspect of the femur.
- The osteotomy is positioned to prevent extension or flexion.
- The blade portion is inserted through the greater trochanter into the neck of the femur.
- The distal femur is then clamped to a plate.
- The distal femur is rotated externally, and the head and neck are placed in decreased valgus.
- The femoral head is centered into the acetabulum, and the femoral anteversion is corrected.
- The proximal screw is inserted, and the ROM is evaluated.
- The goal is to have an approximate 2:1 ratio (60 to 30 degrees) of hip external to internal rotation.
    1. If the desired rotation is achieved, then the remaining screws are inserted.
    2. If not, the proximal screw is removed, and the degree of rotation is modified.

Rehabilitation Overview

- The rehabilitation following a VRO is designed to progressively increase range of joint motion, muscle strength, and the patient's ability to resume lower extremity weight-bearing activities.
- Communication between the physical therapist and the surgeon is imperative. The surgeon will assess bone healing via radiograph and advise the therapist when the healing is sufficient to begin weight-bearing activities in therapy.

Postoperative Rehabilitation of VRO: Phase I (Days 2 to 4) with Spica Cast

GOALS
- Control of postoperative pain/spasm
- Frequent changes of position: side-lying/prone and sitting in a reclining wheelchair (typically days 2 to 3)
- Ensure that the cast fits appropriately and does not impede circulation or cause irritation
- Maintain patient non-weight-bearing status
- Caregiver independent in patient transfers

PRECAUTIONS
- Avoid prolonged periods of lying in supine
- Monitor skin for irritation/breakdown from cast and positioning
- Monitor distal extremities for signs of edema

TREATMENT STRATEGIES
- Caregiver instructed to monitor the cast for fit and skin irritation
- Caregiver education in importance of position changes
  1. Prone
  2. Side-lying
  3. Supine
  4. Sitting
- Caregiver instructed in proper body mechanics for transfers

CRITERIA FOR ADVANCEMENT
- Dependent upon bone healing seen on radiograph; determined by the surgeon

Postoperative Rehabilitation of VRO: Phase I (Days 2 to 4) with Jordan Splints; No Casting

GOALS
- Control of postoperative pain/spasm
- Educate patient/caregivers regarding hip precautions
- Frequent changes of position (maintaining hip precautions) to prevent decubiti and decrease fear of movement
- Develop ability to sit in a reclining wheelchair
- Develop/maintain passive range of motion (PROM) of lower extremities maintaining hip precautions
- Educate caregivers on transfers and importance of maintaining non-weight-bearing status

PRECAUTIONS
- Avoid prolonged periods of lying in supine
- Maintain hip precautions of no adduction or internal rotation past neutral; no flexion past 90 degrees
- Hip external rotation; extension and abduction as tolerated
- The patient is typically non-weight-bearing for at least 3 weeks, but this is dependent on bone healing and clearance by the surgeon

THERAPEUTIC STRATEGIES
- Frequent change of position
  1. From supine to side-lying with pillows to maintain hip abduction and neutral rotation
  2. Reclining wheelchair with knees flexed if tolerated (typically PODs 2 to 3)
- Gentle PROM of the hips, within precautions of hip flexion to 90 degrees, hip internal rotation to neutral, hip adduction to neutral; hip external rotation, extension, and abduction as tolerated
- Gentle PROM of the knees and ankles may begin POD 2
- Active ankle pumps
- Training patient/caregiver regarding hip precautions and the importance of position change

CRITERIA FOR ADVANCEMENT
- Dependent upon bone healing seen on radiograph; determined by the surgeon

Postoperative Rehabilitation of VRO: Phase II (Days 5 to 21) with Spica Cast

GOALS
- Controlling postoperative pain/spasm
- Ensure that cast fits appropriately and does not impede circulation or cause irritation
- Frequent changes of position to side-lying, prone, and up to reclining wheelchair
- Patient maintains non-weight-bearing until clearance from surgeon

PRECAUTIONS
- Avoid prolonged periods of lying in supine
- If patient is allowed to stand in the spica cast at home, supervision and support must be given at all times

TREATMENT STRATEGIES
- Caregiver/patient education and importance of position changes
- Caregiver instructed in transfers
- The surgeon may allow the patient to stand in the spica cast at home

CRITERIA FOR ADVANCEMENT
- Dependent upon the bone healing seen on radiograph; determined by the surgeon

Postoperative Rehabilitation of VRO: Phase II (Days 5 to 21) with Jordan Splints

GOALS
- Control of pain/spasm
- Decrease fear of movement
- Sitting in a wheelchair for longer periods of time
- Active and active-assisted motion of the lower extremities

PRECAUTIONS
- Avoid prolonged periods of lying in supine
- Maintain hip precautions of no adduction or internal rotation past neutral; no hip flexion past 90 degrees

- Hip external rotation; extension and abduction as tolerated
- The patient is typically non-weight-bearing for at least 3 weeks, but this is dependent upon the bone healing and clearance by the surgeon

TREATMENT STRATEGIES

- Control of postoperative pain and swelling
- Frequent change of position
  1. To side-lying with pillows between legs to maintain hip abduction and neutral rotation
  2. Reclining wheelchair, moving the trunk toward an upright position with knees flexed
- Passive, active-assisted, or active range of motion (AROM) of the hips, knees, and ankles as tolerated, to include heel slides, hip abduction with neutral hip rotation, quad sets, ankle pumps
- Review with caregiver/patient the importance of position changes and sitting in wheelchair with the knees flexed

CRITERIA FOR ADVANCEMENT

- Dependent upon the bone healing seen on radiograph; determined by the surgeon

---

Postoperative Rehabilitation of VRO: Phase III (Weeks 3 to 6) with Spica Cast–Cast Removal

Note: If there is adequate bone healing on radiograph at 3 weeks, the orthopedist may choose to remove the cast. Following cast removal, physical therapy will begin when prescribed by the physician.

GOALS

- Control pain and spasm
- Decrease fear of movement
- Upright sitting in wheelchair
- Increase ROM of hips/knees/ankles, maintaining hip precautions
- Initiate weight-bearing
- Begin lower extremity active movement and strengthening

Continued

Postoperative Rehabilitation of VRO: Phase III (Weeks 3 to 6) with Spica Cast–Cast Removal—Cont'd

PRECAUTIONS
- Continue to avoid periods of prolonged static positioning
- Maintain hip precautions
- Weight-bearing to patient's tolerance, with appropriate therapist support and assistive device

TREATMENT STRATEGIES
- Frequent changes of position: prone/supine/sitting/side-lying with pillows between legs to maintain neutral hip abduction and rotation
- Passive, progressing to AAROM and AROM of hips, knees, and ankles as tolerated, maintaining hip precautions
- Gluteal sets
- Quadriceps sets
- AROM/AAROM of the hips, knees, and ankles
  1. Supine hip abduction, adduction to neutral
  2. Heel slides for hip and knee flexion
  3. Ankle dorsiflexion and plantar flexion
- Gentle stretching/elongation of the hip flexors, hamstrings, quadriceps, and gastrocsoleus as tolerated
- Initiation of weight-bearing can be achieved using the therapy ball to move from prone to standing with support. Increasing the amount of time and decreasing the amount of support as the patient progresses
- Weight-bearing with appropriate assistive device to begin as prescribed by surgeon
- Weight-shifting facilitated in sitting/standing to assist body to readjust to new lower extremity orientation
- HEP—warm water bath may aid in relaxation for performance of gentle ROM exercises

CRITERIA FOR ADVANCEMENT
- Dependent upon strength and ROM in the lower extremities as well as patient tolerance

Postoperative Rehabilitation of VRO: Phase III (Weeks 3 to 6) with Jordan Splints

Note: If there is adequate healing on radiograph at 3 weeks, the orthopedist may allow the patient to begin weight-bearing.

GOALS
- Control pain and spasm
- Decrease fear of movement
- Initiate weight-bearing
- Improve ROM of the lower extremities

PRECAUTIONS
- Maintain hip precautions of no adduction or internal rotation past neutral; no hip flexion past 90 degrees
- Weight-bearing to patient's tolerance

TREATMENT STRATEGIES
- Frequent position changes as previously described
- Passive, progressing to AAROM to AROM of the hips, knees, and ankles as tolerated; heel slides for hip and knee flexion, supine hip abduction with neutral rotation, adduction to midline
- Begin lower extremity active-assistive/active movements against gravity if able
- Ankle pumps
- Gluteal sets
- Quadriceps sets
- Ankle dorsiflexion and plantar flexion
- Gentle stretching/elongation of the hip flexors, hamstrings, quadriceps, and gastrocsoleus as tolerated
- Facilitate weight-shifting in sitting forward over feet to assist body to readjust to new lower extremity orientation and begin to accept weight through lower extremities
- Progressive weight-bearing with appropriate assistive device as prescribed by orthopedist

CRITERIA FOR ADVANCEMENT
- Dependent upon strength and ROM in the lower extremities

Postoperative Rehabilitation of VRO: Phase IV (Week 6 to Month 9 or Full Recovery)

GOALS
- Develop/increase lower extremity ROM
- Strengthen lower extremities
- Improve quality of ambulation and progress ability and endurance ambulation with or without assistive device
- Return to or surpass the patient's functional level before surgery

PRECAUTIONS
- Avoid pain with therapeutic exercise and functional activities
- Avoid jumping/ballistic or high impact activities

TREATMENT STRATEGIES
- Core muscle strengthening exercises
- Sit to stand with facilitation; grade assistance as needed
- Qualitative gait training; work toward normalized gait pattern
- Endurance gait training
- Total gym activities (progressive weight-bearing and strengthening)
- Stationary bicycle
- Treadmill walking-forward, sideways, and retroambulation
- Stair negotiation
- Hip abduction in standing
- Single leg stance activities
- Side stepping with neutral rotation
- Return to typical physical therapy routine/program

Hip Flexors Release

- Excessive hip flexion is a common deformity in CP. Most hip flexor deformities are caused by a tight iliopsoas unit.
- A physical exam may reveal hip flexor spasticity or a hip flexion contracture.
  1. Impairments associated with excessive hip flexion are restricted stride length during gait, excessive anterior

pelvic tilt, excessive lordosis, hip dysplasia, subluxation, and dislocation.

2. A hip flexion contracture of more than 20 degrees is clinically significant because it may contribute to hip instability.

- The goal of a hip flexor release is to decrease static contractures, rebalance the muscles around the hip joint to aid in hip stability, allow for functional hip extension during gait in ambulatory children, and preserve the ability of the psoas to function appropriately in a concentric fashion.
- Ambulatory children should have tenotomy of the psoas tendon alone (not the iliacus fibers) performed over the brim of the pelvis.
- Indications for a hip flexor release are
  1. Hip flexion contracture greater than 15 to 20 degrees
  2. Radiographic measurement of the sacrofemoral angle is less than normal (40 to 60 degrees).
  3. Hip flexor contracture associated with hip instability (subluxation)

Surgical Overview

- The surgical procedure for release of the psoas muscles is performed with the patient supine.
- An oblique incision is made 2 cm below the anterior superior iliac spine to visualize the sartorius, tensor fascia lata (TFL), and the lateral femoral cutaneous nerve.
- The TFL is reflected to visualize the anterior inferior iliac spine and rectus femoris.
- The iliacus is retracted to reveal the tendon of the psoas, where it lies under the iliacus muscle.
- The psoas is then transected.
- In selected cases, when applicable, the TFL can be lengthened by incising the aponeurosis through the same incision.

Rehabilitation Overview

- Rehabilitation for a hip flexor release focuses on early ROM, positioning the patient to maintain the new muscle length, mobility out of bed to include ambulation (as functional level permits), and the return of the patient to his or her preexisting therapeutic program as soon as possible.

- No casting or splinting is used postoperatively post–hip flexor release.

Postoperative Rehabilitation of Hip Flexor Release: Phase I (Days 1 to 2)

GOALS
- Control postoperative pain/swelling/spasms
- Full passive hip extension
- Caregiver able to perform gentle passive hip extension in prone
- Early weight-bearing—standing and ambulation as tolerated with appropriate assistive device
- Independence in HEP

PRECAUTIONS
- Avoid prolonged periods of hip flexion (sitting)

TREATMENT STRATEGIES
- Educate patient/caregiver in positioning to promote hip extension, prone-lying positioning
- Teach caregiver gentle passive and active assistive hip extension in prone
- Gait training with assistive device as appropriate. Educate patient/caregiver in importance of good posture; trunk/hip extension in standing/ambulation

CRITERIA FOR ADVANCEMENT
- Discharge from hospital PODs 1 to 2
- Dependent upon level of functioning before surgery

Postoperative Rehabilitation of Hip Flexor Release: Phase II (Day 3 to Week 6)

GOALS
- Promote/maintain full passive and active hip extension in prone and side-lying

- Strengthening gluteals in new end range
- Improve hip extension in stance phase of gait
- Independence in HEP

PRECAUTIONS
- Avoid increased pain with therapeutic exercise and functional activities
- Avoid prolonged periods of hip flexion (sitting)

TREATMENT STRATEGIES
- Gluteal sets
- Passive/active/active-assistive hip extension in prone and side-lying
- Bridging exercises
- Sit to stand with facilitation
- Standing activities that promote gluteal and abdominal co-contraction
- Core muscle activation/exercises
- Stair climbing/step-up activities
- Treadmill walking when able (forward and retroambulation)
- HEP

CRITERIA FOR ADVANCEMENT
- Dependent upon level of functioning before surgery
- Resume preoperative physical therapy program

Hip Adductor Tenotomy

- Hip adductor spasticity is common in many patients with CP, regardless of their ambulatory status. A physical exam may reveal the presence of a true hip adductor contracture.
  1. Impairments associated with hip adductor spasticity or contractures are a scissoring type gait pattern demonstrating a decreased stride length and a decreased base of support, a predisposition to hip dysplasia or subluxation, and the inability of the caregiver to perform adequate perineal care in the more severely involved patient.

   2. It is considered clinically significant if passive hip abduction is limited to 30 degrees or less.
- In the *ambulatory patient*, the goal of surgery is to obtain a base of support during gait, which is similar to that of a normal gait pattern: 5 to 10 cm from heel to heel.
- In the *nonambulatory patient* the goal of surgery may be to balance the muscles about the hip joint to improve or preserve the integrity and stability of the hip and pelvis, aid in an improved sitting posture with a leveled pelvis and neutral lower extremity alignment, and assist the caregiver in performing perineal care.
- Indications for a hip adductor tenotomy are:
  1. Passive hip abduction is 30 degrees or less, with hips and knees flexed or extended
  2. Presence of scissoring gait, which interferes with functional ambulation
  3. Radiographic evidence of hip subluxation (or potential)
  4. The need to facilitate perineal care in patients with total body involvement

Surgical Overview

- Adductor tenotomy is performed with the patient supine.
- A transverse incision is made over the adductor longus tendon.
- The adductor longus and brevis, as well as the gracilis, are identified with blunt dissection.
- The adductor longus is transected.
- Simple percutaneous adductor longus tenotomy may be sufficient to achieve a release in ambulatory patients.
- PROM of hip abduction is then assessed.
  1. The goal of this procedure is to obtain at least 50 to 60 degrees of passive hip abduction on each side, with the hips and knees flexed to 90 degrees or at least 45 degrees of passive abduction, with the hips and knees extended.
  2. Excessive lengthening beyond that leads to pelvic instability.

3. If passive abduction remains limited after the initial adductor longus tenotomy, the adductor brevis and gracilis may also be released.

Rehabilitation Overview

- Rehabilitation for a hip adductor tenotomy is similar to that for the hip flexor release focusing on early mobilization and out-of-bed mobility, including gait training, ROM/positioning to maintain the new muscle length, and return to the preexisting therapeutic program as soon as possible.
- If hip adductor release is the sole procedure performed, there is no postoperative casting or splinting.

Postoperative Rehabilitation of Hip Adductor Tenotomy: Phase I (Days 1 to 2)

GOALS
- Control postoperative pain/swelling/spasms
- Full passive hip abduction in supine
- Caregiver to perform gentle passive and active-assistive hip abduction in supine
- Early weight-bearing-standing and ambulation as tolerated with appropriate assistive device
- Independence in HEP

PRECAUTIONS
- Avoid increased pain with therapeutic exercise and functional activities
- Avoid prolonged periods of hip adduction (side-lying) to maintain lengthened muscle position

TREATMENT STRATEGIES SPECIFIC TO INCREASING HIP ABDUCTION
- Educate patient/caregiver in positioning to promote hip abduction
- Supine/sitting/side-lying positioning; pillow placement between legs to maintain hip abduction
- Teach caregiver gentle passive and active-assistive hip abduction in supine
- Gait training with assistive device as appropriate. Educate patient/caregiver in the importance of proper foot placement and adequate base of support in standing

Continued

Postoperative Rehabilitation of Hip Adductor Tenotomy: Phase I (Days 1 to 2)—Cont'd

CRITERIA FOR ADVANCEMENT
- Discharge from the hospital POD 1-2
- Dependent upon level of functioning before surgery

Postoperative Rehabilitation of Hip Adductor Tenotomy: Phase II (Day 3 to Week 6)

GOALS
- Promote/maintain full passive and active hip abduction in supine
- Strengthening hip abductors in new end range
- Develop a balance between hip adductor/abductor musculature
- Improve hip abductor control in standing/stance phase of gait/unilateral stance
- Independence in home exercise program (HEP)

PRECAUTIONS
- Avoid pain with therapeutic exercise and functional activities
- Avoid prolonged periods of hip adduction (side-lying, sitting)

TREATMENT STRATEGIES SPECIFIC TO INCREASING HIP ABDUCTION
- Supine active hip abduction
- Side-lying A/AA hip abduction
- Clamshell exercises
- Sit to stand while straddling a bolster
- Facilitate single leg stance
- Standing active hip abduction
- Side-stepping/cruising with facilitation
- Treadmill walking sideways, if able
- Step up and down to the side off a step

CRITERIA FOR ADVANCEMENT
- Dependent upon level of functioning before surgery
- Resume preoperative physical therapy program

Rectus Femoris Transfer

- In children with CP, spasticity of the quadriceps muscle leading to continuous rectus femoris activity throughout the swing phase severely limits knee flexion in swing and subsequent foot clearance to take steps.
- Functionally, the child displays a stiff knee gait pattern with decreased ability to step up to negotiate a curb-step or stairs and may frequently trip and drag his or her toes on the floor.
- Distal rectus femoris transfer is a commonly performed operation in children with CP who present with a stiff knee gait. Transferring the distal rectus femoris posterior to the axis of the knee into either the gracilis or semitendinosus enhances knee flexion in the swing phase.
- Clinically, rectus femoris tightness or contracture can be assessed using the Duncan Ely test.
- Indications for a rectus femoris muscle transfer are:
  1. Stiff knee gait pattern (decreased knee flexion in swing) and positive Duncan Ely test.
  2. Poor foot clearance and rectus femoris activity in the swing phase of gait confirmed by 3-D motion analysis with EMG.

Surgical Overview

- Rectus femoris transfer is performed with the patient supine.
- A longitudinal incision is performed at the mid- to distal anterior thigh, and the incision is extended distally.
- The quadriceps tendon is identified, and the rectus femoris tendon is isolated from the tendinous portion of the vastus medialis and lateralis.
- The rectus femoris is further separated from the inter-medialis.
- Next, the rectus femoris tendon is released from its distal insertion at the patella, ensuring that the knee joint is not disturbed.
- The tendon, which is flat, is then surgically "tubed" to have the shape of a typical tendon.

- The tendon is brought from the anterior thigh through a subcutaneous tunnel and is sewn into either the semitendinosus or gracilis, thus making the rectus femoris muscle act as a knee flexor by changing its insertion. The tendon transfer should be fixed with the knee in about 15 to 20 degrees of flexion.

Rehabilitation Overview

- The rehabilitation program following rectus femoris transfer is designed to facilitate increased knee ROM passively and actively immediately after surgery.
- In the immediate postoperative phase, the patient may have significant spasms in the quadriceps muscle.
- Jordan splints are used during ambulation because of quadriceps weakness and decreased ability to maintain knee extension during the stance phase of gait.
- The physical therapist should focus on the neuromuscular reeducation of the transferred muscle and using its new function to facilitate increased knee flexion during ambulation on level surfaces and during stair negotiation.
- Postoperative spasms are very common with rectus femoris transfers.
    1. It is important to stress early knee ROM, into both knee flexion and extension.
    2. The patient will use Jordan splints to maintain knee extension during ambulation, as a result of the initial presentation of knee flexion in stance postoperatively.
    3. The patient is encouraged to remove the splints in sitting to allow for the knee to flex.

Postoperative Rehabilitation of Rectus Femoris Transfer: Phase I (Days 2 to 3)

GOALS
- Control of postoperative spasm, which is common with rectus femoris transfers
- Control of postoperative pain and swelling

- Improve PROM knee extension and active-assistive knee flexion
- Sitting with knees in a flexed position, working toward 45 degrees of knee flexion
- Early weight-bearing for standing and ambulation with the use of Jordan splints and appropriate assistive device
- Educate/train caregiver for independence in HEP
  1. Knee ROM exercises in sitting (passive knee extension and AA knee flexion)
  2. Gentle passive SLR
  3. Positioning-no prolonged periods of knee flexion or extension
  4. Ankle pumps
  5. Ambulation, as tolerated, with appropriate assistive device and Jordan splints

PRECAUTIONS
- Avoid prolonged periods of knee flexion (sitting) or knee extension
- Avoid increased pain with therapeutic exercise and functional activities
- Monitor use/tolerance of Jordan splints application/fit/tolerance/irritation
- Monitor surgical scar for color changes/swelling/discharge/drainage
- Jordan splints must be on at night for sleeping for 6 weeks

TREATMENT STRATEGIES
- Positioning, as noted above
- Training patient in ambulation with improved knee extension in stance phase
- Passive knee extension in supine/sitting
- AAROM knee flexion in sitting at edge of bed; goal is to obtain 45 degrees knee flexion
- Ankle pumps
- Progress ambulation with Jordan splints and appropriate assistive device, as tolerated, with specific focus on quality of gait pattern to gain better control of knee flexion during swing and extension during stance

CRITERIA FOR ADVANCEMENT
- Discharge from the hospital is typically on POD 3, depending on patient comfort level as a result of postoperative pain and spasm

Continued

Postoperative Rehabilitation of Rectus Femoris Transfer: Phase I (Days 2 to 3)—Cont'd

- Active-assistive knee flexion to 45 degrees
- Ability to passively extend the knee in supine
- Dependent upon level of functioning before surgery

Postoperative Rehabilitation of Rectus Femoris Transfer: Phase II (Days 4 to 14)

GOALS

- Control of postoperative spasm, which is common with rectus femoris transfer
- Control of postoperative pain and swelling
- Postoperative weeks 1 to 2 removal of Jordan splints during waking hours
- Emphasis on both passive extension and active-assistive flexion of the knee
- Sitting with knees in a flexed position with a goal of 90 degrees
- Progress ambulation with appropriate assistive device and begin to wean patient out of Jordan splints
- Advance out of Jordan splints if able to actively extend knee during ambulation
- Independence in the HEP
  1. Positioning so as not to be in prolonged periods of knee flexion or extension
  2. Knee ROM exercises-AA flexion, passive extension
  3. Gentle passive SLR
  4. Quadriceps sets
  5. Assisted heel slides in supine
  6. Ambulation as tolerated with appropriate assistive device

PRECAUTIONS

- Avoid prolonged periods of knee flexion (sitting) or knee extension
- Avoid pain with therapeutic exercise and functional activities
- Monitor use/tolerance of Jordan splints application/fit/ tolerance/irritation

- Monitor surgical scar for color changes/swelling/discharge/drainage
- Jordan splints must be on at night for sleeping for 6 weeks

TREATMENT STRATEGIES

- Gait training: improved knee extension in stance phase, improved knee flexion in swing, and ability to co-activate hamstrings and quadriceps for knee stability
- AAROM knee flexion-working toward obtaining active knee flexion
- Passive extension in sitting
- Ankle pumps, quadriceps sets, passive SLR
- Progress ambulation with Jordan splints and appropriate assistive device as tolerated with specific focus on endurance

CRITERIA FOR ADVANCEMENT

- Ability to actively flex the knee to 90 degrees
- The ability to actively extend the knee in standing is very important. Jordan splints may be discontinued when the patient is able to display full knee extension in stance. If there is any lag into knee flexion, the splints should continue to be used
- Dependent upon level of functioning before surgery

Postoperative Rehabilitation of Rectus Femoris Transfer: Phase III (Weeks 2 to 6)

GOALS

- Discontinue use of Jordan splints during waking hours at 2 weeks postoperatively
- Discontinue use of Jordan splints at night 6 weeks postoperatively
- Increase knee flexion passively and actively
- Promote/maintain knee extension passively and actively
- Strengthening lower extremities
- Improved foot clearance during swing phase of gait
- Return to stair/curb negotiation as functional level permits

Continued

Postoperative Rehabilitation of Rectus Femoris Transfer: Phase III (Weeks 2 to 6)—Cont'd

PRECAUTIONS
- Avoid pain with therapeutic exercise and functional activities
- Monitor use/tolerance of Jordan splints application/fit/tolerance/irritation
- Monitor surgical scar for color changes/swelling/discharge/drainage
- Jordan splints must be on at night for sleeping for 6 weeks to maintain knee extension

TREATMENT STRATEGIES
- Active knee flexion in sitting
- Active/active-assisted knee flexion in prone
- Standing activities with facilitation for co-activation of quadriceps and hamstrings
- Activities to promote knee flexion in standing (i.e., low step up, stepping over small obstacles)
- Activities to promote concentric and isometric quadriceps strengthening
- Transitions from sit to and from stand with therapeutic assistance as needed
- Total gym squats, progressing to wall squats
- Ascending stairs emphasizing graded control and progress to descending stairs with control
- Treadmill/gait training
- Weight-shifting in stance progressing toward single limb stance activities-emphasizing knee control
- Continue with HEP: evaluation-based

CRITERIA FOR ADVANCEMENT
- Dependent on the level of functioning before surgery
- Ability to extend knee in stance phase of gait
- Ability to flex knee in swing phase of gait
- Discontinue use of Jordan splints at night 6 weeks postoperatively.

Postoperative Rehabilitation of Rectus Femoris Transfer: Phase IV (Weeks 6 to 14)

GOALS
- Enhance co-activation of quadriceps and hamstrings in single limb stance
- Improve eccentric hamstring activation for deceleration during swing
- Improve eccentric quadriceps control for functional activities (stair descension, stand to sit)
- Increase functional muscle strength
- Continue to improve quality of ambulation
- Return to or surpass functional level before surgery

PRECAUTIONS
- Avoid pain with therapeutic exercise and functional activities

TREATMENT STRATEGIES
- Stair-stretch for increased knee flexion; single-leg stance activities to promote co-activation
- Swing phase activities
- Stand to sit, emphasizing eccentric control of quadriceps
- Total gym progressive
- Wall squats
- Step-ups/step over
- Stair negotiation, emphasizing eccentric control
- Treadmill walking
- Stationary bicycle
- Gait training
- HEP: evaluation-based

CRITERIA FOR ADVANCEMENT
- Dependent on the level of functioning before surgery
- Ability to flex knee in swing phase of gait and allow for heel strike at initial contact
- Resume existing preoperative physical therapy program

Hamstring Lengthening

- Many patients with CP exhibit excessive knee flexion because of spastic or tight hamstring musculature.
- A knee flexion deformity may be the result of a fixed capsular contracture, but, typically, it is caused by simply spastic and tight hamstring muscles.
  1. In ambulatory patients with CP, the hamstrings tend to be active throughout the entire stance phase, thus leading to persistent knee flexion during the stance phase of gait, as well as a shortened stride length during swing phase.
- Additionally, with a knee flexion deformity, there is often an associated hip flexion contracture, and a crouched gait pattern is observed.
- Clinically, hamstring tightness can be assessed by performing a straight leg raise (SLR) or measuring the popliteal angle.
- The normal ROM of an SLR is 90 degrees, and a normal popliteal angle is considered full knee extension to 180 degrees, with the hip flexed to 90 degrees.
- Indications for a hamstring lengthening are:
  1. Knee flexion of 15 degrees or more during the stance phase of ambulation
  2. Decreased stride length
  3. Straight leg raise less than 70 degrees or popliteal angle less than 135 degrees
  4. Knee pain during transfers in nonambulatory patients or patients with limited ambulation ability
  5. Increased posterior pelvic tilt, which impacts postural alignment and/or ability to sit upright

Surgical Overview

- The medial hamstrings are usually the tighter muscle group and are typically surgically addressed first.
- Lengthening of the hamstrings can be performed in supine or prone.
- Lengthening the medial hamstrings is performed by incising the fascial aponeurosis of the semimembranosus muscle at

one or two levels and step-cut lengthening or tenotomizing the semitendinosus and gracilis tendons.

- If adequate ROM is not obtained after these procedures, the lateral hamstrings are addressed and the biceps femoris may then also require aponeurotic lengthening.

Rehabilitation Overview

- Rehabilitation following hamstring lengthening is designed to both maintain and actively use the newly obtained length of the hamstrings in all positions.
- In the initial postoperative phase, the patient will use Jordan splints for ambulation and during sleeping hours to maintain knee extension. Rehabilitation will focus on decreasing the use of the Jordan splints during ambulation based on the patient's ability to extend the knees during the stance phase of gait.
- Additionally, rehabilitation will focus on functionally integrating the newfound hamstring length by facilitation of an upright pelvis in sitting or a greater step length during ambulation.
- Knee ROM and ambulation with an assistive device is begun early, and all activities should be progressed as strength improves.

Postoperative Rehabilitation of Hamstring Lengthening: Phase I (Days 1 to 2)

GOALS
- Control postoperative pain/swelling/spasms
- Emphasis on positioning to increase knee extension when in supine
- Optimize knee extension ROM, emphasizing hip flexion with knee extension
- Maintain knee flexion ROM for function (sitting and gait)
- Early weight-bearing-standing and ambulation WBAT with Jordan splints and appropriate assistive device
- Independence in HEP
  1. Positioning to maintain hamstring muscle length
  2. ROM exercises of hip and knee
  3. Gentle passive SLR
  4. Gait training

Continued

Postoperative Rehabilitation of Hamstring Lengthening: Phase I (Days 1 to 2)—Cont'd

PRECAUTIONS
- Avoid prolonged periods of knee flexion (sitting) or knee extension
- Avoid increased pain with therapeutic exercise and functional activities
- Avoid overstretching lengthened muscle in any position
- Monitor use/tolerance of Jordan splints application/fit/ tolerance/irritation
- Monitor surgical scar for color changes/swelling/ discharge/drainage
- Jordan splints must be on at night for sleeping up to 6 weeks

TREATMENT STRATEGIES
- Training patient/caregiver in positioning to maintain new hamstring muscle length
- PROM knee extension in supine/sitting
- PROM knee flexion in supine/sitting
- Ankle pumps
- In supine, towel roll may be placed under heel to allow for passive stretch of the knee in supine
- Training patient in ambulation with improved knee extension in stance phase (if ambulatory)

CRITERIA FOR ADVANCEMENT
- Discharge from the hospital is typically on PODs 1 to 2
- Dependent on the level of functioning before surgery
- At discharge from the hospital, patient may resume preoperative therapeutic physical therapy program of upper extremity and proximal core musculature strengthening

Postoperative Rehabilitation of Hamstring Lengthening: Phase II (Day 2 to Week 2)

GOALS
- Control postoperative pain/swelling/spasms
- Optimize knee extension ROM emphasizing hip flexion with knee extension

- Optimize/maintain hip extension; stretching of hip flexors may be indicated
- Emphasis on positioning to increase knee extension when in supine
- Maintain knee flexion ROM for function (sitting and gait)
- Strengthen quadriceps for knee extension during stance to allow for removal of Jordan splints
- Progress standing and ambulation WBAT with Jordan splints and appropriate assistive device
- Independence in HEP
  1. As noted in Phase I, add heel slides in supine

PRECAUTIONS
- As noted in Phase I

TREATMENT STRATEGIES
- Training patient and caregiver in positioning optimizing knee extension
- Towel roll may be placed under heel to allow for passive stretch of the knee in supine
- Training patient in ambulation with improved knee extension in stance phase (if ambulatory)
- Gentle SLR
- P/AAROM knee extension in supine/sitting
- PROM knee flexion in supine/sitting
- AAROM hip and knee flexion in supine-heel slides
- Begin AAROM knee flexion in prone if patient can tolerate
- PROM hip extension and stretching of hip flexors if appropriate
- Quad sets
- Ankle pumps
- Resume preoperative therapeutic physical therapy program of upper extremity and proximal/core muscle strengthening
- Progress ambulation with Jordan splints and appropriate assistive device as tolerated. Specific focus should be on the quality of the gait pattern to gain better control of knee extension during stance.

CRITERIA FOR ADVANCEMENT
- Depends on the level of functioning prior to surgery
- Ability to extend knee in stance phase of gait will dictate discontinuation of Jordan splints during ambulation

Postoperative Rehabilitation of Hamstring Lengthening: Phase III (Weeks 2 to 6)

GOALS

- Promote/maintain knee extension passively and actively
- Promote/maintain hip extension passively and actively
- Discontinue use of Jordan splints during waking hours
- Wean patient out of Jordan splints for ambulation: based on ability to extend knee in stance
- Strengthen quadriceps in new end range
- Strengthen hamstrings throughout range of motion
- Return to preoperative ambulatory status
- Return to stair/curb negotiation as functional level permits

PRECAUTIONS

- As noted in Phase I

TREATMENT STRATEGIES

- ROM knee flexion/extension and SLR
- Quad sets
- Prone hamstring curls
- Standing activities with facilitation for co-activation of quadriceps and hamstrings
- Activities to promote concentric and isometric quadriceps strengthening at end range
- Activities to promote concentric and isometric hamstring strengthening throughout ROM
- Emphasize core muscle strength and control
- Sit to stand
- Step-ups and stair negotiation
- Continue with HEP: evaluation-based

CRITERIA FOR ADVANCEMENT

- Depends on the level of functioning prior to surgery
- Ability to extend knee in stance phase of gait
- Discontinue use of Jordan splints at night 6 weeks postoperatively

Postoperative Rehabilitation of Hamstring Lengthening: Phase IV (Weeks 6 to 8)

GOALS FOR THE AMBULATORY PATIENT
- Enhance co-activation of quadriceps and hamstrings
- Develop concentric and eccentric hamstring and quadriceps strengthening
- Maintain or increase passive and active knee extension range of motion
- Maintain passive knee flexion range of motion
- Increase lower extremity functional muscle strength
- Continue to improve quality of ambulation
- Resume full preoperative physical therapy program
- Discontinue use of Jordan splints completely

PRECAUTIONS
- Avoid pain with therapeutic exercise and functional activities

TREATMENT STRATEGIES
- ROM knee flexion/extension and SLR
- Single leg stance activities to promote co-activation
- Swing phase activities to develop improved stride length
- Sit to stand exercises
- Emphasize core muscle strength and control
- Total Gym Progressive Exercises for strengthening of the LEs
- Step-ups
- Stair negotiation
- Treadmill walking
- Stationary bicycle
- HEP: evaluation-based

CRITERIA FOR ADVANCEMENT
- Depends on the level of functioning prior to surgery
- Ability to extend knee in stance phase of gait

Tendo Achilles Lengthening

- Children with CP typically present with spasticity of the ankle plantar flexor muscles, resulting in shortening of the gastrocsoleus musculature and an equinus gait pattern.

- This combination of failure to passively elongate the ankle plantar flexors during gait, with diminished ability to functionally activate the ankle dorsiflexors, inhibits the normal elasticity of the calf muscles.
- Rapid skeletal growth in children may impact the muscle's ability to keep up with bone length, thus contributing to the occurrence of muscle contracture in children with CP.
- Children with spastic ankle plantar flexors typically toe-walk or display a toe-heel gait pattern.
- Though equinus deformity of the ankle is the most common cause for toe-walking or a toe-heel gait pattern, increased knee flexion can also cause this foot contact pattern.
- Treatment of an equinus gait with gastrocsoleus lengthening, when the true problem is knee flexion spasticity or contracture, will universally result in profound weakness and calcaneus gait.
- It is well reported in the literature that a calcaneus deformity is much more functionally debilitating than a moderate degree of equinus.
- Indications for a tendo Achilles lengthening (TAL) are:
  1. Passive ankle dorsiflexion less than zero degrees.
  2. A fixed equinus deformity is present such that the ankle cannot be dorsiflexed to neutral with the hindfoot locked in varus in an ambulatory patient.

Surgical Overview

- The goal of a TAL is to correct an equinus deformity and relieve the contracture without excessively weakening the muscle.
- Excessive lengthening of the gastrocnemius can result in a crouch gait and an actual decrease in functional ambulation over time because of the inability to push-off during the stance phase of gait.
- Although several surgical procedures may be used to lengthen the ankle plantar flexors, only two procedures will be presented: the Vulpius and the Hoke procedures.
- The Silverskiold tests assist the surgeon in determining which procedure to use because it differentiates between

contracture of the gastrocnemius alone or combined contracture of the gastrocnemius and the soleus.

- The *Vulpius procedure* lengthens the gastrocnemius and
  spares the soleus muscle.
  1. It consists of making an inverted V incision in the gas-
     trocnemius tendinous aponeurosis and passively dorsi-
     flexing the ankle with the knee in extension.
  2. The aponeurosis separates and thus lengthens the
     gastrocnemius.
  3. This method is advantageous because it preserves the
     soleus muscle, which can be used as a muscle for
     push-off.
- The *Hoke procedure* is performed by making three incisions, each one half way through the tendon.
  1. Two incisions are made on the medial aspect of the
     Achilles tendon, one proximal and one distal, and a sin-
     gle lateral incision is performed halfway between the
     previous two.
  2. The surgeon then dorsiflexes the ankle to neutral, caus-
     ing a sliding lengthening of the tendon.
  3. No sutures are necessary with the Hoke procedure.
  4. This procedure weakens both the soleus and the gas-
     trocnemius musculature.
- Regardless of the procedure used by the surgeon to lengthen
  the Achilles tendon, the patient is placed in a short leg cast
  for 3 to 6 weeks postoperatively.

Rehabilitation Overview

- The patient is permitted to ambulate immediately postoperatively in the short leg cast, with cast boots and appropriate
  assistive device.
- While in the short leg cast, it is important to position and
  maintain the knee in extension.
- Once the cast is removed the physical therapist will need to
  address the ROM limitations of the ankle as well as strengthening the muscles about the ankle foot complex for functional mobility and control.
- The goal post-TAL is for the patient to display a heel-toe gait
  pattern.

Postoperative Rehabilitation of Tendo Achilles Lengthening: Phase I (Days 1 to 2)

GOALS
- Control postoperative pain/swelling/spasms
- Emphasis on positioning to increase knee extension when in supine
- Maintain overall knee range of motion
- Encourage active toe movements
- Early weight-bearing: standing and ambulation WBAT with appropriate assistive device
- Independence in HEP

PRECAUTIONS
- Avoid prolonged periods of knee flexion (i.e., sitting)
- Monitor skin for signs of irritation or constriction from cast
- Monitor exposed foot/toes for signs of edema

TREATMENT STRATEGIES
- Educate and train patient/caregivers in positioning. Towel roll may be placed under the ankle to allow for passive stretching of the knee in supine. Initially, operated extremity is elevated to control postop edema
- Encourage toe wiggling
- Teach patient/caregivers PROM of knee extension
- Gentle SLR to elongate the hamstrings
- Quad sets may be performed if tolerated
- Gait training emphasizing good posture and knee extension in stance phase (for ambulators)

CRITERIA FOR ADVANCEMENT
- Patient is typically discharged PODs 1 and 2
- Assistance will be necessary for distance mobility (stroller, wheelchair)
- Depends upon level of functioning prior to surgery

Postoperative Rehabilitation of Tendo Achilles Lengthening: Phase II (Day 3 to Cast Removal)

GOALS
- Control postoperative pain/swelling/spasms
- Emphasis on positioning to increase knee extension when in supine

- Maintain overall passive and active knee range of motion
- Encourage active toe movements
- Increase standing and ambulation distance WBAT with appropriate assistive
- Independence in HEP
- Resume preoperative physical therapy program to tolerance

PRECAUTIONS
- Same as in Phase I

TREATMENT STRATEGIES
- Continue with treatment strategies from Phase I
- Active knee extension exercises may be performed
- Resume preoperative physical therapy program to tolerance
- Gentle passive SLR
- Quad sets
- Gait training emphasizing good posture and knee extension in stance phase (for ambulators)

CRITERIA FOR ADVANCEMENT
- Assistance will be necessary for distance mobility (stroller, wheelchair)
- Depends upon level of functioning prior to surgery

Postoperative Rehabilitation of Tendo Achilles Lengthening: Phase III (Day of Cast Removal to 3 Weeks Post–Cast Removal)

GOALS
- Promote/maintain ankle dorsiflexion with knee extension passively and actively
- Strengthening dorsiflexors
- Strengthening plantarflexors in elongated range of motion (with dorsiflexion and knee extension)
- Patient/caregiver education regarding the importance of utilizing AFOs during the day to maintain ankle joint range of motion
- Progress ambulation endurance and independence as appropriate

Continued

Postoperative Rehabilitation of Tendo Achilles Lengthening: Phase III (Day of Cast Removal to 3 Weeks Post–Cast Removal)— Cont'd

PRECAUTIONS
- Avoid pain with therapeutic exercise and functional activities
- Avoid overstretching into dorsiflexion
- Monitor incision/scar for irritation and continued adequate healing

TREATMENT STRATEGIES
- Gentle stretching into dorsiflexion with subtalar neutral, not to exceed normal ROM
- Myofascial release of the plantar fascia if indicated
- Passive great toe extension for push-off
- Ankle pumps (emphasis on dorsiflexion)
- Standing activities to promote isometric contraction of ankle plantar flexion in an elongated position
- Sit to stand activities with emphasis on tibial translation forward over foot with neutral STJ
- Work in step stance-ability to control transition of tibia over foot
- Begin to work on push-off during gait
- Continue with HEP: evaluation-based

CRITERIA FOR ADVANCEMENT
- Assistance may be necessary for distance mobility (stroller, wheelchair)
- Depends upon level of functioning prior to surgery

Postoperative Rehabilitation of Tendo Achilles Lengthening: Phase IV (Weeks 3 to 6 Post Cast Removal)

GOALS
- Enhance co-activation of postural plantarflexors, and dorsiflexors
- Promote appropriate ankle kinematics during gait

• Progress ambulation endurance and independence to level at or greater than presurgery

PRECAUTIONS
• Same as Phase III

TREATMENT STRATEGIES
• Continue with treatment strategies from Phase II
• Single leg stance activities to promote co-activation
• Strengthening of anterior tibialis, and dorsiflexors to improve heel strike during gait (heel walking)
• Eccentric plantar flexion activities (retro ambulation, step-ups, squats)
• Dynamic foot reactions
• Walking balance beam, tandem walking
• HEP: evaluation-based

CRITERIA FOR ADVANCEMENT
• Assistance may be necessary for distance mobility (stroller, wheelchair)
• Depends upon level of functioning prior to surgery
• Progress ambulation endurance/distance as tolerated

Bibliography

Aiona, M.D., Sussman, M.D. Treatment of Spastic Diplegia in Patients with Cerebral Palsy: Part II. *J Pediatr Orthop* 2004;13(3): S13-S38.

Bleck, E.E. Orthopaedic Management in Cerebral Palsy. JB Lippincott, Philadelphia,1987.

Bobroff, E.D., Chambers, H.G., Sartoris, D.J., Wyatt, M.P., Sutherland, D.H. Femoral Anteversion and Neck-shaft Angle in Children with Cerebral Palsy [Section II: Original Articles: Knee]. *Clin Orthop Relat Res* 1999;1(364):194-204.

Delp, S.L. Computer Modeling and Analysis of Movement Disabilities and Their Surgical Corrections. In Harris, G.F., Smith, P.A. (Eds). Human Motion Analysis. IEEE Press, Piscataway, NJ, 1996, pp. 114-132.

Grant, A.D., Feldman, R., Lehman, W.B. Equinus Deformity in Cerebral Palsy: A Retrospective Analysis of Treatment and Function in 39 Cases. *J Pediatr Orthop* 1985;5(6):678-681.

Herring, J.A. Tachdjian's Pediatric Orthopaedics, 3rd ed. WB Saunders, Philadelphia, 2002.

Laplaza, F.J., Root, L. Femoral Anteversion and Neck-shaft Angles in Hip Instability in Cerebral Palsy. *J Pediatr Orthop* 1994;14:719-723.

Magee, D.J. Orthopedic Physical Assessment, 3rd ed. WB Saunders, Philadelphia, 1997.

Morrissy, R.T., Weinstein, S.L. Atlas of Pediatric Orthopedic Surgery, 3rd ed. Lippincott Williams & Wilkins, Philadelphia, 2001.

Murray-Weir, M., Root, L., Peterson, M., Lenhoff, M., Daly, L., Wagner, C., Marcus, P. Proximal Femoral Varus Rotation Osteotomy in Cerebral Palsy: A Prospective Gait Study. *J Pediatr Orthop* 2003;23(3):321-329.

Nelson, K. What Proportion of Cerebral Palsy is Related to Birth Asphyxia? *J Pediatr* 1988;113:572-574.

Novacheck, T.F. Surgical Intervention in Ambulatory Cerebral Palsy. In Harris, G.F., Smith, P.A. (Eds). Human Motion Analysis. IEEE Press, Piscataway, NJ, 1996, pp. 231-254.

Ounpuu, M.S., Davis, R.B., Gage, J.R., DeLuca, P.A. Rectus Femoris Surgery in Children with Cerebral Palsy. Part I: The Effect of the Rectus Femoris Transfer Location on Knee Motion. *J Pediatr Orthop* 1993;13:325-330.

Ounpuu, S.M., DeLuca, P., Davis, R., Romness, M. Long-term Effects of Femoral Derotation Osteotomies: An Evaluation Using Three-dimensional Gait Analysis. *J Pediatr Orthop* 2002;22(2):139-145.

Perry, J. Distal Rectus Femoris Transfer. *Dev Med Child Neurol* 1987;29:153-158.

Personal communication, Dr. Leon Root, Medical Director of Rehabilitation, Hospital for Special Surgery, November 2004; May 2005.

Press Room/Facts and Figures, January 2005. Available online at http://www.ucp.org.

Renshaw, T., Green, N.E., Griffin, P.P., Root, L. Cerebral Palsy: Orthopaedic Management-Instructional Course Lectures. *J Bone Joint Surg Am* 1995;77A(10):1590-1606.

Renshaw, T.S. Cerebral Palsy. In Morrissy, R.T., Weinstein, S.L. (Eds). Lovell and Winter's Pediatric Orthopaedics, 5th ed., vol. 1. Lippincott Williams & Wilkins, New York, 2001, pp. 563-599.

Rinsky, L.A. Surgery for Cerebral Palsy. In Chapman's Orthopaedic Surgery, 3rd ed. Lippincott Williams & Wilkins, New York, 2001, pp. 4485-4506.

Root, L., Siegal, T. Osteotomy of the Hip in Children: Posterior Approach. *J Bone Joint Surg Am* 1980;62:571-575.

Staheli, L.T. Medial Femoral Torsion. *Orthop Clin North Am* 1980; 11:39-50.

Sussman, M.D., Aiona, M.D. Treatment of Spastic Diplegia in Patients with Cerebral Palsy. *J Pediatr Orthop B* 2004;13(2):S1-S128.

Sutherland, D.H., Kaufman, K.R. Human Motion Analysis and Pediatric Orthopaedics. In Harris, G.F., Smith, P.A. (Eds). Human Motion Analysis. IEEE Press, Piscataway, NJ, 1996, pp. 219-230.

Sutherland, D.H., Santi, M.D., Abel, M.F. Treatment of Stiff Knee Gait in Cerebral Palsy: A Comparison by Gait Analysis of Distal Rectus Femoris Transfer vs Proximal Rectus Release. *J Pediatr Orthop* 1990;10:433-441.

Sutherland, D.H., Zilberfarb, J.L., Kaufman, K.R., Wyatt, M.P., Chambers, H.G. Psoas Release at the Pelvic Brim in Ambulatory Patients with Cerebral Palsy: Operative Technique and Functional Outcome. *J Pediatr Orthop* 1997;17(5):563-570.

CHAPTER 26

Spinal Fusion in Adolescent Idiopathic Scoliosis

Loretta Amoroso, DPT

Kelly Ann Sindle, PT

The Scoliosis Research Society defines idiopathic scoliosis as a lateral curvature of the spine of unknown etiology that is greater than or equal to a 10-degree Cobb angle with rotation. Adolescent idiopathic scoliosis (AIS) appears before the onset of puberty and before skeletal maturity.

The degree of curvature and risk of progression will dictate whether treatment will be managed conservatively or surgically. Conservative management of AIS consists of observation and/or bracing. Curves that are 20 degrees or less before the time of skeletal maturity are considered mild and are usually observed every 6 months for progression. Bracing is indicated for individuals with curves of 25 to 45 degrees who have not reached skeletal maturity and/or those curves that progress 5 to 10 degrees in 6 months.

Surgical intervention may be indicated depending on the degree of curvature, the risk for progression, the secondary effects of the scoliosis, and the failure or success of conservative treatment. Surgery is indicated for curves greater than 50 degrees in the skeletally immature patient and 60 degrees in the skeletally mature patient.

Surgical Overview

- The curve fused and levels of fusion are determined by the identification of the primary and secondary curves as well as the severity of the curve.
  1. The first and the last vertebra of the major curve(s) are identified and all included vertebras are fused.
  2. To achieve a neutrally rotated spine, the fusion must often extend one level above the scoliotic curve.

3. The fusion is extended one level below the curve to achieve a stable base.

- The possible surgical approaches for correction of scoliosis include a posterior spinal fusion (PSF), an anterior spinal fusion (ASF), or a combination of both.
- The most common surgical procedure performed for correction of AIS is a posterior spinal fusion in conjunction with posterior instrumentation.
  1. In a PSF, a subperiosteal exposure is made followed by facet excision, and fusion is achieved with bone obtained from the iliac crest or ribs.
  2. Instrumentation is added to the fusion to achieve and maintain correction.
- An anterior approach is often chosen when there is a single lumbar curve or for a thoracolumbar curve.
  1. For this surgical approach, the segments included in the fusion are those central to the structural central area of the curve.
  2. In an ASF, exposure is made on the convex side of the curve with complete disc excision.
  3. The disc space is packed with autologous rib bone graft, then stabilized with compression instrumentation on the convex side.
- A combined anterior/posterior spinal fusion for AIS is indicated for large, stiff curves and/or a progressing curve that demonstrates a rotational deformity, especially in a skeletally immature patient.
- Spinal fusion combined with instrumentation takes between 6 and 12 months to be completely healed. Most patients do not require removal of hardware from this surgery.

Rehabilitation Overview

- At HSS, physical therapy plays a primary role in the postsurgical rehabilitation of AIS. The rehabilitation program following ASF and/or PSF surgery is designed to progressively return patients to their prior level of function.
- The focus of physical therapy is to restore trunk and core abdominal strength, upper and lower extremity flexibility and strength, as well as educate the patient in proper posture and body mechanics.

- Both the anatomy and biomechanics of the spine pre- and post-surgery must be considered throughout the course of treatment. The biomechanics of the fused levels are altered post-surgically as well as those levels just above and below the fusion.
- Continuous communication between the surgeon, therapist, and patient is key for a successful outcome.
- Throughout the rehabilitation course, the patient should play an active role in his or her recovery by setting and working toward functional goals. The patient must be compliant with all spine precautions to protect the healing fusion and be diligent in performing his or her home exercise program (HEP) to ensure carryover and success in the rehabilitative process.

Preoperative Rehabilitation

GOALS
- Patient/caregiver education
- Maximize trunk extensor strength
- Maximize core abdominal strength
- Demonstrate independence in log rolling
- Demonstrate understanding of all spine precautions

TREATMENT STRATEGIES
- Patient/parent education in spine precautions, body mechanics, and proper postural alignment
- Breathing exercises: incentive spirometry
- Log rolling
- Hamstring/hip flexor stretching
- Trunk extension strengthening
- Core abdominal strength: neutral spine stabilization exercises, Physio ball Therex
- LE strengthening: quadriceps sets, bridges, wall squats, total gym
- Endurance training/general conditioning: stationary bike, treadmill, elliptical

Postoperative Rehabilitation Acute/ Inpatient Phase I (Week 1)

GOALS
- Independent with all spine precautions
- Independent or minimally assisted transfers

- Independent ambulation
- Independent stair climbing with one railing
- Independent with proper posture and body mechanics
- Independent with donning/doffing brace, if applicable

Precautions
- No lumbar or thoracic flexion
- No lumbar or thoracic rotation
- No lifting of heavy objects (<8 to 10 pounds)

TREATMENT STRATEGIES

Day 1
- Patient education regarding spine precautions to protect the healing fusion
- Incentive spirometry
- Assisted log rolling for transfers in and out of bed
- Assisted dangle at bedside
- Ankle pumps and quadriceps sets 10 times per hour

Day 2
- Review spine precautions
- Incentive spirometry
- Log rolling for transfers in and out of bed
- Stand and ambulate at bedside with rolling walker and assistance
- Ankle pumps and quadriceps sets 10 times per hour

Days 3 and 4
- Review spine precautions
- Incentive spirometry
- Log rolling for transfers in and out of bed
- Progress ambulation with rolling walker, with emphasis on decreasing use of upper extremities-assess ability to ambulate with hand-held assistance
- Patient comfortable sitting in chair for 20 minutes
- Ankle pumps and quadriceps sets 10 times per hour

Days 5 and 6
- Review spine precautions
- Deep breathing exercises
- Log rolling for transfers in and out of bed
- Ambulation with hand-held assistance to supervised ambulation
- Stairs with supervision and one rail

Continued

Postoperative Rehabilitation Acute/Inpatient Phase I (Week 1)—Cont'd

Day 7—Discharge
- Review all spine precautions and discharge instructions
- Independent with donning/doffing brace, if applicable (caregiver can assist if needed)
- Independent/minimal assistance for log rolling for transfers in and out of bed
- Independent ambulation
- Independent stairs with one rail
- Patient comfortable sitting in chair for all meals
- Independent with HEP (quadriceps sets, ankle pumps, endurance training with walking program)

Postoperative Rehabilitation Outpatient Phase I (Weeks 1 to 6)*

GOALS
- Patient can verbalize and demonstrate spine precautions, proper body mechanics, positioning, and posture
- Maximize core strengthening
- Maximize postural strength
- Maximize flexibility of upper and lower extremities
- Maximize strength of upper and lower extremities
- Maximize endurance
- Independent with HEP

PRECAUTIONS
- No lumbar or thoracic flexion
- No lumbar or thoracic rotation
- No lifting of heavy objects (8 to 10 pounds)
- Sports/gym activities, as per surgeon
- No weights or resistance training
- Hamstring stretching, as per surgeon (reinforce use of abdominal stabilization as to stretch only hamstrings and reduce pull on lumbar spine)

TREATMENT STRATEGIES
- Review log rolling, bed mobility, resting/sleep positioning
- Review and facilitate proper posture in sitting and standing
- Core stabilization (Sahrmann) at appropriate level: neutral spine stabilization exercises with emphasis on abdominal contraction
- Lower extremity flexibility, as per surgeon (gentle stretching only)
- Active shoulder girdle mobilization—shoulder shrugs, forward/backward shoulder rolls, scapular retraction
- Postural strengthening—scapular retraction (progressive), shoulder forward flexion in scapular plane on bench, sitting posture with visual cueing, chin tucks, prone scapular retraction with upper and middle trapezius, shoulder extension, scapular stabilization
- Soft tissue/myofascial to trunk and shoulder girdle
- Endurance/general conditioning: treadmill, stationary bike

ADVANCEMENT CRITERIA
- Patient exhibits symmetrical shoulders and pelvis 50% of the time
- Ambulation with reciprocal arm swing
- Improved core strength, Sahrmann level II
- Independent in log rolling, bed mobility

*Postoperative rehabilitation begins 1 to 6 months after surgery.

Postoperative Rehabilitation Outpatient Phase II (Weeks 6 to 12)

GOALS
- Independent with proper posture and body mechanics during advanced functional activities
- Core strength Sahrmann level III
- Maximize postural strength
- Maximize postural endurance
- Maximize flexibility of upper and lower extremities
- Maximize lower extremity strength, proximal hip strength (5/5)
- Maximize endurance and general conditioning

Continued

Postoperative Rehabilitation Outpatient Phase II (Weeks 6 to 12)—Cont'd

PRECAUTIONS
- Same as phase I
- Hamstring stretching, as per surgeon (reinforce use of abdominal stabilization so as to stretch hamstrings only and reduce pull on lumbar spine)

TREATMENT STRATEGIES
- Body mechanics with regard to squatting to pick objects off floor; use hip flexion not lumbar motion
- Postural strengthening—emphasis on scapular stabilization, scapular retraction, shoulder forward flexion in prone
- Advanced core stabilization—therapeutic ball, quadruped with neutral spine
- Lower extremity flexibility—gentle stretching with abdominals activated
- Continue active shoulder girdle mobility
- Soft tissue/myofascial release
- Continue and progress endurance

CRITERIA FOR DISCHARGE
- Symmetrical shoulders and pelvis 100% of the time
- Proper posture and body mechanics 100% of the time
- Pre-surgical level of endurance
- Sahrmann level III

Bibliography

Lonstein, J., Bradford, D., Winter, R., Ogilvie, J. Moe's Textbook of Scoliosis and Other Spinal Deformities, 3rd ed. WB Saunders, Philadelphia, 1995.

Rowe, D.E., Bernstein, S.M., Riddick, M.F., Adler, F., Emans, J.B., Gardner-Bonneau, D.A. Meta-analysis of the Efficacy of Nonoperative Treatments for Idiopathic Scoliosis. *J Bone Joint Surg* 1997;79: 664-674.

SRS Terminology and Working Group on Spinal Classification (Chair Larry Lenke, MD). Revised Glossary of Terms, 2000. Available online at http://www.SRS.org.

Weinstein, S.L. The Pediatric Spine, Principles and Practice, 2nd ed. Lippincott Williams & Wilkins, Philadelphia, 2001.

CHAPTER 27

Congenital Muscular Torticollis

Deborah Corradi-Scalise, PT, DPT, MA
Amanda R. Sparrow, PT
Loretta Amoroso, DPT

Congenital muscular torticollis (CMT) is defined as a unilateral shortening or contracture of the sternocleidomastoid (SCM) muscle, present at birth. It presents as a persistent tilt of the head toward the involved side with the chin rotated toward the opposite shoulder. The coexistence of CMT with developmental hip dysplasia has been reported with variations of 0 to 20%. The exact etiology of CMT is unknown; however, many causative theories have been postulated, including intrauterine malposition, birth trauma, uterine compression/crowding, possible ischemic event causing a compartment syndrome of the SCM, faulty SCM cell differentiation, or possible entrapment of the spinal accessory nerve due to fibrosis.

An infant with right CMT presents with cervical lateral flexion to the right side and cervical rotation to the left shoulder. Facial asymmetry and plagiocephaly (flattening of the occiput on the contralateral side as the tilt) are also often associated with CMT. Occasionally, a palpable mass or pseudotumor is associated with CMT. This fibrotic mass is within the SCM muscle belly and will gradually resolve.

Differential Diagnosis

- Medical differential diagnosis is important to rule out other causative factors of positional head/neck asymmetry.
- Other causative factors, such as viral infection, muscular strain, postnatal trauma (clavicular fracture), congenital anomalies of the base of the skull, congenital anomalies of the upper cervical spine, ocular pathology, imbalance of

the extraocular muscles, rotary subluxation of the atlantoaxial joints (following URI), tumor of the posterior fossa, brain stem, or cervical spinal cord, all need to be ruled out as the cause of the presenting neck asymmetry.

- Neurologic evaluation may be required to rule out an underlying neurological cause, especially in the event of sudden onset torticollis in the infant.
- Evidence shows that a thorough clinical examination is necessary to assist in differential diagnosis as it relates to CMT.
- If CMT is diagnosed or suspected, specific focus should be placed on assessing neck ROM both passively and actively, using a universal goniometer. Neck measurements of lateral flexion and rotation are performed in supine.

Rehabilitation Overview
Primary Impairments
- The baby postures with a lateral tilt toward the involved side and rotation away from the tight SCM.
- There is limited passive range of motion (PROM) into lateral flexion toward the uninvolved side and decreased rotation toward the involved side.
- The baby with CMT also has decreased active head righting and decreased active rotation toward the involved side in developmental positions.

Secondary Impairments
- Plagiocephaly and facial deformity are also encountered in babies with CMT. This involves flattening on the posterior lateral portion of the skull on the uninvolved side because of the child's positioning in supine; associated facial deformities include posterior displacement of the ear on the same side of the involved SCM, posterior recession of the same side eyebrow and forehead, and the tip of the chin skewed toward the involved side.
- Muscle shortening, which includes tightness in secondary muscle(s) such as the platysma, scalene muscles, trapezius muscles, cervical extensors, pectoral muscles, as well as limitation of scapulohumeral ROM and trunk flexibility

may exist. Shoulder elevation and protraction on the involved side may also be present.

- Developmental delays can also be found in babies with CMT.
  1. The habitual posturing may lead to asymmetrical strength between sides.
  2. Weakness in the ipsilateral trunk and scapular musculature due to the decreased active and controlled weight-bearing to and on that side may also be present.
  3. Delays or asymmetrical movement patterns can develop, which include delayed rolling or rolling toward/over the unaffected side only, decreased weight-bearing and/or use of the arm on the involved side (prone prop and reaching), in sitting asymmetrical weight-bearing that fosters lateral flexion to the involved side, delayed creeping, pull to stand, and ambulation.

Treatment Guidelines

- At HSS, infants are seen for physical therapy intervention two to three times per week for 30 to 45 minute-sessions, depending on the severity of the CMT and the child's tolerance to therapeutic intervention.
- A HEP is recommended to be performed a minimum of four to five times per day or at every diaper change.
- During the initial evaluation, the parent and/or caregiver should be instructed in a home stretching program of lateral flexion toward the uninvolved side and rotation toward the involved side, to be performed at a minimum of four to five times per day.
  1. Each stretching exercise should be held for a minimum of 30 seconds if tolerated.
  2. The parents should be shown various positions in which to perform stretching activities and should be able to demonstrate all of the exercises independently in front of the therapist before beginning them at home.
- Positioning is also an important adjunct to therapy, and family/caregivers should be educated in ways to position the infant, hold/carry the infant, and play/stimulate the infant in ways that encourage rotation toward the involved side and lateral flexion away from the involved side as well as midline orientation.

- Supervised time spent in prone is important for the development of symmetrical neck extension and upper extremity weight-bearing.
- Active neck ROM can also be encouraged through positioning of toys, positioning during feeding, and varying the carrying position.
- This HEP remains in place 3 to 6 months after discharge with decreased frequency.

Precautions

- All patients should have had medical clearance before the physical therapy examination.
- Infants cry to express themselves; they will cry if they are experiencing negative symptoms associated with stretching, such as pain, numbness, or burning; they will also cry if they are afraid, tired, or hungry.
- The therapist should develop a sense of the infant's personality and his or her tolerance for stretching and exercise. Performing gentle stretching and constantly monitoring the baby for signs of discomfort or distress throughout the treatment session are extremely important.
- While passively stretching the SCM into lateral flexion, the neck must be kept in a neutral position within both the sagittal and transverse planes.
- Functional strengthening exercises or positions that promote strengthening (antigravity control) should be age-appropriate and should not be included in the treatment until the infant begins to develop independent head control.

Recommendations

- The best time to work with an infant is when he or she is well fed and rested.
- The therapist should take time to develop a rapport with the infant and to gain the infant's trust through interaction and play before initiating stretching.
- Stretching can typically be accomplished without eliciting crying if the therapist is gentle and can develop strategies to distract the infant, such as using singing and/or sensory stimulating and age-appropriate toys during treatment.

Rehabilitation Phase I (Weeks 1 to 8)

GOALS
- Increase PROM of cervical lateral flexion to the uninvolved side by 10-15 degrees
- Increase PROM of cervical rotation to the involved side by 10-15 degrees
- Actively bring head into midline in supine and hold it there 50% of the time
- Actively rotate head from side to side in supine to visually track a toy in available ROM
- Actively begin to right head to midline against gravity in side-lying and supported sitting positions from the involved side
- Hold head in cervical extension for 10 seconds in the prone position (if infant has head control)
- Prone prop on forearms with good weight-bearing on the UE on the affected side
- Demonstrate head righting reactions 50% of the ROM during facilitated rolling
- Caregiver is independent and compliant with HEP

PRECAUTIONS
- Keep the infant's neck in a neutral position; do not stretch in a flexed or hyperextended position
- Keep the stretching gentle
- Look for signs of discomfort or pain throughout the treatment session

TREATMENT STRATEGIES
- Parent education of positioning, gentle manual stretching, and HEP
- Passive manual stretching of the SCM in cervical lateral flexion to the uninvolved side
- Passive manual stretching of the SCM in cervical rotation to the involved side
- Myofascial/soft tissue techniques to the SCM, upper chest, shoulder girdle, and scapulohumeral muscles Maintain distance/mobility between neck and shoulders
- Positioning of musical or visually attractive toys to promote active rotation to the involved side
- If independent head control is beginning, start strengthening of the uninvolved side to bring the head

Continued

Rehabilitation Phase I (Weeks 1 to 8)—Cont'd

into midline through hands on facilitation and the use of the righting reactions if present
- Mild vestibular activities to encourage eyes horizontal in space
- Facilitation of all age-appropriate developmental skills, such as rolling, prone prop on forearms and extended elbows, reaching in prone, midline orientation in supine as appropriate

CRITERIA FOR ADVANCEMENT
- Increase in neck PROM of lateral flexion toward the uninvolved side and rotation toward the involved side
- Increase in neck active range of motion (AROM), with observation of midline head control

Rehabilitation Phase II (Weeks 8 to 16)

GOALS
- Full PROM of both cervical lateral flexion and cervical rotation (to equal the ROM of the uninvolved side)
- Midline head control in supine 100% of the time
- Midline head control in highest age-appropriate developmental position 50%-75% of the time
- Actively rotate head to both sides within full ROM in supine
- Actively hold head in midline against gravity for 10-15 seconds in side-lying and supported sitting positions on both sides
- Hold head in cervical extension in prone for an appropriate amount of time to play with a toy
- Prone prop on forearms or extended elbows with good weight-bearing on the UE on the affected side
- Bring head into midline in supported sitting and hold it there to play with a toy for 20 seconds
- Visually track an object 180 degrees in the horizontal plane in supine and if developmentally appropriate supported sitting

- Demonstrate head righting reactions during facilitated rolling over/on either side
- Head in midline and chin tuck evident in pull to sit
- Demonstrate the ability to reach forward for a toy with two hands in supported sitting, without head tilt
- Caregiver is independent and compliant with HEP.

PRECAUTIONS
- Same as noted in Phase I

TREATMENT STRATEGIES
- Passive manual stretching of the SCM muscle into cervical lateral flexion to the uninvolved side and rotation to the involved side
- Myofascial/soft tissue techniques to maintain mobility of the upper chest and shoulder girdle musculature
- Promote active cervical rotation toward the involved side in all-age appropriate developmental positions via toy placement and manual facilitation
- Manual facilitation and/or positioning of toys to promote head in midline in supine, supported/ unsupported sitting
- Vestibular input and manual facilitation to elicit appropriate head righting reactions in all planes
- Therapeutic ball activities to grade antigravity head control
- Facilitation of all age-appropriate developmental skills such as rolling, prone prop on forearms and extended elbows, reaching in prone, midline orientation in supine, hand to hand, hand to mouth, hands to feet, and feet to mouth focusing on active head control and midline orientation without compensations. Facilitation of sitting and creeping with midline head control if appropriate

CRITERIA FOR ADVANCEMENT
- Increase in neck PROM of lateral flexion toward the uninvolved side and rotation toward the involved side
- Increase in neck AROM, with observation of midline head control

Rehabilitation Phase III: Discharge (Weeks 16 to 24)

GOALS
- Full passive and active ROM of both cervical lateral flexion and rotation
- Head is in midline 95%-100% of the time in all age-appropriate developmental positions
- Able to hold head in midline and play with a toy in all age-appropriate developmental positions
- Full active cervical rotation in highest developmental positions without compensations
- Demonstrates no preference when performing functional activities such as rolling, reaching, and UE weight-bearing
- Age-appropriate antigravity neck strength
- Parents are independent with and understand the importance of continuing the HEP

PRECAUTIONS
- Same as noted in Phase 1

TREATMENT STRATEGIES
- Same as noted in Phase II

CRITERIA FOR ADVANCEMENT
- Physical therapy discontinued if the child has met all phase III goals

Surgical Management

- Stretching and conservative intervention is effective in greater than 90% of CMT cases; however, conservative treatment is usually unsuccessful after age 12 months.
- When conservative methods fail, surgery may be indicated. Indications for surgical intervention include facial deformity or cervical ROM limitations of 30 degrees or more.
- Typically, a unipolar release is performed at the distal or clavicular end of the SCM muscle. If this muscle remains tight, a bipolar release is performed with the second lengthening performed at the proximal or mastoid end.
- Depending on physician recommendation, physical therapy may begin immediately or within the first 2 weeks postoperatively.

- The postoperative patient is typically placed in a soft cervical collar for comfort, which is removed for physical therapy treatment. The collar begins to be removed during the day as the patient develops sufficient neck strength and endurance to maintain midline head control.
- The HEP is kept in place after discharge from physical therapy and is performed once a day for 4 to 8 weeks after discharge.

Postoperative Phase I (Weeks 1 to 8)

GOALS
- Patient and caregiver education
- Control of postoperative pain, as per physician recommendation
- Monitor healing of surgical incision
- Maintain/gain passive range of all cervical motions
- Develop head and neck midline postural awareness and control
- Develop active head righting reactions in all planes
- Maximize cervical muscle strength
- Scar management
- Patient/caregiver is independent with HEP

PRECAUTIONS
- Same as noted in Phase I, Conservative Treatment
- Keep the child's neck in a neutral position; do not stretch in a flexed or hyperextended position
- Keep the stretching gentle
- Look for signs of discomfort or pain throughout the treatment session
- Do not cause irritation to the incision

TREATMENT STRATEGIES
- Parent education of positioning and instruction of HEP for gentle manual stretching
- Caregiver and patient education in wear schedule for soft cervical collar
- Caregiver and patient education in monitoring incision site

Continued

Postoperative Phase I (Weeks 1 to 8)—Cont'd

- Upon physician approval, use of silicon-based patch to aid in flattening and softening of the scar
- Passive manual stretching of the SCM in cervical lateral flexion to the uninvolved side
- Passive manual stretching of the SCM in cervical rotation to the involved side
- Myofascial/soft tissue techniques to the SCM, upper chest, shoulder girdle, and scapulohumeral muscles. Maintain distance/mobility between neck and shoulders.
- Facilitate midline head orientation through visual and vestibular cues/feedback
- Develop head righting reactions in all planes, especially in antigravity positions
- Develop ability to chin tuck in pull to sit or sit up with head in midline, with emphasis on symmetrical muscle activation into flexion
- Develop ability to extend the cervical spine against gravity in midline, with emphasis on symmetrical muscle activation into extension
- Strengthening of the uninvolved side via active lateral cervical flexion against gravity in side-lying
- Therapeutic ball activities to grade antigravity head control, and develop functional head righting skills in all planes

DISCHARGE CRITERIA
- Functional integration of midline head orientation without soft cervical collar
- Symmetrical neck ROM
- Symmetrical neck muscle strength

Take Home Message

- Physical therapy is the "Gold Standard" of care for the initial treatment of CMT.
- Differential diagnosis is extremely important in dictating type of treatment.
- Early diagnosis of CMT and initiation of physical therapy treatment are the key to the success of conservative management.

- HEP and caregiver compliance/participation is critical for the optimal results.
- Infants are unable to fully express themselves; *remember precautions at all times.*
- When conservative methods fail, surgical intervention may be indicated in children over age 1 year.

Bibliography

Cheng, J.C., Tang, S.P. Outcome of Surgical Treatment of Congenital Muscular Torticollis. *Clin Orthop Relat Res* 1999;1(362):190–200.

Emery, C. The Determinants of Treatment Duration for Congenital Muscular Torticollis. *Phys Ther* 1994;74:921–929.

Loder, R.T. The Cervical Spine. In Morrissy, R.T., Weinstein, S.L. (Eds). Lovell and Winter's Pediatric Orthopaedics, 5th ed., vol. 2. Lippincott Williams & Wilkins, New York, 2001, pp. 811–815.

Stanger, M. Orthopedic Management. In Tecklin, J.S. (Ed). Pediatric Physical Therapy, 3rd ed. Lippincott Williams & Wilkins, New York, 1999, pp. 394–396.

Taylor, J.L., Stamos, N.E. Developmental Muscular Torticollis: Outcomes in Young Children Treated by Physical Therapy. *Pediatr Phys Ther* 1997;9:173–178.

Tein, Y.C., Su, J.Y. Ultrasonographic Study of the Coexistence of Muscular Torticollis and Dysplasia of the Hip. *J Pediatr Orthop* 2001;21(3):343–347.

Verbal Conversation with Dr. Daniel Green, Attending Pediatric Orthopedic Surgeon, Hospital for Special Surgery, May 2005.

Weiner, D.S. Congenital Dislocations of the Hip Associated with Congenital Muscular Torticollis. *Clin Orthop* 1976;121–163.

Yu, C., Wong, F.H., Lo, L.J., Chen, Y.R. Craniofacial Deformity in Patients with Uncorrected Congenital Muscular Torticollis: An Assessment from Three-dimensional Computed Tomography Imaging. *Plast Reconstr Surg* 2004;113(1):24–33.

SPINE REHABILITATION

Holly Rudnick, PT, Cert MDT

C H A P T E R *28*

Lumbar Microdiscectomy

Todd Gage, PT, CSCS

Lumbar Disc Herniation

- Lumbar disc herniation (LDH) is one of the most common injuries to the lumbar spine. LDH most commonly occurs between ages 30 and 50. Approximately 95% of LDH occur at the L4/L5 and L5/S1 levels.
- Disc herniations are broken into two classifications: contained and sequestered.
  1. Contained herniations include protruded/bulging discs, in which the nucleus has not perforated the annulus fibrosis, and prolapsed discs, in which the nucleus has perforated the annulus but is contained by the posterior longitudinal ligament (PLL).
  2. A sequestered disc is described as perforation of the PLL by the disc, with a fragment in the epidural space.
- Flexion/rotation of the lumbar segments has been shown to lead to an increase in intradiscal pressure and LDH.
  1. The greatest amount of lumbar flexion/extension range of motion (ROM) occurs at the L4/L5 and L5/S1 segments, which creates an increased risk for herniation at these levels.
  2. Because combined motions are a part of activities of daily living (ADL), there is the potential for breakdown

of the annulus and migration of nuclear material beyond the confines of the disc and surrounding ligaments leading to mechanical or chemical irritation of the nerve roots or spinal cord.

- Many herniations will spontaneously disappear or decrease in size over the course of several months.
- Less than 2% of disc herniations require surgery and less than 15% of patients with disc herniations will have underlying nerve root compression.
- Indications for microdiscectomy include evidence of cauda equina syndrome, significant motor weakness, or intractable pain. In addition, the patient will have failed conservative treatment, which includes nonsteroidal anti-inflammatory drugs (NSAIDs), physical therapy for 8 to 12 weeks, and epidural steroid injections.

Surgical Overview

- A lumbar microdiscectomy (LMD) is performed in the reverse Trendelenburg's position.
- A small incision (ranging from 3 to 6 cm) is made along the midline, over the interspace of the affected level.
- The paraspinal musculature is stripped subperiosteally, and a retractor with a 5-pound weight is placed over the facet to open the interspace. The interspinous ligament is kept intact.
- The microscope is then introduced, part of the lateral aspect of the ligamentum flavum is resected, and a foraminotomy is performed. The nerve root is then retracted medially.
- The PLL and nucleus are cut laterally to the nerve root, and a nucleotomy is performed.
- Insult to the ligamentum flavum and paraspinal musculature is routinely not repaired; however, the lumbar fascia is closed with absorbable sutures.

Rehabilitation Overview

- The rehabilitation program following an LMD begins on the day of surgery. Patients who undergo an LMD are hospitalized for approximately 1 to 2 days.
- The treatment in the acute stage is primarily one of education. Patients must have a basic understanding of the

mechanism of injury for disc herniations, to avoid the risk of reherniation following microdiscectomy.

- The recurrence rate following LMD is reported as being between 3% and 19%. Morgan-Hough et al. performed a retrospective analysis of 531 patients who underwent primary microdiscectomy over a 16-year period. They calculated a revision rate of 7.9% and reported that contained protrusions were almost three times more likely to require revision surgery compared to extruded or sequestered discs. Seventy-six percent of the recurrent herniations occurred between 3 and 48 months following primary LMD.

- The physical therapist must consider the work done by Nachemson on intradiscal pressure and loads when educating the patient on body mechanics, posture, and exercise.

- At the Hospital for Special Surgery (HSS), all patients are instructed in log-roll transfers, when performing supine to sit, and a basic home exercise program consisting of abdominal setting, gluteal sets, and ankle pumps, before leaving the hospital.

- Patients are discharged from the hospital on the first or second postoperative day. Criteria for discharge include patient demonstration of proper supine-sit transfers, a basic understanding of body mechanics during ADL to avoid lumbar flexion, independent ambulation, with or without an assistive device, and demonstration of independence with donning/doffing a lumbar orthosis.

- Patients are provided with an activity guide upon discharge from the hospital, to provide a basic framework for the progression of activity following LMD before initiating formal physical therapy.

- During the first 4 weeks postoperatively, patients are encouraged to walk and continue with the basic exercise program described previously. Patients must continue to avoid lifting, bending, twisting, and prolonged sitting during this period in an attempt to allow healing and diminish postoperative pain.

- Patients begin formal outpatient physical therapy between 4 and 6 weeks postoperatively and are seen two to three times per week for 8 to 14 weeks.

- The phases of tissue healing, along with symptom behavior, recovery of motor deficits, and the restoration of muscle imbalances, will dictate the progression in the rehabilitation program following LMD.
- Ahlgren et al. looked at the effect of annular repair on the healing strength of the intervertebral disc in sheep spines following a partial discectomy. They determined that at 6 weeks following partial discectomy, disc strength ranged between 60% and 75% of the control values. As a result, patients must make every attempt to minimize intradiscal pressures during the first 6 weeks post-LMD.
- A systematic review of randomized controlled trials was conducted by Ostelo et al. to determine the effectiveness of active treatments following primary lumbar disc surgery. After looking at 13 studies that fulfilled the inclusion criteria, they determined that there is strong evidence that intensive exercise programs initiated 4 to 6 weeks postoperatively are more effective on functional status and faster return to work.

Preoperative Phase: Conservative Management

GOALS
- Education
  1. Anatomy/biomechanics of lumbar disc
  2. Patients are educated on proper body mechanics during transfers
  3. Mechanism of injury
  4. Proper sitting posture to avoid loss of lumbar lordosis
  5. Instruct on pain-relieving positions
  6. Educate patient on the principles of centralization
- Decrease pain/centralize/abolish symptoms
- Patient to demonstrate proper abdominal setting with activation of transversus abdominis during spinal stabilization exercise
- Independent with home exercise program

PRECAUTIONS
- Avoid prolonged sitting/driving (>20 min) or flexed postures
- Avoid lifting and carrying

- Avoid flying
- Avoid activities that involve repetitive loading of the spine (i.e., jogging)

TREATMENT STRATEGIES
- Relative rest
- Soft tissue mobilization/joint mobilization
- Modalities for pain control (US, TENS, Ice)
- Repeated movement of the lumbar spine (direction determined by evaluation) to decrease, abolish, or centralize symptoms
- Lumbar stabilization initiated in unloaded position progressing to loaded positions as tolerated
- Neural mobilization

CRITERIA FOR SURGERY
- Failed conservative management
- Intractable pain
- Neurologic signs that have worsened or do not respond to conservative therapy
- Cauda equina syndrome

Postoperative Phase I: Protected Mobilization (Weeks 4 to 6)

GOALS
- Education
  1. Anatomy/biomechanics of lumbar disc
  2. Patients are educated on proper body mechanics during transfers.
  3. Mechanism of injury
  4. Proper sitting posture to avoid loss of lumbar lordosis
  5. Instruct on pain-relieving positions
  6. Educate patient on the surgical procedure
- Decrease pain/centralize symptoms
- Patient to demonstrate proper abdominal setting with activation of transversus abdominis
- Improve neural mobility
- Independent with home exercise program

Continued

Postoperative Phase I: Protected Mobilization (Weeks 4 to 6)—Cont'd

PRECAUTIONS
- Avoid prolonged sitting/driving (>20 min) or flexed postures
- Avoid lifting and carrying >10 pounds
- Avoid flying
- Avoid activities that involve repetitive loading (i.e., jogging) and/or repetitive flexion of the lumbar spine in a loaded position
- Avoid all sporting activities at this time

TREATMENT STRATEGIES
- Relative rest—walking, unloaded cycling
- Soft tissue mobilization/joint mobilization
- Education on sitting posture, avoiding prolonged lumbar flexion
- Modalities for pain control (US, TENS, Ice)
- Basic lumbar stabilization initiated in unloaded position (supine/prone)
- Neural mobilization (sciatic and/or femoral nerve)

CRITERIA FOR ADVANCEMENT
- Patient demonstrates understanding of proper sitting posture, body mechanics during transfers, and pain-relieving positions
- Patient to demonstrate understanding of LDH mechanism of injury
- Patient demonstrates basic principles of abdominal stabilization in an unloaded position

Postoperative Phase II: Neutral Stabilization (Weeks 6 to 10)

GOALS
- Patient to demonstrate improved tolerance to loaded positions (sitting, standing, and walking)
- Increase the time between peripheralization of symptoms and/or decrease frequency and intensity of pain
- Improve myotomal weakness, if present

- Patient to demonstrate proper squatting mechanics
- Patient to demonstrate good segmental lumbar control and proprioceptive awareness during unloaded lumbar stabilization exercises
- Improve muscle imbalances that contribute to patient symptoms
- Restore lumbar ROM

PRECAUTIONS
- Avoid prolonged sitting/driving or flexed postures
- Avoid activities that involve repetitive loading of the spine (i.e., jogging)

TREATMENT STRATEGIES
- Continue with repetitive movement that centralizes symptoms
- Instruct subject in proper squatting mechanics (beginning in quadruped and progressing to standing)
- Verbal/manual cueing during unsupported spinal stabilization exercise (i.e., quadruped)
- Address muscle imbalances that contribute to patient symptoms (movement imbalance principles developed by Sahrmann)
- Manual techniques to improve restricted segmental ROM of the lumbar spine
- Initiate AROM lumbar spine in unloaded position (always ending with lumbar extension)
- Continue to progress supine, prone, and quadruped neutral stabilization exercise
- Standing isotonic UE and LE strengthening in cardinal planes while maintaining neutral lumbar spine
- Modalities for pain control (US, TENS, Ice)
- Aerobic conditioning

CRITERIA FOR ADVANCEMENT
- Full AROM of lumbar spine
- Patient to demonstrate proper squatting mechanics
- Lower extremity strength >4/5 throughout
- Patient to demonstrate ability to maintain neutral spine during quadruped and standing stabilization exercise

Postoperative Phase III: Dynamic Stabilization (Weeks 10 to 14)

GOALS
- Patient to tolerate standing repeated motion of the lumbar spine in all planes, pain-free
- Patient to perform dynamic stabilization activities without pain
- Patient to demonstrate 5/5 lower extremity strength
- Patient to demonstrate proper body mechanics with bending/lifting and activities that involve diagonal planes of motion
- Improve muscle imbalances that contribute to patient symptoms

PRECAUTIONS
- Avoid exacerbation of symptoms

TREATMENT STRATEGIES
- Continue with repetitive movement that centralizes symptoms
- Perform dynamic stabilization exercises
- Address muscle imbalances that contribute to patient symptoms (movement imbalance principles developed by Sahrmann)
- Manual techniques to improve restricted segmental ROM of the lumbar spine
- Initiate AROM lumbar spine in loaded position (always ending with repeated motion that has been determined to centralize symptoms)
- Continue to progress supine, prone, and quadruped neutral stabilization exercise
- Standing isotonic UE and LE strengthening in cardinal planes while maintaining neutral lumbar spine, beginning on stable surfaces, progressing to unstable surfaces
- Progress aerobic conditioning

CRITERIA FOR ADVANCEMENT
- Full pain-free AROM of lumbar spine in standing
- Patient to demonstrate dynamic stabilization activities, pain-free with good body mechanics
- Lower extremity strength 5/5 throughout
- Patient to have no lower extremity neural tension signs
- Patient to demonstrate normal flexibility in bilateral LE

Postoperative Phase IV: Sport-Specific Activities (Weeks 14 to 18)

GOALS
• Patient to return pain-free to prior sport participation
• Patient to demonstrate good mechanics during functional/sporting activities so as to minimize lumbar motion
• Patient to demonstrate understanding of appropriate progression to return to sport

PRECAUTIONS
• Avoid participation in sport if symptoms exacerbated by sporting activities

TREATMENT STRATEGIES
• Perform sport-specific activities
• Continue to progress dynamic stabilization activities
• Progress cardiovascular training
• Progress upper and lower extremity strengthening

CRITERIA FOR RETURNING TO SPORT
• Patient to perform sport-specific activities pain-free
• Patient to demonstrate good mechanics during sport-specific activities

Bibliography

Ahlgren, B.D., Lui, W., Herkowitz, H.N., Panjabi, M.M., Guiboux, J.P. Effect of Annular Repair on the Healing Strength of the Intervertebral Disc: A Sheep Model. *Spine* 2000;25(17):2165-2170.

Daneyemez, M., Sali, A., Kahraman, S., Beduk, A., Seber, N. Outcome Analyses in 1072 Surgically Treated Lumbar Disc Herniations. *Minim Invas Neurosurg* 1999;42:63-68.

Deyo, R.A., Tsui-Wu, Y.J. Descriptive Epidemiology of Low-back Pain and Its Related Medical Care in the United States. *Spine* 1987;12 (3):264-268.

Ito, T., Takano, Y., Yuasa, N. Types of Lumbar Herniated Disc and Clinical Course. *Spine* 2001;26:548-551.

Javedan, S., Sonntag, V. Lumbar Disc Herniation: Microsurgical Approach. *Neurosurgery* 2003;52(1):160-164.

Keskimaki, L., Seitsalo, S., Osterman, H., Rissanen, P. Reoperations after Lumbar Disc Surgery. *Spine* 2000;25:1500-1508.

Komori, H., Shinomiya, K., Nakai, O., Yamaura, I., Takeda, S., Furuya. The Natural History of Herniated Nucleus Pulposus with Radiculopathy. *Spine* 1996;21(2):225-229.

Lewis, P.J., Weir, B.K., Broad, R.W., Grace, M.G. Long Term Prospective Study of Lumbosacral Discectomy. *J Neurosurg* 1987;67:49-53.

Mooney, V. Where Is the Pain Coming From? *Spine* 1987;12:754-759.

Morgan-Hough, C.V., Jones, P.W., Eisenstein, S.M. Primary and Revision Lumbar Discectomy: A 16-year Review from One Centre. *J Bone Joint Surg Br* 2003;85B(6):871-874.

Nachemson, A. Disc Pressure Measurements. *Spine* 1981;6:93-96.

Nachemson, A. The Load on Lumbar Disks in Different Positions of the Body. *Clin Orthop* 1966;45:107-122.

Ostelo, R.W., de Vet, H.C., Waddell, G., Kerckhoffs, M.R., Leffers, P., van Tulder, M. Rehabilitation Following First-time Lumbar Disc Surgery: A Systematic Review Within the Framework of the Cochrane Collaboration. *Spine* 2003;28(3):209-218.

Weir, B.K., Jacobs, G.A. Reoperation Rate Following Lumbar Discectomy: An Analysis of 662 Lumbar Discectomies. *Spine* 1980;5:366-370.

CHAPTER 29

Osteoporosis (Including Kyphoplasty)

Holly Rudnick, PT, Cert MDT

Kataliya Palmieri, PT, MPT

Osteoporosis is a relatively new diagnosis, although the disease process is not. Before 1994, a clinical syndrome of low trauma fracture amongst the elderly was noted but no cause identified. In 1994 the World Health Organization (WHO) defined the threshold for the diagnosis of osteoporosis as being a bone mineral density (BMD) of more than 2.5 standard deviations below average of a normal 25- to 30-year-old Caucasian woman. "Sometimes referred to as the *silent thief*, osteoporosis is a disease that robs the skeleton of its resources and causes microarchitectural deterioration of bone as people, especially post-menopausal women, age." This compromised bone strength often predisposes the osteoporotic person to an increased risk of fracture.

There are approximately 1.5 million osteoporosis-related fractures annually. Today, in the United States, more than 44 million men and women age 50 and older have low bone mass or osteoporosis, accounting for over $47 million a day spent on the medical care of osteoporosis-related fractures. The primary goal for the osteoporotic patient is to prevent fracture. At the Hospital for Special Surgery (HSS), the approach to the treatment of osteoporosis is multidisciplinary and multifactorial.

Anatomy Overview

- Two types of bone are found in the body: cortical and trabecular.
  1. Cortical bone comprises 80% of the skeletal mass and is primarily responsible for skeletal strength. The cortical bone has a slow turnover rate and high resistance to bending and torsion.

2. The trabecular bone comprises only 20% of the skeletal mass but accounts for 80% of the skeletal surface area. It has a high turnover rate and is the interior scaffolding, able to maintain skeletal shape despite compressive forces.

- There are three primary types of bone cells.
    1. Osteoblasts synthesize new bone.
    2. Osteoclasts are active in resorption of bone.
    3. Osteocytes direct bone to form where it is most needed.
- Bone remodeling is a continuous process of bone resorption and bone formation. Osteoporosis can result from an imbalance in the normal remodeling process.
- Skeletal factors, such as low bone density and impaired bone quality, as well as non-skeletal factors, including poor balance and falls, play an important role in the development of osteoporosis and osteoporotic fractures.
- Bone density is by far the best measure of fracture risk. It accounts for almost 70% of bone strength.
    1. Peak bone density is nearly attained by age 18 and fully attained by age 40.
    2. Bone loss occurs at a rate of 0.5% per year and can increase up to 3% during the perimenopausal period to 7 years postmenopause and then slows down to a steady rate of 0.5% to 1% per year.
- Bone strength is affected by changes in bone quality (impaired mineralization, increased bone turnover, and diminished trabecular microarchitecture). Because trabecular bone has high metabolic activity, it is more affected by bone turnover, resulting in greater resorption, weakening the microstructure of the bone and increasing susceptibility to fracture.

Differential Diagnosis

- Osteoporosis is broken down into two classifications: primary and secondary.
- Primary osteoporosis is age-related.
    1. It is largely caused by estrogen deficiency, which results in high turnover bone loss. subsequently, areas that are high in trabecular bone are more affected.
    2. Vertebral, distal radius, and intertrochanteric fractures tend to be more common in this population.

- Secondary osteoporosis is bone loss related to chronic disease, medication therapy, or lifestyle.
  1. A wide variety of medical conditions have been linked to the development of osteoporosis, including rheumatoid arthritis, multiple myeloma, hyperparathyroidism, hyperthyroidism, inflammatory bowel disease, chronic kidney disease, and transplantation.
  2. Oral glucocorticoids are by far the most common pharmaceutical associated with drug-induced osteoporosis; however, inhaled glucocorticoids, anticonvulsant medications, neuroleptic agents, methotrexate, and lithium have all been known to have detrimental effects on bone.
  3. Secondary osteoporosis affects both cortical and trabecular bone. Therefore, femoral neck, proximal humerus, tibial, and pelvic fractures can occur in addition to vertebral, distal radius, and intertrochanteric fractures.
- The diagnosis of osteoporosis is made via both laboratory tests and physical exam.
  1. Bone pain, kyphosis, loss of height, and x-ray findings are all factors that may lead to further testing to rule in or out the diagnosis of osteoporosis.
  2. The single most widely used test for diagnosing osteoporosis is bone densitometry.
- Several technologies are available for measuring BMD; however, central dual-energy x-ray absorptiometry (DXA) is the gold standard.
- Generally, the hip is the preferred site of BMD measurement and has been shown to be the best predictor of fracture risk.
- Three key pieces of information are obtained from the bone densitometry report: actual BMD, T score, and Z score.
  1. The BMD is used to determine the effectiveness of drug therapy.
  2. The T score is a comparison of the patient's measured BMD with the mean BMD of a healthy, young (25- to 30-year-old) sex matched reference population. The purpose of using a young, matched population is to compare the BMD with that of a population at peak bone mass. This number is reported as the number of standard deviations from the mean.

- The WHO uses T scores to derive the thresholds for the diagnosis of osteopenia and osteoporosis.
- The T score is also used by the National Osteoporosis Foundation (NOF) to determine treatment thresholds.
  1. The Z score is the comparison of the patient's BMD to that of a healthy age- and sex-matched population that can be helpful in identifying secondary causes of osteoporosis.

Rehabilitation Overview

- The evaluation of the osteoporotic patient should be comprehensive and include a detailed history, including prior history of fractures and falls, BMD scores, as well as any of the other risk factors that may contribute to the diagnosis of osteoporosis (Box 29-1). It is also important to obtain a detailed exercise history, paying special attention to the amount of weight-bearing activity that the patient participates in on a daily basis.
- The objective examination should include *five major areas of assessment:* patient posture and body mechanics, flexibility, strength, balance, and weight-bearing (Box 29-2). Addressing these five key areas during the evaluation and

---

BOX 29-1

Risk Factors Associated with Osteoporosis

Gender: women > men
Age: > with age
Body size: small frame, <127lbs
Ethnicity: Caucasian, Asian
Family history
Personal history: fractures or falls
Dementia
Poor health/frailty
Cigarette smoking
Excessive alcohol: >2 drinks/day
Estrogen/testosterone deficiency
Low calcium intake
Sedentary lifestyle or prolonged bedrest
Use of high-risk medications

BOX 29-2

Key Areas of Assessment for Osteoporosis

POSTURE/BODY MECHANICS
FlexiCurve measurement of kyphosis

FLEXIBILITY
Hamstring (°SLR)
Quadriceps (°PKF)
Psoas (Thomas Test)
Gastrocnemius (°DFKE)
Pectoralis minor (cm from the table)
Spinal ROM

STRENGTH
UE/LE strength via MMT
Lower abdominals (Sahrmann levels 1-5)
Trunk extension (time held in secs)

BALANCE
Unilateral stance time (eyes open/eyes closed in secs)
Functional reach (average of 3 trials in inches)
Timed get-up and go (average of 3 trials in secs)

then subsequent rehabilitation is the basis of the *five-point program* for osteoporosis at HSS.

1. The severity of thoracic kyphosis has been associated with the occurrence of vertebral fractures, most likely as a result of the loss of vertebral height. A measurement of the thoracic kyphosis can be taken with a FlexiCurve ruler and documented.

2. The measurement of strength and flexibility is fairly straightforward in this population; however, special attention should be paid to back extensor strength, in particular. Back extensor strength has been shown to be inversely proportional to both kyphosis and vertebral fracture.

3. Strength measurements of hip extensors, scapular, and lower abdominal stabilizers are also important.

4. Flexibility of the anterior chest musculature, hip flexors, and ankle plantar flexors is required to allow for

correct posture and body mechanics and should be evaluated.

5. The assessment of balance is crucial because falls prevention in this population is a primary goal. Unilateral stance time with eyes opened and closed, functional reach, and "timed get-up and go test" are the tools used at HSS to measure balance, because the results can easily be correlated to falls risk.

6. Balance and falls risk can also be used to determine which patients are appropriate for group exercise and which may require individual instruction and balance training.

Posture and Body Mechanics

GOALS
- Maintain neutral spinal posture
- Prevent vertebral fracture
- Education
- Maintain proper alignment with lifting

PRECAUTIONS
- Current fracture

TREATMENT STRATEGIES (AREAS TO FOCUS)
- Standing posture
- Sitting posture
- Hip hinge
- Sleeping position
- Lifting boxes or crates
- Golfers lift (for patients with uncompromised balance only)
- Getting out of bed (log roll)

Flexibility

GOALS
- Maintain ROM
- Prevent postural deformity
- Spinal extension
- Maintain extensibility of soft tissue

PRECAUTIONS
- Spinal stenosis
- Spondylolysis
- Spondylolisthesis
- Shoulder pathology
- Hip pathology

TREATMENT STRATEGIES
- Pectoralis stretch in supine or sitting
- Doorway stretch
- Corner stretch
- Prone press-up
- Quadruped rock back and forth
- AROM cervical spine
- SCM, upper trap stretching
- Dorsiflexion stretch
- STM to lumbar spine

Strengthening

GOALS
- Maintain strength
- Improve postural muscles
- Abdominal stabilization
- Improve balance

PRECAUTIONS
- Current fracture

TREATMENT STRATEGIES
Level I: Normal BMD
- Mat exercises, including prone extension, lower abdominals
- Closed chain exercises, including squats and/or lunges with free weights
- Progressive resistive exercises (PREs): dumbbells as appropriate
- Exercise machine: hoist (row, triceps, biceps, lats), total gym, multihip, treadmill, upper body ergometer (UBE), bike

Continued

Strengthening—Cont'd

Level II: Osteopenia
- Level I exercises
- Postural exercises
  1. Scapular retraction with Thera-Band
  2. Prone scapular retraction
  3. Lower traps prone
  4. Latissimus dorsi
  5. Cervical retraction
  6. Standing lower trap

Level III: Osteoporosis
- Postural exercises
  1. Scapular retraction
  2. UE PNF sitting
  3. Wall slide (arc 0 to 70 degrees)
  4. Sitting/standing abdominal sets with UE lift
- Mat exercises
  1. Lower abdominal stabilization
  2. Prone on elbows
  3. Leg raises with resistance
  4. Quadruped upper extremity lifts
- Low resistance aerobic
  1. Bike (with resistance)
  2. Treadmill

IV: Osteoporosis with fracture
- Gentle introduction to exercise
  1. Abdominal setting/gluteal setting
  2. Scapular retraction
  3. UE PNF in sitting
  4. Bent knee fallout
  5. Heel slides

Weight-Bearing

GOALS
- Increase BMD
- Promote bone growth
- Strengthening

PRECAUTIONS
- Problematic or painful walking
- Weight-bearing status

TREATMENT STRATEGIES
- Walking program/treadmill
- Squats
- Sitting weight shifts
- Step-ups
- Sitting pushups to wall to floor
- Contralateral hip extension/abduction support to unsupported with Thera-Band

Balance

GOALS
- Decrease risk for falls
- Decease risk for fracture

PRECAUTIONS
- Environmental hazards
  1. Shoes
  2. Carpets
  3. Nightlights
  4. Inclement weather
- Physical disabilities/decreased functional mobility
- Visual deficits
- Sensory deficits
- Vestibular deficits
- Mental impairments/judgments

TREATMENT STRATEGIES
- Single-leg balance
- Heel walking
- Braiding
- Tandem walking
- Reaching
- Timed get-up and go
- Quick feet

Continued

Balance—Cont'd

- Balance board
- Obstacle course (closed and open spaces)
- Education on falls

Rehabilitation Following Vertebral Kyphoplasty

- The treatment of vertebral compression fractures (VCFs) has traditionally been limited to bed rest, bracing, analgesic medications, narcotic medications, and activity modification. These methods have had varying degrees of success and often require prolonged immobilization.
- In 1984 an innovative new technique for the treatment of VCFs was developed in France, called *percutaneous vertebroplasty.*
  1. The procedure involves transpedicular, percutaneous bone cement injections into the collapsed vertebral bodies.
  2. This offers the patient reduced pain, prevention of further collapse, return to function, and eliminates the complications of bed rest.
- Kyphoplasty was developed several years later as a progression of the vertebroplasty procedure.
  1. Kyphoplasty combines vertebroplasty and balloon catheter technology developed for angioplasty.
  2. It involves the placement of a cannula and inflatable bone tamp under fluoroscope into the collapsed vertebral body.
  3. The balloon is then inflated and the cavity filled with bone cement.
  4. Kyphoplasty, unlike vertebroplasty, restores vertebral body height and addresses spinal deformity, as well as reduces pain and restores the patient to a normal functional level.
  5. Kyphoplasty is a relatively safe procedure; however, complications can occur.
  6. The most severe complications of kyphoplasty involve cement embolization and cement extravasation. This

can happen as a result of the cement leaking into either the venous system or spinal canal.

- Not all VCFs are appropriate for a kyphoplasty procedure.
  1. Fractures that are nonpainful and have minimal deformity rarely require treatment beyond activity modification.
  2. If the VCF is painful, has associated deformity, or has failed traditional nonoperative treatment, kyphoplasty may be indicated.
  3. The level and number of VCFs also play a role in determining the appropriateness of kyphoplasty.
- Rehabilitation considerations following a kyphoplasty procedure are not unique.
  1. The same precautions are taken, as with any patient who has severe osteoporosis, with or without untreated VCF.
  2. Typically, rehabilitation is not initiated for a range of a few days to a week following the procedure.
  3. The post-kyphoplasty patient may have some post-procedure pain, which can be addressed with modalities; however, in general, most patients should have considerably less pain than pre-procedure.
  4. Exercise should be based upon level IV of the five-point program and tailored to the patient's functional and balance impairments, as outlined in previous sections.

Bibliography

Bohannon, R.W., Larken, P.A., Cook, A.C., Gear, J., Singer, J. Decrease in Timed Balance Test Scores with Aging. *Phys Ther* 1984;64:1067-1070.

Cummings, S.R., Black, D.M., Nevitt, M.C., Browner, W., Cauley, J., Ensrud, K., Genant, H.K., Palermo, L., Scott, J., Vogt, T.M. Bone Density at Various Sites for Prediction of Hip Fractures. *Lancet* 2000;341:72-75.

Delmas, P.D., Eastell, R., Garnero, P., Seibel, M.J., Stepan, J. (Committee of Scientific Advisors of the International Osteoporosis Foundation). The Use of Biochemical Markers of Bone Turnover in Osteoporosis. *Osteoporos Int* 2000;11(Suppl 6):S2-S17.

Duncan, P.W., Weiner, D.K., Chandler, J., Studenski, S. Functional Reach: A Clinical Measuring of Balance. *J Gerontol Soc* 1990;45:194-197.

Fitzpatrick, L.A. Secondary Causes of Osteoporosis. *Mayo Clin Proc* 2002;77:453-468.

Follin, S.L., Hansen, L.B. Current Approaches to the Prevention and Treatment of Post Menopausal Osteoporosis. *Am J Health Sys Pharm* 2003;60(9):883-901.

Kanis, J.A., Gluer, C.C. International Osteoporosis Foundation: An Update on the Diagnosis and Assessment of Osteoporosis with Densitometry. *Osteoporos Int* 2000;11:192-202.

Lieberman, I., Reinhardt, M. Vertebroplasty and Kyphoplasty for Osteolytic Vertebral Collapse. *Clin Orthop* 2003;1(415S):S176-S186.

Lipworth, B.J. Systemic Adverse Effects of Inhaled Corticosteroid Therapy: A Systemic Review and Meta-analysis. *Arch Intern Med* 1999;159:941-955.

Marshall, D., Johnell, O., Wedel, H. Meta Analysis of How Well Measures of Bone Mineral Density Predict Occurrences of Osteoporotic Fractures. *Br Med J* 1996;312:1254-1259.

North American Menopause Society. Management of Postmenopausal Osteoporosis: Position Statement of the North American Menopause Society. *Menopause* 2002;9:84-101.

Posadillo, D., Richardson, S. The Tmied Up and Go: A Test of Basic Functional Mobility for Frail Elderly Persons. *J Am Geriatr Soc* 1991;39:142-148.

Pouilles, J.M., Tremollieres, F., Ribot, C. Effect of Menopause on Femoral and Vertebral Bone Loss. *J Bone Miner Res* 1995;10:1534-1536.

Sinaki, M., Itoi, E., Rogers, J.W., Bergstralh, E.J., Wahner, H.W. Correlation of Back Extensor Strength with Thoracic Kyphosis and Lumbar Lordosis in Estrogen Deficient Women. *Am J Phys Med Rehabil* 1996;75:370-374.

Sinaki, M., Wollan, P.C., Scott, R.W., Gelczer, R.K. Can Strong Back Extensors Prevent Vertebral Fractures in Women with Osteoporosis? *Mayo Clin Proc* 1996;71(10):951-956.

Star, V., Hochberg, M. Osteoporosis: Treat Current Injury, Retard Future Loss. *Intern Med* 1993;113(14):32-42.

Tannirandorn, P., Epstein, S. Drug-Induced Bone Loss. *Osteoporosis Int* 2000;11:637-659.

Vellas, B.J., Wayne, S.J., Romero, L., Baumgartner, R.N., Rubenstein, L.Z., Garry, P.J. One-leg Balance is an Important Predictor of Injurious Falls in Older Persons. *J Am Geriatr Soc* 1997;45:735-738.

Woolf, A.D., Dixon, A.S. Osteoporosis: A Clinical Guide, 2nd ed. Livery House, London,1998.

CHAPTER *30*

Adult Lumbar Spinal Fusion

Charlene Hannon, PT, MBA

More than 200,000 spinal fusions are performed each year in the United States. Controversy exists as to whether spinal fusion is the treatment of choice for patients with various types of low back pain. Some of the reasons for this controversy are that there is a 10% to 40% pseudarthrosis (failure of fusion) rate; improved function, particularly return to work, does not always occur; and many patients experience continued postoperative pain. Furthermore, in some cases, additional surgery is necessary and adds to health care costs. In the United States alone, total health care expenditures incurred by individuals with back pain reached an estimated 90.7 billion dollars, and, on average, individuals with back pain incurred 60% higher expenditures than individuals without back pain. Careful patient selection and choice of the appropriate surgical procedure seem to generate the best surgical outcomes.

Fusions can be classified into two categories: instrumented and noninstrumented. *Noninstrumented fusions* do not use any hardware. They are much less commonly performed and are usually done for single-level fusions only. The two most common *instrumented lumbar spinal fusion* procedures are posterior lumbar interbody fusion (PLIF) and circumferential fusion. Both procedures have a very good rate of fusion. Bono and Lee showed that PLIF has a fusion rate of 85%, and circumferential yielded 91% fusion. For the purpose of this guideline, only the PLIF will be described. It is important, however, that the physical therapist be aware that there are many spinal fusion techniques. The principles of rehabilitation following lumbar spinal fusion remain the same, regardless of the procedure.

One of the most important concepts for the physical therapist to understand is the concept that the hardware is merely a temporary scaffold until biological healing is complete. Biological healing can be affected by many factors including smoking, poor surgical technique, and mechanical stress across the fusion mass (movement during the phases of healing). It is the mechanical stress with which the physical therapist is to be most concerned when developing a rehabilitation program. Careful consideration must be made of the forces generated by lever arms, such as the upper and lower extremities and their effects on the lumbar spine. Although there is a paucity of research examining the in vivo forces generated across a healing fusion site, Rohlmann et al. did show that lifting both legs in the supine position generated the highest loads on the fixation devices as compared to most other lumbar stabilization exercises.

Osteoporosis is a relative precaution and does not preclude complete healing from occurring. Additional precautions, such as bracing, may be required in patients with osteoporosis.

In summary, the following are generally accepted indications for spinal fusion:

- When decompression (laminectomy) is warranted because of spinal stenosis, spondylosis or degenerative disc disease, and more than half of the lamina is removed, creating an unstable segment.
- Without decompression to stabilize a motion segment that is unstable (defined as >4mm excursion on bending X rays).
- To stabilize a motion segment with spondylolisthesis and thus prevent further slippage or possibly correct for slippage.
- After the surgical removal of various types of bony sarcomas (this will not be addressed in this guideline).
- Intractable pain.
- Neurological signs.
- Failed conservative management.

Surgical Overview

- PLIF describes a technique that is indicated to treat various spinal pathologies, as listed previously.

- The primary goal of the technique is to provide a solid interbody fusion with decompression of the surrounding neural structures and restoration of vertebral alignment.
- In addition, the procedure should provide global spinal balance that protects adjacent normal segments. Global spinal balance is the concept that when alignment is corrected at a given intervertebral segment, total spinal alignment is preserved. In other words, a new misalignment is not created.
- The PLIF is a four-stage procedure, as follows:

  Stage 1: Exposure and decompression

  Stage 2: Spinal instrumentation and preliminary fixation

  Stage 3: Anterior column reconstruction and interbody fusion

  Stage 4: Internal stabilization and completion of surgery
- Stage 1: The area is decompressed, taking care to preserve normal tissues and structures at adjacent levels, particularly the posterior spinous processes and the interspinous ligaments, as well as the facet joints to prevent late adjacent segment instability. Also, care is taken so as not to denervate the paraspinal muscles.
- Stage 2: The instrument system is also referred to as "hardware" and is essentially internal spinal fixation. The components may consist of rods, plates, hooks, wires, and/or screws and are available in both stainless steel and titanium (the main advantage of titanium is its magnetic resonance imaging compatibility). Instrumentation is placed in the pedicles to prepare for stage 3.
- Stage 3: Numerous distraction techniques may be used to restore normal disc height. Care is taken so as not to place the neural structures under excessive tension. Once the ideal height is attained, the screws on the plates are tightened to maintain the gains. Next, the disc space is prepared. A complete discectomy is performed, and the end plate is scraped to create bleeding. If bleeding becomes excessive, it must be controlled. The ultimate goal is to ensure a good bone graft to vertebral bone contact, a large surface area of bleeding bone, and no interposition of soft tissue. The bone graft is then placed. Graft material may be the bone chipped away

from the decompression procedure, iliac crest bone graft, or allograft material.

- Stage 4: The working hardware is replaced with the final implants, and the incision is closed. The procedure described can be repeated for multiple segments, as necessary.

Rehabilitation Overview

- The rehabilitation program begins postoperatively at the bedside and is progressed to achieve short-term goals for discharge to the home.
- Patients continue a basic home exercise program for the first 4 to 6 weeks and then begin outpatient therapy.
  1. Careful consideration is given to provide a protective environment for the healing fusion.
  2. Outpatient therapy is typically provided from 6 weeks to as long as 6 months, depending on the individual and the surgeon.
  3. Generally, for a one-level procedure, fusion should occur within 4 months of the surgery. For more complex, multilevel spinal fusions biological healing of the fusion reaches a peak at 1 year but continues to mature from 1 to 2 years.
- Goals are set individually and are functionally based, targeting return to full activities of daily living (ADL) and return to full-time employment.

Preoperative Phase

GOALS
- Patient education: pain management, logrolling, concept of bending from the hips, and importance of avoiding lumbar movement
- Maximize strength/functional capabilities: Upper body strength becomes important for bed mobility, hamstring flexibility in the absence of neural tension signs
- General conditioning: Improvements in preoperative endurance will benefit patients in the postoperative phase

PRECAUTIONS
- Avoid movements that increase pain (patient may be flexion, neutral, or extension-biased)
- Avoid loaded positions if load-sensitive
- Avoid exercises that aggravate neural tissue in the presence of neural tension signs

TREATMENT STRATEGIES
- Neutral-biased lumbar stabilization
- Functional tests—squatting, lunging, transitions to/from floor
- Gait training (educate in progression from walker to cane)
- Home program:
  1. Preoperative conditioning
  2. Endurance training: stationary bicycle, treadmill, elliptical
  3. Strength training: wall squats, wall push-ups
- Postoperative therapeutic exercise instruction:
  1. Quadriceps sets
  2. Gluteal sets
  3. Abdominal sets
  4. Ankle pumps
- Pain relief modalities: electrical stimulation
- Criteria for surgery:
  1. Failed conservative management
  2. Intractable pain
  3. Neurological signs

Postoperative Phase I (Days 1 to 14)

USE LOGROLLING FOR TRANSFERS
- Progress from walker to cane to no device
- Balance activity with rest

GOALS
- Patient education
- Provide the most protective environment for the healing fusion
- Maximize function
- Control postoperative pain

Continued

Postoperative Phase I (Days 1 to 14)—Cont'd

- Independence in home therapeutic exercise program
- Improve endurance and tolerance to daily activities

PRECAUTIONS
- Avoid all lumbar movements (absolutely no lumbar flexion, extension, sidebending, or rotation)
- Avoid sitting more than 20 to 30 minutes
- May or may not be wearing a brace, depending on the surgeon's advice
- No lifting more than 5 pounds (a gallon of milk is 8 pounds)
- No prone positioning or quadruped

TREATMENT STRATEGIES
- Transfer training
- Gluteal set, quadriceps set, dorsiflexion for neural gliding
- Walking in the home or community
- Pain modalities, activity modification to control pain, communication with MD regarding activity and pain medications
- Home therapeutic exercise program: as previous
- Emphasize patient compliance to home therapeutic exercise program and protective environment, body mechanics, use of assistive devices, such as reacher, elastic shoelaces, long-handled shoe horn

CRITERIA FOR ADVANCEMENT
- Pain well controlled
- Tolerating sitting for 30 minutes
- Progression to cane
- Independent in logroll transfers

Postoperative Phase II (Weeks 2 to 6)

- Use logrolling for transfers
- Continue progression from walker to cane to no device
- Progress outdoor activity

GOALS
- Patient education
- Provide the most protective environment for the healing fusion

- Maximize function: patients are usually independent in all ADL by week 6
- Control postoperative pain
- Independence in home therapeutic exercise program
- Improve endurance and tolerance to daily activities

PRECAUTIONS
- Avoid all lumbar movements (absolutely no lumbar flexion, extension, sidebending, or rotation)
- Progress sitting tolerance to between 30 and 45 minutes
- May or may not be wearing a brace, depending on the surgeon's advice
- No lifting more than 5 pounds (a gallon of milk is 8 pounds)
- No prone positioning or quadruped
- No progressive resistive exercises (PREs), no use of ankle cuff weights or upper extremity weights

TREATMENT STRATEGIES
- Transfer training
- Gentle submaximal abdominal sets, abdominal sets with heel slide, abdominal sets with bent knee fallout, total body extension isometric, dorsiflexion for neural gliding
- Use of stationary bicycle, treadmill
- Pain modalities, activity modification to control pain, communication with physician regarding activity and pain medications
- Home therapeutic exercise program: as previous
- Emphasize patient compliance to home therapeutic exercise program and protective environment, body mechanics, use of assistive devices, such as reacher, elastic shoelaces, long-handled shoe horn

CRITERIA FOR ADVANCEMENT
- Pain well controlled
- Tolerating sitting for 45 minutes
- Progression to ambulation without device
- Increased independence in ADL

Postoperative Phase III (Weeks 6 to 14)

- Use logrolling for transfers
- Continue progression from cane to no device
- Progress outdoor activity
- Patients getting stronger overall, progressing lumbar stabilization, improving endurance, striving toward return to work if they haven't already

GOALS

- Patient education
- Provide the most protective environment
- Maximize function: patients may return to work during this phase, depending on their occupation. Counseling and problem solving with the PT for return to work is a key component of this phase. Return part-time is ideal, if possible
- Control postoperative pain, decreasing medications, especially if returning to work
- Independence in home therapeutic exercise program
- Improve endurance and tolerance to daily activities

PRECAUTIONS

- Avoid all lumbar movements (absolutely no lumbar flexion, extension, sidebending, or rotation)
- Progress sitting tolerance to that which is necessary to perform their work
- May or may not be wearing a brace, depending on the surgeon's advice
- No lifting more than 5 pounds (a gallon of milk is 8 pounds)
- No PREs, no use of ankle cuff weights or upper extremity weights

TREATMENT STRATEGIES

- Progressive lumbar stabilization: Gentle submaximal abdominal sets, abdominal sets with heel slide, abdominal sets with bent knee fallout, total body extension isometric
- Prone on pillows protecting the neutral lumbar spine may be initiated
- Quadruped may be initiated

- Upright and loaded resistive exercises in a spine safe neutral position may be initiated if patient demonstrates good trunk control
- Use of stationary bicycle, treadmill
- Pain modalities, activity modification to control pain, communication with MD regarding activity and pain medications
- Hamstring stretching may be initiated in supine with a stretching strap
- Home therapeutic exercise program: as previous
- Emphasize patient compliance to home therapeutic exercise program and protective environment, body mechanics, use of assistive devices, such as reacher, elastic shoelaces, long-handled shoe horn

CRITERIA FOR ADVANCEMENT
- Pain well controlled
- Tolerating sitting for 45 minutes
- Return to work if indicated
- Ability to tolerate exercise in multiple positions: prone, quadruped, supine, upright
- Ability to perform resistive exercises with adequate abdominal control

Postoperative Phase IV (Weeks 14 to 22)
- Use logrolling for transfers
- Continue progression from cane to no device if still using a cane
- Progress outdoor activity
- Patients getting stronger overall, progressing lumbar stabilization; most have resumed normal daily activities and will need reminders about lifting precautions
- Communicate with surgeon regarding progression and weight limits

GOALS
- Patient education
- Provide a spine-safe environment
- Maximize function: patients may return to limited gym if they demonstrate good understanding of spine-safe activity

Continued

Postoperative Phase IV (Weeks 14 to 22)—Cont'd

- Independence in home therapeutic exercise program
- Improve endurance and tolerance to daily activities

PRECAUTIONS

- Avoid all lumbar movements (absolutely no lumbar flexion, extension, sidebending, or rotation)
- Progress sitting tolerance to that which is necessary to perform their work
- Wean from brace with surgeon's permission if patient is still wearing one
- Increased lifting depending on surgeon
- Light upper extremity PREs with short lever arms (biceps curls) to improve daily function, no use of ankle cuff weights

TREATMENT STRATEGIES

- Progressive lumbar stabilization: advance lower abdominal stabilization using lower extremities as longer lever arms (no cuff weights)
- Prone on pillows protecting the neutral lumbar spine
- Quadruped using resistive bands
- Use of stationary bicycle, treadmill
- Pain modalities, activity modification to control pain, communication with MD regarding activity and pain medications
- Hamstring stretching may be initiated in supine with a stretching strap
- Home therapeutic exercise program: as previous
- Set discharge goals

CRITERIA FOR ADVANCEMENT

- Pain well controlled
- Tolerating sitting for 45 minutes
- Ability to perform resisted, loaded upright exercise with good trunk control

Postoperative Phase V: Return to Sport

- Use logrolling for transfers
- Patients getting stronger overall, progressing lumbar stabilization; most have resumed normal daily activities and will need reminders about lifting precautions
- Communicate with surgeon regarding gradual return to sport and progression

GOALS

- Patient education: form may need to be modified (e.g., golf swing)
- Gradual return to sport
- Independence in home therapeutic exercise program
- Minimize excessive forces at the segment adjacent to the fusion

PRECAUTIONS

- Assess active range of motion (AROM) of nonoperated spinal segments and add gentle ROM exercises as necessary
- Surgeon may suggest wearing brace as a reminder for certain sports
- Increased lifting according to surgeon's recommendations
- Light upper extremity PREs with short lever arms (biceps curls) to improve daily function, no use of ankle cuff weights

TREATMENT STRATEGIES

- Use of equipment and resistance to simulate sport
- Upright and loaded resistive exercises in a spine safe neutral position with spinal motion, including rotation, are initiated if patient demonstrates good trunk control
- Refine discharge goals
- Maintenance of home exercise program

Bibliography

Boden, S.D. Overview of the Biology of Lumbar Spine Fusion and Principles for Selecting a Bone Graft Substitute. *Spine* 2002; 27 (Suppl 16S):S26–S31.

Bono, C.M., Lee, C. Critical Analysis of Trends in Fusion for Degenerative Disc Disease Over the Past 20 Years: Influence of

Technique on Fusion Rate and Clinical Outcome. *Spine* 2004;29 (4):455-463.

Glassman, S., Anagonost, S.C., Parker, A., Burke, D., Johnson, J., Dimar, J. The Effect of Cigarette Smoking and Smoking Cessation on Spinal Fusion. *Spine* 15 October 2000;25(20):2608-2615.

Hu, S. Internal Fixatio in the Osteoporotic Spine. *Spine* 1997; 22(24S):43S-48S.

Keppler, I., Steffee, A.D., Biscup, R.S. Posterior Lumbar Interbody Fusion with Variable Screw Placement and Isola Instrumentation. In Bridwell, K., DeWald, R. (Eds). The Textbook of Spinal Surgery, 2nd ed., Lippincott Raven, Philadelphia, 1997.

Luo, X., Pietrobon, R., Sun, S.X., Liu, G.G., Hey, L. Estimates and Patterns of Direct Health Care Expenditures Among Individuals with Back Pain in the United States. *Spine* 2004;29(1):79-86.

Parker, L.M., Murrell, S., Boden, S., Horton, W. The Outcome of Posterolateral Fusion in Highly Selected Patients with Discogenic Low Back Pain. *Spine* 1996;21(16):1909-1916.

Rohlmann, A., Graichen, F., Bergmann, G. Loads on an Internal Spinal Fixation Device During Physical Therapy. *J Am Phys Ther Assoc* 2002;82(1):44-52.

SPORTS MEDICINE REHABILITATION

John I. Cavanaugh, PT, MEd, ATC

CHAPTER *31*

Hip Arthroscopy

Theresa A. Chiaia, PT

Matthew D. Rivera, PT, MPT, CSCS

Hip arthroscopy has gained increased popularity over the past decade; however, it has undergone slow development compared to arthroscopy of the knee and shoulder. Knee and shoulder arthroscopy has evolved from open techniques, whereas the hip has not benefited from such early procedures. The advent of hip arthroscopy has led to improved recognition of intra-articular pathologies, which facilitated improved soft tissue diagnostic imaging techniques. This, in turn, has led to advances in hip arthroscopy techniques as a treatment for intra-articular lesions, including repair or excision of a torn labrum, removal of loose bodies, or repair of chondral lesions.

Injuries to the labrum are the most common source of hip pain identified at arthroscopy. The primary causes of these injuries are the result of femoral acetabular impingement or capsular laxity/hypermobility. Labral injury often results from repetitive motion in sports, such as golf, hockey, and soccer. Although traumatic tears are significantly less common, they are most common in high level athletes who participate in sports, such as football and skiing. The rehabilitation guidelines following hip arthroscopy for a torn labrum are presented here by the Hospital for Special Surgery.

Surgical Overview

- The labrum is a fibrocartilaginous rim that runs circumferentially around the perimeter of the acetabulum to the base of the fovea and becomes attached to the transverse acetabular ligament posteriorly and anteriorly.
- The labrum has many functions. It creates a seal enhancing joint lubrication, reinforces the acetabular rim contributing to joint stability, and plays a role in load distribution.
- The labrum is distinctively thinner in the anterior inferior portion and thicker posteriorly. The majority of labral tears occurs anteriorly.
- The labrum is predominately avascular, except the outermost layer that limits intrinsic healing.
- Free nerve endings and sensory organs have been identified within the labral tissue, which contributes to nociceptive and proprioceptive input.
- The goal of arthroscopic debridement of a torn labrum is to relieve the pain by removing the unstable flap that causes hip discomfort and addressing the underlying pathology.
  1. The surgeon seeks to remove only torn labral tissue, leaving as much healthy intact labrum as possible.
  2. If the underlying pathology is capsular laxity, thermal capsulorrhaphy and plication is indicated, whereas with femoral acetabular impingement, bony resection is recommended.
- The architectural constraints of the hip joint, as well as the proximity of the neurovascular structures, make arthroscopy of the hip more challenging than the shoulder.
  1. Recent adaptations of flexible scopes and instruments designed for the hip have led to improved safety, visualization, and accessibility of this joint.
  2. Distraction of the femoral head from the acetabulum, using 25 to 50 pounds of traction force, is necessary to visualize the articular surfaces.
- Typically, a three-portal approach is used.
  1. The anterolateral portal is directly off the anterosuperior portion of the greater trochanter and penetrates the gluteus medius before entering the lateral capsule.

2. The anterior portal penetrates the sartorius and the rectus femoris and then enters the capsule. It presents the greatest risk to the lateral femoral neurovascular bundle.

3. The posterolateral portal is posterior to the tip of the greater trochanter, placing the sciatic nerve at risk of injury.

- A flexible chisel is used to cut the torn labrum, then a motorized shaver is used to complete the debridement.
- If the labrum is detached from the bone, a bioabsorbable suture anchor is placed on the rim of the acetabulum, and suture material is passed twice through the labrum.
- With femoral acetabular impingement, sequential removal of the osteophyte is performed, using the anterior scoping portal and distal lateral accessory portal.
- For capsular laxity, arthroscopic capsular plication of the iliofemoral ligament is performed following thermal modification of the capsule.

Rehabilitation Overview

- The rehabilitation program following hip arthroscopy for a torn labrum is initiated between 0 and 2 weeks postoperatively. The surgeon's preference, the surgical procedure, and the intraoperative findings will guide the postoperative course.
- The rate of progression through rehabilitation will depend on the underlying condition of the joint and the chronicity of the impairments.
- A period of restrictive weight-bearing with an assistive device followed by progressive weight-bearing as tolerated is recommended to allow for adequate healing, decreased inflammation, and pain control.
- Control of pain and inflammation through activity modification is necessary for progression of function, especially in the early phase of rehabilitation.
- Hip range of motion (ROM) will be progressed within the surgeon's designated parameters to allow for adequate healing and should be monitored to reduce joint compression forces and symptom provocation.

- The patient will follow a functionally-based progression with criteria for discharge, largely depending on the goals of the patient.
- The phases of rehabilitation represent a continuum rather than discrete, well-defined phases.

Postoperative Phase I (Day 1 to Week 4)

GOALS
- Communication with surgeon to gain understanding of intraoperative findings of the joint and provide insight into underlying causative factors
- Provide patient with understanding of etiology
- Patient education
- Compliance with self-care, home management, activity modification
- Normalize gait with appropriate assistive device
- 0/10 pain at rest
- 0/10 pain with ambulation

PRECAUTIONS
- Capsular irritation
- Ambulation to fatigue
- Pivoting during ambulation
- Symptom provocation during ambulation, activities of daily living (ADL), therapeutic exercise
- External rotation, bridging, gluteal sets following capsular procedure
- Active hip flexion with long lever arm, such as straight leg raising
- Weight-bearing as per surgeon's guidelines
- ROM as per surgeon's guidelines: capsular procedure

TREATMENT STRATEGIES
- Home exercise program, as instructed: abdominal setting, plantar flexion with elastic bands, gluteal setting, quadriceps setting, knee extension
- Patient education
  1. Activity modification
  2. Bed mobility
  3. Positioning

- Gait training with appropriate assistive device on level surfaces and stairs
  1. Following capsular procedure, instruct in a step to gait pattern
- Training in transitional movements with support from nonoperative leg
- Hydrotherapy when adequate wound healing for
  1. Gait
  2. Pain-free active-assisted ROM (AAROM)
  3. Single-leg standing
- Open chain strengthening for knee extension, flexion; gastrocnemius strengthening
- Initiate core control: heel slides, upper extremity forward flexion, hip extension to neutral
- Balance training: double-limb support

CRITERIA FOR ADVANCEMENT
- Control of pain
- Normalized gait with appropriate assistive device

Postoperative Phase II (Weeks 5 to 10)

GOALS
- Normalize gait without an assistive device
- 0/10 pain during ADL
- Ascend/descend 8-inch step with good control
- Core control during low demand exercises
- Adequate pelvic stability to meet demands of ADL
- ROM within functional limits
- Patient education and independence with home therapeutic exercise program, as instructed

PRECAUTIONS
- Premature discharge of assistive device. Continue to use assistive device until non-antalgic gait
- Symptom provocation
- Pain during ADL
- Pain during therapeutic exercise: abduction and flexion to tolerance
- Faulty movement patterns, posture

Continued

Postoperative Phase II (Weeks 5 to 10)— Cont'd

- Active hip flexion until pain subsides
- Capsular and soft tissue irritation

TREATMENT STRATEGIES

- Home exercise program, as instructed: evaluation-based
- Underwater treadmill
- Hydrotherapy: buoyancy assisting to buoyancy resisting exercises
- Hip strengthening progression
  1. Multihip machine: hip extension with knee extension, knee flexion to neutral
- Functional strengthening: leg press, squats, step-ups/step-downs
- Hip ROM with a stable pelvis
  1. Quadruped rocking backward
  2. Bent knee fallout
  3. Heel slides
- Core control progression
- Gluteal strengthening: clam shell, hip extension with knee flexion
- Postural reeducation to control at neutral pelvis
- Bicycle ergometry: progress from short crank as needed, to a standard cycle
- Proprioception and balance exercises: progress from double-limb to single-limb support
- Flexibility: evaluation-based

CRITERIA FOR ADVANCEMENT

- ROM within functional limits
- Ascend/descend 8-inch step with good pelvic control
- Good pelvic control during single-limb stance
- Normalized gait without an assistive device

Postoperative Phase III (Weeks 11 to 13)

GOALS

- Independent home exercise program, as instructed
- Optimize ROM
- Core control: levels II-III/V, based on Sahrmann scale

- 5/5 LE strength
- Good, dynamic balance
- Pain-free ADL

PRECAUTIONS
- Symptom provocation
- Ignoring functional progression
- Sacrificing quality for quantity

TREATMENT STRATEGIES
- Home exercise program, as instructed: evaluation-based to incorporate treatment strategies
- Instruction of ROM at end range
- Demonstration of moderate level core exercises
  1. Level II Sahrmann
  2. Quadruped extremity lifts
  3. Diagonal patterns
- Cross-training: elliptical trainer, bicycle, stair stepper, cross-country ski machine
- Initiate gym routine to include hip strengthening machines as tolerated
- Initiate plyometrics

CRITERIA FOR ADVANCEMENT
- Good, dynamic balance
- 5/5 LE strength
- Levels II-III/V core control (Sahrmann progression)
- ROM to meet demands of activities
- Pelvic control with single-limb activities is also necessary

Postoperative Phase IV (Weeks 14 to 16)

GOALS
- Independent home exercise program, as instructed
- Minimize postexercise soreness

PRECAUTIONS
- Symptom provocation
- Ignoring functional progression
- Maintaining adequate strength base

Continued

Postoperative Phase IV (Weeks 14 to 16)—Cont'd

TREATMENT STRATEGIES
- Home exercise program, as instructed: strength training and flexibility exercises
- Advance plyometric training
- Initiate running program: interval training
- Dynamic balance activities
- Cutting/agility skills
- Advance training of core
- Address muscle imbalances
- Endurance

CRITERIA FOR RETURN TO SPORT
- Gluteal strength to maintain pelvic control
- 0/10 pain with advanced activities
- Optimal ROM

Bibliography

Baber, Y.F., Robinson, A.H., Villar, R.N. Is Diagnostic Arthroscopy of the Hip Worthwhile? A Prospective Review of 328 Adults Investigated for Hip Pain. *J Bone Joint Surg* 1999;81:600–603.

Byrd, T., Jones, K. Hip Arthroscopy in Athletes. *Clin Sports Med* 2001;4:749–778.

Byrd, T. Hip Arthroscopy the Supine Position. *Clin Sports Med* 2001;4:703–731.

Kelly, B., Draovitch, P., Enseki, K., Martin, R., Ernhardt, R., Philippon, M. Hip Arthroscopy and the Management of Non-arthritic Hip Pain. University of Pittsburgh Medical Center.

Kelly, B., Shapiro, G., Digiovanni, C.W., Buly, R., Potter, H., Hannafin, J.A. Vascularity of the Hip Labrum: A Cadaveric Investigation. *Arthroscopy*, 2005;21(1):3–11.

Kim, Y., Azusa, H. The Nerve Endings of the Acetabular Labrum. *Clin Orthop* 1995;310:60–68.

Konrath, G.A., Hamel, A.J., Olson, S.A., Bay, B., Sharkey, N.A. The Role of the Acetabular Labrum and the Transverse Acetabular Ligament in Load Transmission in the Hip. *J Bone Joint Surg* 1998;80A(12):1781–1788.

Lavinge, M., Parvizi, J., Beck, M., Siebenrock, K., Ganz, R., Leunig, M. Anterior Femoroacetabular Impingement Part I. Techniques of Joint Preserving Surgery. *Clin Orthop* 2004;418:61–66.

Mason, J.B. Acetabular Labral Tears in the Athlete. *Clin Sports Med* 2001;4:779-790.

McCarthy, J., Barsoum, W., Puri, L., Lee, J., Murphy, S., Cooke, P. The Role of Hip Arthroscopy in the Elite Athlete. *Clin Orthop Relat Res* 2003;406:71-74.

CHAPTER *32*

Microfracture Procedure of the Knee

John T. Cavanaugh, PT, MEd, ATC

Heather A. Williams, PT, DPT

Rehabilitation following articular cartilage repair continues to evolve with advances in the understanding of articular cartilage structure and function. Mechanisms of injury to articular cartilage can include direct trauma, indirect impact loading, or torsional loading at the knee joint. Injury to the articular cartilage in the knee decreases mobility and commonly causes pain with movement, eventually progressing to deformity and constant pain. An awareness of acute lesions of the articular surfaces of the knee joint has increased in recent years because diagnostic application of magnetic resonance imaging and arthroscopy techniques have improved.

An estimated 385,000 procedures for repairing articular cartilage defects were performed in the United States in 1995. Nonsurgical treatment may have satisfactory outcomes for some patients. However, as these defects may eventually progress to degenerative arthritis, a heightened interest among orthopedists to surgically repair these lesions has evolved. One such procedure is a *microfracture chondroplasty* introduced by Steadman et al. The goal of this procedure is to enhance chondral resurfacing by providing an enriched environment for tissue regeneration, using the body's own healing capabilities. Indications for the microfracture procedure generally include a full-thickness articular cartilage lesion on either a weight-bearing surface (femur or tibia) or a contact lesion on either the patella or trochlear surfaces of the patellofemoral joint. Other indications include unstable cartilage overlying subchondral bone and degenerative changes in knees that present with normal axial alignment. Contraindications for this procedure include axial misalignment, patient's potential for noncompliance, partial thickness defects, any systemic immune-mediated disease, disease-induced arthritis, or cartilage disease.

Surgical Overview

- Articular cartilage plays a crucial role in the function of the musculoskeletal system by permitting nearly frictionless motion to occur between the articular surfaces of synovial joints.
  1. Its unique structure allows a joint to withstand high compressive and shear loads throughout a lifetime.
  2. Articular cartilage is avascular in nature and therefore has minimal potential to regenerate after injury.
- Several studies have demonstrated the medial femoral condyle to be the most common location for full-thickness focal chondral defects. These lesions are commonly found in the area that contacts the tibia between 30 and 70 degrees of flexion.
- The microfracture procedure begins with an arthroscopic assessment of the articular cartilage defect.
  1. A debridement of the base of the defect is then performed to fully expose the subchondral bone with a standard arthroscopic shaver or curved curette.
  2. Any unstable cartilage is removed and a stable boundary is defined.
  3. The walls of the perimeter of the defect should be perpendicular to the subchondral plate so that the marrow elements to follow will be optimally contained within the defect.
  4. Arthroscopic angled awls are then used to make multiple perforations, or microfractures, in the exposed subchondral plate. These awls produce essentially no thermal necrosis of the bone compared with hand-driven or motorized drills.
  5. The microfracture holes are approximately 3 to 4 mm apart and are typically made to a depth of 3 to 4 mm. These perforations serve as an access channel for blood and mesenchymal stem cells from cancellous bone

and the marrow cavity to migrate into the prepared defect.

6. The eventual aim of the procedure is to establish a reparative granulation superclot that will proliferate and differentiate into a fibrous or fibrocartilage mosaic repair tissue.

Rehabilitation Overview

- Rehabilitation of the patient following any articular cartilage procedure of the knee presents a challenging task for the rehabilitation specialist.

- The rehabilitative process is typically several months following microfracture surgery.

- The rehabilitation specialist should instill the importance of compliance to the patient early in the rehabilitation period because adherence to weight-bearing restrictions and home therapeutic exercise assignments will have a direct influence on functional outcomes.

- The clinician should appreciate the healing response throughout the rehabilitative course by continually providing an optimal environment where the articular cartilage lesion can heal.

- Using a working knowledge of the structure and function of articular cartilage, combined with an appreciation of the forces induced upon the articular surfaces of the knee during specific exercises and activities, will permit the clinician to protect and progress the patient toward an optimal outcome.

- Communication with the surgeon throughout the rehabilitative process is important because the size and location of the lesion will have a direct effect on the rehabilitation program.

- A therapeutic exercise program addressing a medial femoral condyle lesion on a weight-bearing surface will differ from a non-weight-bearing femoral surface or a patellofemoral defect.

- Postoperative "guidelines" should be individualized for each patient. The rehabilitative course should be advanced via a criteria-based approach.

- The ultimate goal of rehabilitation is to restore the range of motion (ROM), flexibility, strength, and proprioception needed for the functional demands of daily living and/or sports activity while protecting the healing cartilage and applying appropriate stresses.

Postoperative Phase I (Weeks 0 to 6)

GOALS
- Control postoperative pain/swelling
- ROM 0 to 120 degrees
- Prevent quadriceps inhibition
- Normalize proximal musculature muscle strength
- Independence in home therapeutic exercise program

PRECAUTIONS
- Maintain weight-bearing restrictions: postoperative brace locked at 0 degrees; 0 to 20 degrees for patellofemoral lesion
- Avoid neglect of ROM exercises

TREATMENT STRATEGIES
- Continuous passive motion (CPM)
- Active-assisted ROM (AAROM) exercises (pain-free ROM)
- Towel extensions
- Patellar mobilization
- Toe-touch weight-bearing with brace locked at 0 degrees, with crutches
- Partial weight-bearing progressing to weight-bearing as tolerated; brace 0 to 20 degrees for patellofemoral lesion
- Quadriceps reeducation (quadriceps sets with electrical muscle stimulation or electromyography)
- Multiple angle quadriceps isometrics (bilaterally to submaximal)
- Short crank ergometry to standard ergometry
- Straight leg raises (SLRs) (all planes)
- Hip progressive resisted exercises
- Pool exercises
- Plantar flexion Thera-Band
- Lower extremity flexibility exercises
- Upper extremity cardiovascular exercises, as tolerated
- Cryotherapy
- Home therapeutic exercise program: evaluation-based

Continued

Postoperative Phase I (Weeks 0 to 6)—Cont'd

- Emphasize patient compliance to home therapeutic exercise program and weight-bearing restrictions

CRITERIA FOR ADVANCEMENT

- Physician direction for progressive weight-bearing (week 6)
- ROM 0 to 120 degrees
- Proximal muscle strength 5/5
- SLRs (supine) without extension lag

Postoperative Phase II (Weeks 6 to 12)

GOALS

- ROM 0 to within normal limits (WNL)
- Normal patellar mobility
- Restore normal gait
- Ascend 8-inch stairs with good control without pain

PRECAUTIONS

- Avoid descending stairs reciprocally until adequate quadriceps control and lower extremity alignment is demonstrated
- Avoid pain with therapeutic exercise and functional activities

TREATMENT STRATEGIES

- Progressive weight-bearing/gait training with crutches
  1. D/C crutches when gait is non-antalgic
- Postoperative brace discontinued as good quadriceps control (ability to SLR without lag or pain) is demonstrated
- Unloader brace/patella sleeve per physician preference
- Computerized forceplate (NeuroCom) for weight-bearing progression/patient education
- Underwater treadmill system (gait training) if incision benign
- Gait unloader device
- AAROM exercises
- Leg press (60- to 0-degree arc)
- Mini-squats/weight shifts
- Retrograde treadmill ambulation

- Proprioception/balance training
  1. Proprioception board/contralateral Thera-Band exercises/balance systems
- Initiate forward step-up program
- StairMaster
- SLRs (progressive resistance)
- Lower extremity flexibility exercises
- Open kinetic chain (OKC) knee extension to 40 degrees (tibiofemoral lesions)—closed kinetic chain (CKC) exercises preferred
- Home therapeutic exercise program: evaluation-based

CRITERIA FOR ADVANCEMENT
- ROM 0 to WNL
- Normal gait pattern
- Demonstrate ability to ascend 8-inch step
- Normal patellar mobility

Postoperative Phase III (Weeks 12 to 18)

GOALS
- Demonstrate ability to descend 8-inch stairs with good leg control without pain
- 85% limb symmetry on isokinetic testing (tibiofemoral lesions) and forward step-down test
- Return to normal ADL
- Improve lower extremity flexibility

PRECAUTIONS
- Avoid pain with therapeutic exercise and functional activities
- Avoid running until adequate strength development and physician clearance

TREATMENT STRATEGIES
- Progress squat program
- Initiate step-down program
- Leg press (emphasizing eccentrics)
- OKC knee extensions 90 to 40 degrees (CKC exercises preferred)
- Advanced proprioception training (perturbations)
- Agility exercises (sport cord)

Continued

Postoperative Phase III (Weeks 12 to 18)—Cont'd

- Elliptical trainer
- Retrograde treadmill ambulation/running
- Hamstring curls/proximal strengthening
- Lower extremity stretching
- Forward step-down test (NeuroCom) at 4 months
- Isokinetic test at 4 months
- Home therapeutic exercise program: evaluation-based

CRITERIA FOR ADVANCEMENT
- Ability to descend 8-inch stairs with good leg control without pain
- 85% limb symmetry on Isokinetic testing (tibiofemoral lesions) and forward step-down text

Postoperative Phase IV: Return to Sport (Week 18 and Beyond)

GOALS
- Lack of apprehension with sport-specific movements
- Maximize strength and flexibility as to meet demands of individual's sport activity
- Hop test $\geq$ 85% limb symmetry

PRECAUTIONS
- Avoid pain with therapeutic exercise and functional activities
- Avoid sport activity until adequate strength development and physician clearance

TREATMENT STRATEGIES
- Continue to advance lower extremity strengthening, flexibility, and agility programs
- Forward running
- Plyometric program
- Brace for sport activity (physician preference)
- Monitor patient's activity level throughout course of rehabilitation
- Reassess patient's complaints (i.e., pain/swelling daily-adjust program accordingly)

- Encourage compliance to home therapeutic exercise program
- Home therapeutic exercise program: evaluation-based

CRITERIA FOR DISCHARGE
- Hop test ≥ 85% limb symmetry
- Lack of apprehension with sport-specific movements
- Flexibility to accepted levels of sport performance
- Independence with gym program for maintenance and progression of therapeutic exercise program at discharge

Bibliography

Blevins, F.T., Steadman, J.R., Rodrigo, J.J., Silliman, J. Treatment of Articular Cartilage Defects in Athletes: An Analysis of Functional Outcome and Lesion Appearance. *Orthopedics* 1998;21:761–768.

Bobic, V. Current Status of Articular Cartilage Repair. E-BioMed, 2000.

Buckwalter, J.A., Mankin, H.J. Articular Cartilage II. Degeneration and Osteoarthritis, Repair, Regeneration and Transplantation. *J Bone Joint Surg* 1997;79A(4):612–632.

Buckwalter, J.A., Mankin, H.J. Articular Cartilage. I. Tissue Design and Chondrocyte-matrix Interactions. *J Bone Joint Surg* 1997; 79A(4):600–611.

Curl, W.W., Krome, J., Gordon, E.S., Rushing, J., Smith, B.P., Poehling, G.G. Cartilage Injuries: A Review of 31,516 Knee Arthroscopies. *Arthroscopy* 1997;13(4):456–460.

Hjelle, K., Austgulen, O., Muri, R. Full-thickness Chondral Defects: A Prospective Study of 1000 Knee Arthroscopies. Paper presented at Third International Cartilage Repair Society Symposium, April 27-29, 2000, Gothenburg, Sweden.

Mankin, H.J. The Response of Articular Cartilage to Mechanical Injury. *J Bone Joint Surg* 1982;64A:460–466.

Rodrigo, J.J., Steadman, J.R., Silliman, J.F., Fulstone, H.A. Improvement of Full-thickness Chondral Defect Healing in the Human Knee after Debridement and Microfracture Using Continuous Passive Motion. *Am J Knee Surg* 1994;7:109–116.

Rosenberg, T.D., Paulos, L.E., Parker, R.D., Coward, D.B., Scott, S.M. The Forty-five-degree Posteroanterior Flexion Weight-bearing Radiograph of the Knee. *J Bone Joint Surg* 1988;70A(10):1479–1483.

Sgaglione, N.A., Miniaci, A., Gillogly, S.D., Carter, T.R. Update on Advanced Surgical Techniques in the Treatment of Traumatic Focal Articular Cartilage Lesions in the Knee. *Arthroscopy* 2002; 18(2 Suppl 1):9-32.

Steadman, J.R., Rodkey, W.G., Rodrigo, J.J. Microfracture: Surgical Technique and Rehabilitation to Treat Chondral Defects. *Clin Orthop* 2001;391(Suppl):S362-S369.

Steadman, J.R., Rodkey, W.G., Singleton, S.B., Briggs, K.K. Microfracture Technique for Full-thickness Chondral Defects: Technique and Clinical Results. *Oper Tech Orthop* 1997; 7:300-304.

Terry, G.C., Flandry, F., van Manen, J.W., Norwood, L.A. Isolated Chondral Fractures of the Knee. *Clin Orthop* 1988;234:170-177.

Wright, J.M., Millett, P.J., Steadman, J.R. Osteochondral Injury: Acute Management. In Callahan, J., Rosenberg, A.G., Rubash, H.E., Simonian, P.T., Wickiewicz, T.L. (Eds). The Adult Knee. Lippincott, Williams & Wilkins, Philadelphia, 2003, pp. 885-893.

CHAPTER 33

Patellar and Quadriceps Tendon Repair

Greg Fives, PT, MSPT, SCS

Patellar and quadriceps tendon ruptures are both rare events in the general population. The incidence of isolated patellar tendon ruptures is fairly low. Typically, this injury occurs in the male population younger than age 40. Quadriceps tendon ruptures are also relatively infrequent, occurring more in the older population around the sixth or seventh decade of life. Patellar tendon ruptures occurred about one-third as often as quadriceps tendon ruptures.

The mechanism of injury for both quadriceps and patellar tendon ruptures is usually a violent eccentric contraction of the quadriceps resisted by a fixed position of the leg and foot with the knee in hyperflexion. More commonly, patellar tendon ruptures occur during sports or events that require significant extensor mechanism activation, such as basketball, volleyball, soccer, football, high jump, and gymnastics. Non-sports-related mechanisms of injury are usually the result of a trip-and-fall accident.

A force of approximately 17.5 times body weight can cause a rupture of the patellar tendon. Research has shown that the quadriceps tendon may be able to withstand up to 30 kg/mm of tensile force before rupturing. Spontaneous patellar or quadriceps tendon rupture can occur in patients with systemic or inflammatory conditions, such as systemic lupus erythematosus, gouty arthritis, psoriatic arthritis, hyperparathyroidism, diabetes mellitus, chronic renal failure, and rheumatoid arthritis, which weakens the involved soft tissue structures. Other risk factors include previous knee surgery, such as anterior cruciate ligament reconstruction with patellar tendon autograft and total knee replacement. Corticosteroid injections into the tendon and anabolic steroid use have also

303

been implicated as predisposing factors to isolated patellar tendon rupture.

Progressive patellar tendonitis (jumper's knee) and end-stage degenerative tendinopathy are also common mechanisms by which patellar tendon ruptures occur.

Some partial patellar or partial quadriceps tendon ruptures can be treated with immobilization in full extension for 4 to 6 weeks, but the treatment of choice for complete tendon rupture (quadriceps or patellar) is immediate operative repair. Immediate repair enhances postoperative outcomes for both patellar and quadriceps tendon rupture. The deleterious effects associated with delayed diagnosis and therefore delayed repairs include knee flexion ROM deficits, quadriceps atrophy, and a decreased functional outcome for the patient.

The Hospital for Special Surgery's postoperative rehabilitation guidelines and approach to knee extensor mechanism repairs are presented here.

Surgical Overview

- The extensor mechanism of the knee consists of the quadriceps, quadriceps tendon, patella, and patellar tendon.
- The quadriceps musculature is composed of the rectus femoris, vastus medialis, vastus lateralis, and vastus intermedius, which unite distally to form the common quadriceps tendon.
- Aponeurotic slips from both the vastus lateralis and vastus medialis form the lateral and medial retinaculi, respectively.
- The fibers of the quadriceps tendon traverse the anterior surface of the patella to form the patellar tendon.
- The patellar tendon is primarily composed of the distal central fibers of the rectus femoris, which terminate and insert into the tibial tubercle.

Patellar Tendon Repair

- Most patellar tendon ruptures occur at the osteotendinous junction, where the tendon inserts at the distal pole of the patella.
- A palpable defect is usually present below the distal pole of the patella, and the patella itself may be displaced as much as 5 cm proximally.

- Midsubstance patellar tendon tears are less common and can be more difficult to repair.
- Avulsion repairs are made by placing nonabsorbable sutures into the medial and lateral halves of the tendon.
  1. A bony trough is made across the distal patella and drill holes are made into the inferior and superior patella.
  2. The sutures are then passed through the inferior drill holes and are tied off at the superior pole of the patella.
  3. Midsubstance repairs can be repaired with interlocking sutures that tie the proximal and distal ends of the tendon together.
  4. Repairs may be reinforced or augmented, if needed, with either cerclage sutures, allograft, or surrounding knee musculature.

Quadriceps Tendon Repair

- Ruptures of the quadriceps tendon may occur at the osteo-tendinous junction or through the midsubstance of the tendon.
- Ruptures occur more frequently at the osteotendinous junction near the proximal pole of the patella.
  1. With this scenario, the superior pole of the patella is débrided of residual tendon, and the distal end of the rectus femoris and vastus intermedius are débrided of all chronic inflammatory tissue.
  2. A bony trough is made horizontally across the proximal pole of the patella.
  3. Drill holes are made near the base of the trough, and sutures are passed from the tendon through the drill holes to reattach the tendon.
- Acute midsubstance tears are made by direct repair.
  1. A midline incision is made and the proximal and distal ends are débrided.
  2. The two ends are then approximated and tied together with nonabsorbable sutures.
- After quadriceps or patellar tendon repair, intraoperative ROM is assessed, as is patellar position (alta or baja) and tracking. Intraoperatively, 0-degree knee flexion should be obtained without significant stress to the repair.

- Postoperatively, the patient's lower extremity is placed in a hinged rehabilitative brace locked at 0-degree extension.
- With an uncomplicated, acute extensor mechanism repair, patients are allowed to progressively weight-bear, as tolerated, with the brace locked in full extension.

Rehabilitation Overview

- Rehabilitation after quadriceps or patellar tendon repair should be initiated soon after surgery.
- Communication with the referring surgeon is essential in the care of these patients.
  1. The clinician should discuss with the surgeon specific postoperative range of motion (ROM) limitations and the patient's weight-bearing status.
  2. The clinician and the surgeon need to inform the patient that the rehabilitative process is extensive following quadriceps or patellar tendon repair.
- Other factors to be considered are the patient's age, bone and tissue quality, and the time from injury to surgery.
- Patient education on protection of the repair is vital and needs to be reinforced in the outpatient setting to ensure successful fixation of the repair.
  1. The clinician should educate the patient to specific time frames and goals involved in the rehabilitative process.
  2. The patient should realize that he or she is an active participant in the rehabilitative process and not the passive recipient of care from the clinician.
  3. Also, the goals of the rehabilitation program should match those of the patient. Goals will be different for the older patient with a quadriceps tendon repair rupture as compared to the younger athlete with a patellar tendon repair.
  4. Progress is based on individualized treatment guidelines that are functional and criteria-based.
  5. Postoperative precautions should be stressed to the patient.
- Increases in knee flexion ROM and quadriceps strengthening should be gradual during the early part of the rehabilitative process, to prevent failure of the repair.

- Postoperative rehabilitation may also be modified if the cause of injury is secondary to any of the aforementioned underlying disease states.

Postoperative Phase I: Maximum Protection (Weeks 0 to 6)

GOALS
- Control postoperative pain and swelling
- Patient independent in understanding strict protection of repair
- Gradually increase knee flexion ROM (physician directed)
  Example: 0 to 45 degrees at 0 to 3 weeks, 45 to 90 degrees at 4 to 6 weeks
- Prevent quadriceps inhibition
- Independent in therapeutic home exercise program

PRECAUTIONS
- Avoid active knee extension
- Maintain proper alignment of brace
- Avoid ambulation without brace locked at 0 degrees
- Avoid aggressive flexion; adhere to ROM limits set by physician

TREATMENT STRATEGIES
- Cryotherapy
- Patient education on brace use (locking and unlocking for ROM exercises only)
- Continuous passive motion machine (home and clinic)
- Seated active and active-assisted knee flexion exercises, passive extension
- Short crank ergometry if ROM >85 degrees
- Quadriceps reeducation (submaximal quadriceps setting with neuromuscular electrical stimulation or biofeedback)
- Multiangle quadriceps isometrics
- Straight leg raises (SLRs) (hip flexion) with brace locked at 0 degrees
- Scar mobilization
- Patellar mobilization
- Gait training-progressive weight-bearing as tolerated with crutches with brace locked in full extension, progress to weight bearing as tolerated (WBAT) with cane, brace locked in extension

Continued

Postoperative Phase I: Maximum Protection (Weeks 0 to 6)—Cont'd

- Proximal/distal strengthening, SLR other planes
- Upper body ergometry for cardiovascular exercise as needed

CRITERIA FOR ADVANCEMENT
- ROM 0 to 90 degrees
- Good patellar mobility
- Ability to SLR without extensor lag
- Pain-free WBAT with cane, brace locked at 0-degree extension

Postoperative Phase II: Moderate Protective (Weeks 6 to 11)

GOALS
- Minimize pain and swelling
- Patient understanding of activity modification
- Restore knee flexion ROM to 125 degrees
- Normalize gait without assistive device
- Patient able to ascend 8-inch step

PRECAUTIONS
- Avoid aggressive strengthening
- Avoid excessive activity levels that increase knee effusion and pain
- Avoid aggressive flexion ROM exercises

TREATMENT STRATEGIES
- Cryotherapy
- Patient education on brace use (locking and unlocking, setting dial hinge)
- Gait training-brace unlocked with flexion stop at 60 degrees once the patient demonstrates good quadriceps control
- Discharge brace (good quadriceps control, communicate with physician)
- Pool ambulation or underwater treadmill system
- Active/active-assisted ROM knee flexion exercises
- Continue patellar mobilization

- Progress to regular bike (standard crank length) as knee flexion approaches 110 to 115 degrees
- Leg press machine (bilateral); if ROM >90 degrees progress to eccentric and unilateral
- Initiate forward step-up program
- Initiate squat program—wall slide exercise within comfortable range
- Advance proprioceptive activities
- Retro-ambulation
- Progress resistive exercise/flexibility program for proximal and distal muscle groups
- Initiate quadriceps flexibility exercises

CRITERIA FOR ADVANCEMENT
- Minimal to no joint effusion
- Knee flexion ROM to at least 125 degrees
- Normal patellar mobility
- Good lower extremity control—*no* extensor lag present
- Able to perform 8-inch forward step-up
- Normal and symmetrical gait pattern

Postoperative Phase III: Early Functional (Weeks 11 to 16)

GOALS
- Full knee ROM
- Improve quadriceps and lower extremity flexibility
- Ability to descend 8-inch step with good eccentric leg control
- Return to normal activities of daily living (ADL)
- 85% limb symmetry on forward step down (FSD) test
- Independent in therapeutic home/gym exercise program

PRECAUTIONS
- Avoid pain with daily activities and therapeutic exercise
- Avoid stair descent until adequate quadriceps strength and lower extremity control
- Avoid high-level sport activity until adequate ROM, muscle strength, and flexibility is achieved

Continued

Postoperative Phase III: Early Functional (Weeks 11 to 16)—Cont'd

TREATMENT STRATEGIES
- Continue knee flexion ROM exercises
- Incorporate flexibility exercises for quadriceps musculature
- Soft tissue massage, myofascial release, contract-relax techniques
- Advance closed chain exercise program-advance step program
- Initiate forward step-down program
- Progress squat program
- Incorporate open kinetic chain knee extension exercises (isokinetic/isotonic) as tolerated
- Advanced proprioception exercises
- Agility training
- Elliptical training
- Retrograde running
- FSD test (NeuroCom) at 4 months
- Patient to replicate and comply with treatment program at home/gym

CRITERIA FOR ADVANCEMENT
- Full knee ROM
- Adequate quadriceps strength and lower extremity flexibility
- Ability to descend 8-inch step with good eccentric control (85% limb symmetry on FSD test)
- No pain with ADL-ambulation, reciprocal stair negotiation
- Compliance with home/gym exercise program

Postoperative Phase IV: Late Functional/ Return to Sport (Weeks 16 to 24)

GOALS
- Lack of apprehension with sport-specific movements
- Maximize strength and flexibility as to meet demands of individual's sport activity
- ≥85% limb symmetry with hop test and isokinetic testing
- Independent in therapeutic home/gym exercise program

PRECAUTIONS
- Avoid pain with therapeutic exercise and functional activities
- Avoid sport activity until adequate strength development and physician clearance

TREATMENT STRATEGIES
- Continue to advance lower extremity strengthening, flexibility, and agility programs
- Plyometric program
- Forward running
- Agility and sport-specific training
- Home/gym therapeutic exercise program: evaluation-based

CRITERIA FOR DISCHARGE
- 85% to 90% limb symmetry on functional and isokinetic tests
- Pain-free running
- Lack of apprehension with sport-specific movements
- Patient understands proper progression of home and gym exercise program

Bibliography

Anzel, S.H., Covey, K.W., Weiner, A.D., Lipscomb, P.R. Disruptions of Muscles and Tendons: An Analysis of 1014 Cases. *Surgery* 1959;45:406.

Casey, M.T. Jr., Tietjens, B.R. Neglected Ruptures of the Patellar Tendon. A Case Series of Four Patients. *Am J Sports Med* 2001; 29(4):457-460.

Enad, J.G., Loomis, L.L. Patellar Tendon Repair: Postoperative Treatment. *Arch Phys Med Rehabil* 2000;81(6):786-788.

Enad, J.G. Patellar Tendon Ruptures. *South Med J* 1999;92(6): 563-566.

Kasten, P., Schewe, B., Maurer, F., Gosling, T., Krettek, C., Weise, K. Rupture of the Patellar Tendon: A Review of 68 Cases and a Retrospective Study of 29 Ruptures Comparing Two Methods of Augmentation. *Arch Orthop Trauma Surg* 2001;121(10):578-582.

Kelly, D.W., Carter, V.S., Jobe, F.W., Kerlan, R.K. Patellar and Quadriceps Tendon Ruptures-Jumper's Knee. *Am J Sports Med* 1984;12(5): 375-380.

Kuechle, D.K., Stuart, M.J. Isolated Rupture of the Patellar Tendon in Athletes. *Am J Sports Med* 1994;22(5):692–695.

Marder, R.A., Timmerman, L.A. Primary Repair of Patellar Tendon Rupture Without Augmentation. *Am J Sports Med* 1999;27(3): 304–307.

Rasul, A.T. Jr., Fischer, D.A. Primary Repair of Quadriceps Tendon Ruptures. Results of Treatment. *Clin Orthop* 1993;289:205–207.

Richards, D.P., Barber, F.A. Repair of Quadriceps Tendon Ruptures Using Suture Anchors. *Arthroscopy* 2002;18(5):556–559.

Siwek, C.W., Rao, J.P. Ruptures of the Extensor Mechanism of the Knee Joint. *J Bone Joint Surg Am* 1981;63(6):932–937.

Zernicke, R.F., Garhammer, J., Jobe, F.W. Human Patellar-Tendon Rupture. *J Bone Joint Surg Am* 1977;59(2):179–183.

CHAPTER 34

Proximal and Distal Realignment

Theresa A. Chiaia, PT

Patellofemoral pain comprises 25% of all knee pathologies and is the most common knee complaint in adolescents and young adults. The source of pain in patients with patellofemoral disorders is multifactorial; therefore, numerous therapeutic interventions have been advocated: taping, bracing, foot orthoses, quadriceps strengthening, vastus medialis oblique (VMO) strengthening, timing of muscular contractions, flexibility training, and/or proximal strengthening.

Surgery for patellofemoral pain is an option only after the patient has exhausted nonoperative therapies. Surgical realignment has been divided into proximal and distal procedures. A *proximal realignment* is a soft tissue procedure indicated in the presence of recurrent subluxation/dislocation radiographic lateral patellar subluxation, and moderate or severe patellar tilt with minimal bony malalignment. *Distal realignment* is a bony procedure, an osteotomy of the tibial tubercle, indicated in patellofemoral arthrosis and instability (subluxation/dislocation) with underlying malalignment in a skeletally mature individual. The Hospital for Special Surgery guidelines for rehabilitation following proximal realignment and distal realignment are presented.

Surgical Overview
Proximal Realignment

- Proximal realignment is a soft tissue balancing procedure that involves the lateral retinaculum and/or the medial retinaculum or the distal portion of the vastus medialis.
- The medial patellofemoral ligament (MPFL), a discrete component of the medial retinaculum, provides the majority of passive medial restraint to lateral displacement of the

patella, and the distal portion of the vastus medialis (commonly referred to as the vastus medialis oblique), through its insertion onto the medial side of the patella, is the major dynamic stabilizer of the patella.

- A dysplastic VMO inserts more vertically near the proximal pole of the patella.
- MPFL reconstructions utilize allograft or autograft tissue fixed at the adductor tubercle tensioned to balance the patella within the trochlea and fixed on the patellar side.
- In the *medial imbrication* procedure, the medial stabilizing structures (VMO and medial retinaculum) are dissected free along its insertion into the patella, leaving a small cuff of tissue and then sutured more centrally onto the patella, functionally tightening the redundant tissue with sutures.

Distal Realignment

- Distal realignment is an osteotomy of the tibial tubercle, with subsequent transfer of the tibial tubercle, either medially, anteriorly, anteromedially, or distally.
- Fulkerson Anteromedialization Osteotomy is a combination of the uniplanar tibial tubercle transfer procedures, medialization (Elmslie-Trillat Osteotomy), and anteriorization (Maquet Osteotomy).
  1. The tibial tubercle is osteotomized by angling a single straight cut in anteromedial to posterolateral direction, whereby both medialization and elevation can be obtained.
  2. The tibial tubercle transfer is fixed with two cortical bone screws.
  3. Complications with this procedure are related to fixation, fracture through the osteotomy or through the screw hole, wound healing, and possible deep venous thrombosis.
  4. In cases with severe patella alta, the procedure is combined with distalization. Distal transfer of the tibial tuberosity allows the articular surface of the patella to engage in the trochlea earlier in knee flexion. The tibial tubercle osteotomy is performed, freeing it up circumferentially, and then transferred distally.

- Lateral retinacular release is commonly performed in combination with a proximal realignment or distal realignment. It can be performed as an open procedure with an incision at the lateral border of the patella, or, more commonly, arthroscopically.
  1. The lateral retinaculum is released from the superior pole of the patella to the inferior pole.
  2. The superior geniculate vessels are located at the superior pole of the patella just deep to the retinaculum and are responsible for one of the postoperative complications: hemarthrosis in the joint.

Rehabilitation Overview

- Avoidance of provoking signs and symptoms, such as joint effusion, active inflammation, and pain, should guide the rehabilitation process.
- In the early phases, attention must be paid to the healing process of the involved structures/soft tissues following proximal realignment and bony fixation following distal realignment.
- No healing constraints follow release of the lateral retinaculum; however, control of postoperative hemarthrosis is emphasized.
- Joint hemarthrosis is a concern with lateral retinacular release because of the proximity of the suprageniculate artery as it can lead to scarring and muscular inhibition. Bleeding in the joint will cause quadriceps inhibition, have a deleterious effect on joint proprioception, as well as the articular cartilage, and, ultimately, delay progression of rehabilitation.
- Pain has also been shown to decrease muscle activity of the quadriceps.
- Emphasis is on controlling hemarthrosis and pain, and initiating voluntary quadriceps control.
- Quadriceps strengthening is an essential component of patellofemoral rehabilitation and must be performed in a pain-free arc of motion.
  1. Knowledge of the location of the lesion as well as the patient's subjective complaints will help determine this range.

2. As a result of the origin of the vasti on the linea aspera, gross quadriceps strengthening results in compressive forces through the patellofemoral joint altering contact location and pressure distribution.

- An understanding of the biomechanics of the patellofemoral joint is essential.
  1. Articulation begins on the inferior patella with knee extension and moves proximally as the knee flexes.
  2. Patellofemoral joint reaction force is a measurement of compression of the patella against the femur and is dependent on the knee flexion angle and muscle tension.

- Another important consideration is the patellofemoral contact area. The contact load (force) divided by the contact area will determine the patellofemoral stress (stress = force/area).

- Quadriceps force and contact area vary according to knee flexion angles and thus has implications in prescribing quadriceps strengthening exercises. In closed chain activities, the stress increases from 0 to 90 degrees (force and contact area increase), whereas in open chain activities the stress increases as the knee extends (force increases as contact area decreases).

- Rehabilitation following these procedures is initiated immediately postoperatively.

- The rehabilitation potential will be dependent on the indications for surgery (instability vs arthritis) and the chronicity of the condition, premorbid status, and prior surgical history.

- Exercise should be performed in an optimal loading zone, the level of activity that neither overloads nor underloads the affected tissues.

- Therapeutic exercise and activities of daily living (ADL) must be within the envelope of function, the safe range of painless loading compatible with tissue homeostasis.

- Rehabilitation must respect the healing process and the individual knee's tolerance to imposed stresses. In short, at any given time each knee has an optimal window of function. If the knee is continually asked to work outside of this window, the window of function will become smaller. This philosophy underscores the importance of patient education. Understanding this concept will encourage compliance.

- The rehabilitation phases represent a continuum of rehabilitation rather than discrete, well-defined phases. Progression through the phases is dependent on the factors mentioned earlier, such as premorbid status and the chronicity of the condition.

Proximal Realignment
Postoperative Phase I: Healing (Weeks 0 to 6)

GOALS
- Patient education
- Control effusion
- Control pain
- Range of motion (ROM): 0-degree knee extension to 60-degree knee flexion (4 weeks); 90 degrees (6 weeks)
- Avoid quadriceps inhibition
- Promote healing
- Independent ambulation weight-bearing as tolerated (WBAT) with brace locked in extension
- Independence in a home exercise program (HEP), as instructed

PRECAUTIONS
- Symptom provocation: quadriceps shut down, joint effusion, active inflammation
- Knee flexion ROM, as per surgeon's guidelines
- Lateralization of the patella
  1. Avoid lateral patella glides
  2. Terminal knee extension exercises
- Active knee extension

TREATMENT STRATEGIES
- HEP, as instructed
- Educate patient
- Activity modification
- Cryotherapy
- Modalities, as needed for pain, effusion
- Quadriceps reeducation (submaximal): biofeedback, electrical stimulation, quadriceps sets performed with a

Continued

Proximal Realignment
Postoperative Phase I: Healing (Weeks 0 to 6)—Cont'd

    towel roll, multiangle open chain isometrics, closed chain quadriceps isometrics in sitting at 60-degree knee flexion
- ROM exercises
  1. Passive ROM (PROM) knee extension with a towel roll under heel
  2. Active ROM (AROM) knee flexion and PROM knee extension in sitting
- Patellar mobilization (medial direction: tilt and glide; cephalad and caudal)
- Gait training progressive WBAT, with appropriate assistive device and brace locked in extension
- Initiate proximal strengthening: straight leg raise (SLR) series; in supine, hip flexion can be performed with 20-degree knee flexion
- Address flexibility: gastrocnemius (towel stretch); hamstring stretch
- Initiate distal strengthening: elastic bands for triceps surae
- Initiate balance and proprioceptive training: double-limb support on progressively challenging surfaces

CRITERIA FOR ADVANCEMENT
- Good quadriceps contraction (pain-free)
- Good patellar mobility
- ROM: 0-degree knee extension to 90-degree knee flexion
- 0/10 pain at rest

Proximal Realignment
Postoperative Phase II: Functional-Gait, Motion, and Strengthening (Weeks 7 to 12)

GOALS
- Patient education
- Control effusion, inflammation, and pain
- 0/10 pain with ADL, therapeutic exercise
- ROM: 0-degree knee extension to 110 degrees (8 weeks), 130 degrees (12 weeks)
- Promote healing
- Normalize gait without an assistive device

- Lower extremity postural alignment and the ability to support and control knee in single-limb stance
- Independence in a HEP, as instructed

PRECAUTIONS
- Sign and symptom provocation: pain, inflammation, quadriceps shutdown, joint effusion
- Knee flexion ROM, as per surgeon's guidelines through 8 weeks
- Progression of weight-bearing
- Pathological gait pattern
- "Too much, too soon" progression of strengthening exercises

TREATMENT STRATEGIES
- HEP, as instructed
- Educate patient
- Activity modification
- Cryotherapy
- Quadriceps strengthening: AROM knee extension in a limited arc, bilateral leg press, forward step-up progression
- ROM exercises: progressing to active-assisted ROM (AAROM) knee flexion in sitting
- Patellar mobilization (medial direction: tilt and glide; cephalad and caudal)
- Cycle ergometry: progressing from short crank to standard crank
- Gait training
  1. Hydro-treadmill
  2. Treadmill with a low incline 3% to 5%
- Balance activities: single-limb support from stable to unstable surfaces
- Flexibility exercises: evaluation-based: gastrocnemius, AROM knee flexion with hip extension, hip adductors
- Advance proximal strengthening to include hip extension with knee flexion and closed chain activities, such as contralateral exercises

CRITERIA FOR ADVANCEMENT
- Normalized gait without an assistive device
- 0/10 pain with ADL, therapeutic exercise

Continued

Proximal Realignment
Postoperative Phase II: Functional-Gait, Motion, and Strengthening (Weeks 7 to 12)—Cont'd

- Lower extremity postural alignment and the ability to support and control knee in single-limb stance
- Able to ascend a 6-inch/8-inch step with good control
- ROM 130 degrees

Proximal Realignment
Postoperative Phase III: Advanced Strengthening and Endurance (Weeks 13 to 17)

GOALS
- Patient education
- Control effusion and inflammation
- 0/10 pain with ADL, as recommended by the therapist and therapeutic exercise
- ROM: within normal limits (WNLs)
- Normalize gait
- Lower extremity postural alignment and the ability to support and control knee in single-limb dynamic balance
- Independence in a HEP, as instructed

PRECAUTIONS
- Sign and symptom provocation: pain and active inflammation
- Gait deviations
- "Too much, too soon" progression of strengthening exercises

TREATMENT STRATEGIES
- HEP, as instructed: evaluation-based
- Educate patient
- Activity modification
- Cryotherapy
- Quadriceps strengthening
  1. AROM knee extension, eccentric leg press, forward step-down progression, squat progression

- ROM exercises
  1. AROM to AAROM knee flexion in sitting and supine wall slides
- Gait training
  1. Retro-treadmill with a 5% to 10% incline
- Advance proximal strengthening
- Balance activities progressing to single-limb static balance to dynamic activities
- Address muscle imbalances: evaluation-based: prone figure of four, hip adduction stretch
- Cross training: elliptical trainer, bicycle, stair machine

CRITERIA FOR ADVANCEMENT
- ROM WNLs
- Normalized gait
- Ability to support control knee in dynamic single-limb stance
- Able to ascend an 8-inch step with good control
- Able to descend an 8-inch step with good control, and alignment
- Lower extremity alignment during dynamic single-limb stance

Proximal Realignment
Postoperative Phase IV: Advanced Functional, Return to Sport (Weeks 18 to 25)

GOALS
- Patient education
- 0/10 pain with ADL and advanced therapeutic exercise
- Muscular endurance and flexibility to meet demands of sport
- Independence in a HEP, as instructed
- Strength: 85% limb symmetry via testing

PRECAUTIONS
- Sign and symptom provocation
- Volume of training

TREATMENT STRATEGIES
- HEP, as instructed: incorporate rest
- Educate patient
- Cryotherapy

Continued

Proximal Realignment
Postoperative Phase IV: Advanced
Functional, Return to Sport (Weeks 18 to 25)—
Cont'd

- Continue functional quadriceps strengthening
- Patellar mobilization (medial direction: tilt and glide), as needed
- Dynamic balance activities
- Continue to address muscle imbalances: evaluation-based
- Advance proximal strengthening through functional activities
- Plyometrics training
- Initiate running program: retro to forward running intervals
- Cutting and deceleration training
- Endurance training: cross training
- Strength testing and functional testing

RETURN TO SPORT/CRITERIA FOR DISCHARGE
- 85% limb symmetry with
  1. Strength testing: isokinetics, if appropriate
  2. Functional testing: single-leg hop
- Muscular endurance and flexibility to meet demands of sport

Distal Realignment
Postoperative Phase I (Weeks 0 to 6)

GOALS
- Patient education
- Control effusion
- Control pain
- ROM: 0-degree knee extension to 60-degree knee flexion (2 weeks); 90 degrees (6 weeks)
- Avoid quadriceps inhibition
- Promote healing
- Independent ambulation non–weight-bearing (NWB) with crutches and brace locked in extension on level surfaces and stairs
- Independence in a HEP, as instructed

PRECAUTIONS
- Symptom provocation: quadriceps shut down, joint effusion, active inflammation
- Progression of weight-bearing
- Knee flexion ROM, as per surgeon's guidelines
- Active knee extension
- Wound healing, patella position

TREATMENT STRATEGIES
- HEP, as instructed
- Educate patient
- Activity modification
- Cryotherapy
- Modalities, as needed for pain, effusion
- Quadriceps reeducation: biofeedback, electrical stimulation, quadriceps sets performed with a towel roll
- Continuous passive motion
- ROM exercises
  1. PROM knee extension with a towel roll under heel
  2. AROM knee flexion in sitting, PROM knee extension with noninvolved extremity upon return from flexion in sitting
- Patellar mobilization: emphasize cephalad direction
- Gait training NWB with crutches and brace locked in extension
- Initiate proximal strengthening: SLR series, gluteals, comply with NWB status
- Address flexibility: gastrocnemius (towel stretch); hamstring stretch
- Initiate distal strengthening: elastic bands for triceps surae

CRITERIA FOR ADVANCEMENT
- Radiographic evidence of adequate healing
- Good quadriceps contraction
- Good patellar mobility
- ROM: 0-degree knee extension to 90-degree knee flexion
- 0/10 pain at rest

Distal Realignment
Postoperative Phase II (Weeks 7 to 14)

GOALS
- Patient education
- Control effusion, inflammation, and pain
- Establish pain-free arc of motion
- 0/10 pain with ADL, therapeutic exercise
- ROM: 0-degree knee extension to 120 degrees (8 weeks), WNL at 14 weeks
- Promote healing
- Normalize gait
- Independence in a HEP, as instructed

PRECAUTIONS
- Sign and symptom provocation: pain, inflammation, quadriceps shut down, joint effusion
- Knee flexion ROM as per surgeon's guidelines
- Progression of weight-bearing
- Pathological gait pattern
- Pain-free arc of motion during exercise

TREATMENT STRATEGIES
- HEP, as instructed
- Educate patient
- Activity modification
- Cryotherapy
- Quadriceps strengthening
  1. Submaximal multiangle closed and open chain isometrics
  2. Bilateral leg press: monitor arc of motion
  3. Open chain knee extension: monitor arc of motion
  4. Initiate forward step-up progression
- ROM exercises
  1. AAROM knee extension with noninvolved extremity upon return from flexion in sitting in a pain-free arc
  2. AROM to AAROM knee flexion in sitting
- Patellar mobilization (medially and cephalad)
- Cycle ergometry: progressing from short crank to standard crank
- Gait training
  1. Hydro-treadmill
  2. Unweighted treadmill

- Flexibility exercises: evaluation-based: AROM knee flexion with hip extension
- Advance proximal strengthening: hip extension with knee flexion, and closed chain activities
- Initiate balance and proprioceptive training: double-limb support on progressively challenging surfaces

CRITERIA FOR ADVANCEMENT
- Normalize gait
- 0/10 pain with ADL, therapeutic exercise
- Ability to support and control knee in single-limb stance
- Able to ascend an 8-inch step with good control
- Good postural alignment during single-limb stance

Distal Realignment
Postoperative Phase III (Weeks 15 to 22)

GOALS
- Patient education
- Control effusion and inflammation
- 0/10 pain with ADL, therapeutic exercise
- ROM: WNLs
- Normalize gait
- Good single-leg dynamic balance
- Good eccentric quadriceps control
- Pelvic control during step down
- Independence in a HEP, as instructed

PRECAUTIONS
- Sign and symptom provocation: pain and active inflammation
- Gait deviations
- Overloading the joint

TREATMENT STRATEGIES
- HEP, as instructed
- Educate patient
- Activity modification
- Cryotherapy
- Quadriceps strengthening: monitor arc of motion
  1. Forward step-up progression
  2. Eccentric leg press

Continued

Distal Realignment
Postoperative Phase III (Weeks 15 to 22)—
Cont'd

3. Forward step-down progression
4. Squat progression
- ROM exercises
  1. PROM knee extension with a towel roll under heel
  2. AROM to AAROM knee flexion in sitting and supine wall slides
- Gait training
  1. Treadmill
  2. Retro-treadmill
- Advance proximal strengthening through functional activities
- Balance activities: single-limb static balance to dynamic activities
- Address muscle imbalances: evaluation-based
- Cross training: elliptical trainer, bicycle, stair machine

CRITERIA FOR ADVANCEMENT
- ROM WNLs
- Normalize gait
- Ability to support control knee in dynamic single-limb stance
- Able to descend an 8-inch step with good control, and alignment
- Good postural alignment during dynamic single-limb stance

Distal Realignment
Postoperative Phase IV (Weeks 36 to 44)

GOALS
- Patient education
- 0/10 pain with ADL, advanced therapeutic exercise
- Good dynamic balance
- Muscular endurance and flexibility to meet demands of ADL, and sport
- Independence in a HEP, as instructed
- Strength: 85% limb symmetry

PRECAUTIONS
- Sign and symptom provocation
- Volume of training

TREATMENT STRATEGIES
- HEP: evaluation-based
- Educate patient
- Activity level should be within envelope of function
- Cryotherapy
- Continue functional quadriceps strengthening
- Dynamic balance activities
- Continue to address muscle imbalances: evaluation-based
- Cutting drills and deceleration training
- Endurance training: cross training
- Initiate plyometrics
- Initiate running program: retro to forward running intervals
- Strength testing and functional testing

RETURN TO SPORT/CRITERIA FOR DISCHARGE
- 85% limb symmetry with
  1. Strength testing: isokinetics, if appropriate
  2. Functional testing: single-leg hop
- Muscular endurance and flexibility to meet demands of ADL, and physician clearance must be obtained prior to participation in sport

Bibliography

Clement, D.B., Taunton, J.E., Smart, G.W. A Survey of Overuse Running Injuries. *Phys Sportsmed* 1981;9(5):47-58.

deAndrade, J.R., Grant, C., Dixon, A.S. Joint Distension and Reflex Muscle Inhibition in the Knee. *J Bone Joint Surg* 1965;47A(2): 313-322.

Devereaux, M.D., Lachmann, S.M. Patellofemoral Arthralgia in Athletes Attending a Sports Injury Clinic. *Br J Sports Med* 1984;18:18-21.

Dye, S.F. Patellofemoral Pain Current Concepts: An Overview. *Sports Med Arthrosc Rev* 2001;9:264-272.

Fulkerson, J.P. Anteromedialization of the Tibial Tuberosity for Patellofemoral Malalignment. *Clin Orthop* 1983;177:176.

Goodfellow, J., Hungerford, D.S., Zindel, M. Patello-femoral Joint Mechanics and Pathology: Functional Anatomy of the Patello-femoral Joint. *J Bone Joint Surg* 1976;58B:291-299.

Grelsamer, R.P., McConnell, J. The Patella. A Team Approach. Aspen Publishers, Gaithersburg, MD, 1998.

Hungerford, D.S., Lennox, D.W. Rehabilitation of the Knee in Disorders of the Patellofemoral Joint: Relevant Biomechanics. *Orthop Clin North Am* 1983;14(2):397-402.

Porterfield, J.A., DeRosa, C. Mechanical Low Back Pain. WB Saunders, Philadelphia, 1991.

Powers, C.M. The Effects of Anatomically Based Multiplanar Loading of the Extensor Mechanism on Patellofemoral Joint Mechanics. *Clin Biomech* 1998;13:608-615.

Shubin Stein, B.E., Ahmad, C.S. Patellofemoral Disorders in Athletes. In Essentials of Orthopaedic Surgery Sports Medicine, 2005.

Spencer, J.D., Hayes, K.C., Alexander, I.J. Knee Joint Effusion and Quadriceps Reflex Inhibition in Man. *Arch Phys Med Rehabil* 1984;65:171-177.

Steinkamp, L.A., Dillingham, M.F., Market, M.D., Hill, J.A., Kaufman, K.R. Biomechanical Considerations in Patella Femoral Joint Rehabilitation. *Am J Sports Med* 1993;21(3):438-444.

Young, A., Stokes, M., Shakespeare, D.T., Sherman, K.P. The Effect of Intra-articular Bupivacaine on Quadriceps Inhibition after Meniscectomy. *Med Sci Sports Exerc* 1983;15(2):154.

CHAPTER 35

Anterior Cruciate Ligament Reconstruction

John T. Cavanaugh, PT, MEd, ATC

The anterior cruciate ligament (ACL) is one of the more commonly injured knee ligaments in the general population. An estimated 1 out of 3000 people will suffer an ACL injury in any given year. The majority of these injuries occur during sport activities, which involve rapid change of direction and jumping (basketball, soccer, football, skiing, lacrosse).

The pathomechanics of ACL injury can include contact and noncontact mechanisms. It is estimated that more than 100,000 ACL reconstructions are performed annually in the United States.

Graft choices for reconstruction include autograft (patellar tendon or hamstring tendon) or allograft tissue. The Hospital for Special Surgery ACL reconstruction guideline following autogenous patellar tendon graft is presented.

Surgical Overview

- ACL reconstruction using a patellar tendon graft is performed using a combination of open and arthroscopic surgery.
- The central third of the patellar tendon is harvested along with a segment of bone from the patella above and the tibia below.
- Remnants of the native ACL tissue is arthroscopically débrided.
- Drill holes are created in the tibia and femur in preparation for graft placement.
- The graft is passed through the tibial tunnel, through the central part of the knee joint and into the femoral tunnel.
- The graft is fixated by placing interference screws (one in the femur and one in the tibia) between the bone block and respective walls of the femoral and tibial tunnels.

- The skin incisions are reapproximated with sutures.
- Postoperatively, the patient is placed in a hinged brace locked at 0 degrees of extension.

Rehabilitation Overview

- The rehabilitation program following ACL reconstruction is begun immediately after surgery.
- Care must be given by the rehabilitation specialist to protect the ACL graft substitute.
- The clinician must consider ACL biology throughout the progression of the postoperative rehabilitation program.
- The graft is at its strongest at the time of reconstruction.
- Over time the graft undergoes periods of necrosis, revascularization, and remodeling.
- Graft strength decreases during the period of necrosis and gradually increases as it revascularizes and remodels.
- Graft fixation techniques are an important consideration, as well as biological fixation, and replace mechanical fixation over a 3- to 6-week time frame.
- The patient is progressed via a criteria-based functional progression. Criteria for discharge are targeted between 4 and 6 months after surgery.

Preoperative Rehabilitation

GOALS
- Patient education
- Restore normal range of motion (ROM)
- Normalize gait
- Maximize strength/functional capabilities
- Demonstrate ability to ascend/descend stairs without assistive device

PRECAUTIONS
- Avoid heat application
- Avoid prolonged standing/walking/deceleration and rotary sport activity

- Avoid valgus stress during therapeutic exercise and functional activities with concomitant medial collateral ligament injury

TREATMENT STRATEGIES
- KT1000 exam
- Isokinetic tests/functional tests/balance test
- Measure for postoperative brace; don/doff instruction
- Cryotherapy instruction
- Gait training (progressive)
- Partial weight bearing (PWB) to weightbearing as tolerated (WBAT) (patella tendon) w/crutches, brace locked at 0 degrees
- Home program: postoperative therapeutic exercise instruction
- Quadriceps sets
- Straight leg raise (SLR) (brace locked at 0 degrees)
- Patella mobilization
- Passive (towel) extensions
- Active flexion/active-assisted extension 90 to 0 degrees exercise
- Active ROM (AROM) and active-assisted ROM (AAROM) exercises
- Progressive resistive exercises and functional activities
- Electrical stimulation/biofeedback (muscle reeducation)

CRITERIA FOR SURGERY
- Normal ROM
- Normalize gait
- Demonstrate ability to ascend/descend stairs without assertive device
- Demonstrate independence in postoperative therapeutic exercise program

Postoperative Phase I (Weeks 0 to 2)

GOALS
- Emphasis on full passive extension
- Control postoperative pain/swelling
- ROM 0 to 90 degrees

Continued

Postoperative Phase I (Weeks 0 to 2)—Cont'd

- Early progressive weight-bearing
- Prevent quadriceps inhibition
- Independence in home therapeutic exercise program

PRECAUTIONS

- Avoid active knee extension 40 to 0 degrees
- Avoid ambulation without brace locked at 0 degrees
- Avoid heat application
- Avoid prolonged standing/walking

TREATMENT STRATEGIES

- Towel extensions, prone hangs, etc.
- Quadriceps reeducation (quadriceps sets with electrical muscle simulator or electromyography)
- Progressive weight-bearing PWB to WBAT (patella tendon) with brace locked at 0 degrees with crutches
- Patellar mobilization
- Active flexion/active-assisted extension 90 to 0 degrees exercise
- SLRs (all planes)
- Brace locked at 0 degrees for SLR (supine)
- Short crank ergometry
- Hip progressive resisted exercises
- Proprioception board (bilateral weight-bearing)
- Leg press (bilateral/70- to 5-degree arc) (if ROM >90 degrees)
- Upper extremity cardiovascular exercises as tolerated
- Cryotherapy
- Home therapeutic exercise program: evaluation-based
- Emphasize patient compliance to home therapeutic exercise program and weight-bearing precautions/progression

CRITERIA FOR ADVANCEMENT

- Ability to SLR without quadriceps lag
- ROM 0 to 90 degrees
- Demonstrate ability to unilateral (involved extremity) weight bear without pain

Postoperative Phase II (Weeks 2 to 6)

GOALS
- ROM 0 to 125 degrees
- Good patellar mobility
- Minimal swelling
- Restore normal gait (non-antalgic)
- Ascend 8-inch stairs with good control without pain

PRECAUTIONS
- Avoid descending stairs reciprocally until adequate quadriceps control and lower extremity alignment
- Avoid pain with therapeutic exercise and functional activities

TREATMENT STRATEGIES
- Progressive weight-bearing/WBAT (patellar tendon) with crutches brace opened 0 to 50 degrees, if good quadriceps control (good quadriceps set/ability to SLR without lag or pain)
- Discontinue crutches when gait is non-antalgic
- Brace changed to surgeon's preference (Off-the-shelf [OTS] brace, patella sleeve, etc.)
- Standard ergometry (if knee ROM >115 degrees)
- Leg press (80- to 0-degree arc)
- AAROM exercises
- Mini squats/weight shifts
- Proprioception training: prop board/biomechanical ankle platform system/contralateral Thera-Band exercises
- Initiate forward step-up program
- StairMaster
- AquaCiser (gait training) if incision benign
- SLRs (progressive resistance)
- Hamstring/calf flexibility exercises
- Hip/hamstring PRE
- Active knee extension to 40 degrees
- KT1000 knee ligament arthrometer exam at 6 weeks (no max manual test)
- Home therapeutic exercise program: evaluation-based

CRITERIA FOR ADVANCEMENT
- ROM 0 to 125 degrees
- Normal gait pattern
- Demonstrate ability to ascend 8-inch step

Continued

Postoperative Phase II (Weeks 2 to 6)—Cont'd

- Good patellar mobility
- Functional progression pending KT1000 and functional assessment

Postoperative Phase III (Weeks 6 to 14)

GOALS
- Restore full ROM
- Demonstrate ability to descend 8-inch stairs with good leg control without pain
- Improve ADL endurance
- Improve lower extremity flexibility
- Protect patellofemoral joint

PRECAUTIONS
- Avoid pain with therapeutic exercise and functional activities
- Avoid running and sport activity until adequate strength development and surgeon's clearance

TREATMENT STRATEGIES
- Progress squat program
- Initiate step-down program
- Leg press
- Lunges
- Isotonic knee extensions 90 to 40 degrees (closed kinetic chain [CKC] exercises preferred)
- Advanced proprioception training (perturbations)
- Agility exercises (sport cord)
- VersaClimber
- Retrograde treadmill ambulation/running
- Quadriceps stretching
- Forward Step-Down Test (NeuroCom)
- KT1000 knee ligament arthrometer exam at 3 months
- Home therapeutic exercise program: evaluation-based

CRITERIA FOR ADVANCEMENT
- ROM to WNL
- Ability to descend 8-inch stairs with good leg control without pain
- Functional progression pending KT1000 and functional assessment

Postoperative Phase IV (Weeks 14 to 22)

GOALS
- Demonstrate ability to run pain-free
- Maximize strength and flexibility as to meet demands of ADL
- Hop test ≥75% limb symmetry

PRECAUTIONS
- Avoid pain with therapeutic exercise and functional activities
- Avoid sport activity until adequate strength development and surgeon's clearance

TREATMENT STRATEGIES
- Start forward-running (treadmill) program when 8-inch step-down satisfactory
- Continue lower extremity strengthening and flexibility programs
- Advance agility program/sport-specific
- Start plyometric program when strength base sufficient
- Isotonic knee extension (full arc/pain and crepitus free) (CKC exercises preferred)
- Isokinetic training (fast to moderate velocities) (CKC exercises preferred)
- KT1000 knee ligament arthrometer exam at 3 months
- Home therapeutic exercise program: evaluation-based

CRITERIA FOR ADVANCEMENT
- Symptom-free running
- Hop test ≥75% limb symmetry
- Functional progression pending and functional assessment

Postoperative Phase V (Week 22 and Beyond)

GOALS
- Lack of apprehension with sport-specific movements
- Maximize strength and flexibility as to meet demands of individual's sport activity
- Hop test ≥85% limb symmetry

Continued

Postoperative Phase V (Week 22 and Beyond)—Cont'd

PRECAUTIONS
- Avoid pain with therapeutic exercise and functional activities
- Avoid sport activity until adequate strength development and surgeon's clearance

TREATMENT STRATEGIES
- Continue to advance lower extremity strengthening, flexibility, and agility programs
- Advance plyometric program
- Brace for sport activity (surgeon's preference)
- Monitor patient's activity level throughout course of rehabilitation
- Reassess patient's complaint's (i.e., pain/swelling daily-adjust program accordingly)
- Encourage compliance to home therapeutic exercise program
- KT1000 knee ligament arthrometer exam at 6 months
- Home therapeutic exercise program: evaluation-based

CRITERIA FOR DISCHARGE
- Hop test ≥85% limb symmetry
- Lack of apprehension with sport-specific movements
- Flexibility to accepted levels of sport performance
- Independence with gym program for maintenance and progression of therapeutic exercise program at discharge

Bibliography

Clancy, W.G., Narechania, R.G., Rosenberg, T.D., Gmeiner, J.G., Wisnefske, D.D., Lange, T.A. Anterior and Posterior Cruciate Ligament Reconstruction in Rhesus Monkeys. *J Bone Joint Surg* 1981;63A:1270-1284.

Drez, D.J., DeLee, J., Holden, J.P., Arnoczky, S., Noyes, F.R., Roberts, T.S. Anterior Cruciate Ligament Reconstruction Using Bone-patella Tendon-bone Allografts. A Biological and Biomechanical Evaluation in Goats. *Am J Sports Med* 1991;19:256-263.

Falcoiero, R.P., DiStefano, V.J., Cook, T.M. Revascularization and Ligamentization of Autogenous Anterior Cruciate Ligament Grafts in Humans. *Arthroscopy* 1998;14(2):197-205.

Miyasaka, K.C., Daniel, D.M., Stone, M.L., Hirschman, P. The Incidence of Knee Ligament Injuries in the General Population. *Am J Knee Surg* 1991;4:3–8.

Rougraff, B.T., Shelbourne, K.D. Early Histologic Appearance of Human Patella Tendon Autografts Used for Anterior Cruciate Ligament Reconstruction. *Knee Surg Sports Traumatol Arthrosc* 1999;7(1): 9–14.

CHAPTER *36*

Posterior Cruciate Ligament Reconstruction

John T. Cavanaugh, PT, MEd, ATC

The posterior cruciate ligament (PCL) functions as the primary restraint to posterior displacement of the tibia relative to the femur. Injury to the PCL accounts for approximately 3% of all knee injuries in the general population. In patients who present to trauma centers with knee injuries, the incidence has reported as high as 37%. Isolated PCL injuries may occur at a rate of 40%.

The most frequent mechanism of injury in isolated PCL tears is a direct blow on the anterior tibia with the knee flexed position. Injury to the PCL is often associated with concomitant pathology. Additional knee structures may be injured as a result of hyperextension, hyperflexion, or rotational mechanisms associated with valgus/varus stress.

Management following PCL injury remains controversial. Some investigators have reported successful outcomes in patients treated without surgery who have developed excellent quadriceps strength. Other long-term follow-up studies of PCL injuries treated conservatively have demonstrated degenerative changes accompanied by pain in the patellofemoral joint and the medial compartment of the tibiofemoral joint. Whether reconstruction of the PCL will alter the natural history of the PCL-deficient knee continues to be studied. Clinical results following PCL reconstruction have not been as predictable as those after anterior cruciate ligament reconstruction.

Posterior cruciate ligament reconstructions may be performed using various surgical techniques and graft substitutes. Traditional techniques use a transtibial technique, whereas, more recently, PCL reconstructions have used the posterior inlay technique as well as a two-femoral tunnel (double bundle) procedure. Achilles tendon allograft and bone-patella, tendon-bone autografts are commonly used as graft substitutes. The technique of choice at the Hospital for Special Surgery (HSS) is a transtibial fixation double-bundle PCL reconstruction with an Achilles tendon allograft. The rehabilitation program following this procedure is presented.

Surgical Overview

- The PCL is the stronger and larger of the cruciate ligaments. The ligament has a broad, fan-shaped femoral attachment and a narrower insertion to the posterior tibia.
- The PCL is composed of two separate bundles: the anterolateral and posteromedial.
  1. The anterolateral bundle is taut when the knee is flexed, and the posteromedial bundle is taut when the knee is near extension.
  2. The anterolateral bundle is stronger, stiffer, and has a higher ultimate load to failure than the posteromedial bundle.
  3. Traditionally, the anterolateral bundle has been the focus of PCL reconstructive surgery.
- In recent years, a double-bundle PCL reconstruction has been used to better replicate knee anatomy and biomechanics.
  1. The transtibial fixation double-bundle PCL reconstruction is performed using an all arthroscopic technique.
  2. A split Achilles tendon allograft is used as the graft substitute because it allows for excellent tibial fixation with the bone block and sufficient soft tissue for two femoral bundles.
  3. The bundles are split to make bundles of 8 mm (anterolateral) and 7 mm (posteromedial).
  4. The tibial tunnel is prepared first for the transtibial fixation. A PCL tibial guide is placed through an anteromedial portal and the tibial tunnel is then reamed.
  5. The femoral tunnels are then created after an anteromedial incision is made for exposure of the anteromedial femoral condyle. A double femoral tunnel guide is used to place the guide pins for the two tunnels.

6. The tunnels are drilled using an outside-in technique. The two bundles are then passed up the tibial tunnel and pulled through their respective femoral tunnels and tensioned appropriately.

7. A metal interference screw placed between the bone block and the tunnel is used for tibial fixation.

8. The individual bundles are fixated into the femoral tunnels, using bioabsorbable interference screws and an outside-in technique.

- Postoperatively, the patient is placed in a double upright hinged brace locked at 0 degrees of extension.

Rehabilitation Overview

- The rehabilitation program following PCL reconstruction is designed to progressively restore knee range of motion (ROM) and lower extremity strength while at the same time protect the graft replacement and fixation from deleterious forces.

- The rehabilitation specialist needs to consider and apply his or her knowledge of knee biomechanics and the altered biomechanics inherent of the PCL-deficient and reconstructed knee throughout the rehabilitative process.

- Communication between the surgeon and rehabilitation specialist is vital. Additional structural involvement identified during surgery will have a direct effect on program design and progression.

- The patient is progressed via a criteria-based functional progression. The patient should be made aware of his or her role in the rehabilitative process. The patient's compliance to prescribed therapeutic exercises and activity modifications is vital for a successful outcome.

Posterior Cruciate Ligament Reconstruction: Preoperative Phase

GOALS
- Patient education
- Restore normal ROM
- Normalize gait

- Maximize strength/functional capabilities and demonstrate ability to ascend/descend stairs without assistive device
- Independent with postoperative therapeutic exercise program
- Independent with crutches toe touch weight bearing on all surfaces

TREATMENT STRATEGIES
- Knee ligament arthrometer exam
- Isokinetic test/functional tests/balance testing as appropriate
- Measure for postoperative brace; don/doff instruction
- Cryotherapy instruction
- Gait training: TTWB w/crutches, brace locked at 0 degrees
- Therapeutic exercise instruction
  1. Passive (pillow under calf) extensions
  2. Quadriceps sets
  3. SLR (brace locked at 0 degrees)
  4. Patellar mobilization
  5. Active-assisted knee extension/passive flexion exercise (ROM 0 to 70 degrees)

Postoperative Phase I (Weeks 0 to 6)

GOALS
- Control postoperative pain/swelling
- ROM 0 to 90 degrees
- Prevent quadriceps inhibition
- Improve patellar mobility
- Independence in home therapeutic exercise program

PRECAUTIONS
- Avoid active knee flexion
- Avoid heat application
- Avoid ambulation without brace locked at 0 degrees
- Avoid exceeding ROM and weight-bearing limitations
- Avoid pain with therapeutic exercise and functional activities

Continued

Postoperative Phase I (Weeks 0 to 6)—Cont'd

TREATMENT STRATEGIES
- Passive extension (pillow under calf)
- Quadriceps reeducation (quadriceps sets with electrical muscle stimulator [EMS] or electromyography [EMG])
- Gait: weight-bearing TTWB with brace locked at 0 degrees with crutches
  1. Progressive weight-bearing at weeks 2 to 6 to 75%
- Patellar mobilization
- Active-assisted knee extension/passive flexion exercise (ROM 0 to 70 degrees)
  1. Progress to 90 degrees, as tolerated, weeks 4 to 6
- SLRs (supine/prone), brace locked at 0 degrees
- SLRs (all planes)/progressive resistance
- Multiple angle quadriceps isometrics (ROM 60 to 20 degrees)
- Leg press (ROM 60- to 0-degree arc) (bilaterally)
- Proximal (hip) strengthening PREs
- Proprioception training (bilateral weight-bearing)
- Hamstring/calf flexibility exercises
- Short crank ergometry
- Cardiovascular exercises (UBE, Airdyne, etc.), as tolerated
- Cryotherapy
- Emphasize patient compliance to home therapeutic exercise program and weight-bearing precautions

CRITERIA FOR ADVANCEMENT
- ROM 0 to 90 degrees
- Ability to bear 75% weight on involved extremity
- Ability to SLR without quadriceps lag
- Continued improvement in patellar mobility and proximal strength

Postoperative Phase II (Weeks 6 to 12)

GOALS
- ROM 0 to 130 degrees
- Restore normal gait
- Demonstrate ability to ascend 8-inch stairs with good leg control without pain

- Demonstrate ability to descend 6-inch stairs with good leg control without pain
- Improve ADL endurance
- Improve lower extremity flexibility
- Protect patellofemoral joint

PRECAUTIONS
- Avoid exceeding ROM limitations in therapeutic exercises
- Avoid resistive knee flexion exercises
- Avoid pain with therapeutic exercise and functional activities
- Monitor activity level (prolonged standing/walking)

TREATMENT STRATEGIES
- Discontinue crutches when gait is non-antalgic (weeks 6 to 8)
- Brace changed to surgeon's preference (OTS brace, patellar sleeve, unloader brace, etc.)
- Standard ergometry (if knee ROM >115 degrees)
- Leg press/mini-squats (ROM 60- to 0-degree arc)
- AAROM exercises
- Proprioception training: multiplanar support surfaces
  1. Progress to unilateral support/contralateral exercises (elastic band)
  2. Perturbation training
- Forward step-up program
- Step machine
- Underwater treadmill system/pool (gait training)
- Retrograde treadmill ambulation
- Active knee extension: PRE (OKC) 60 to 0 degrees (monitor patellar symptoms)
- NO active (OKC) hamstring exercises
- Initiate step-down program when appropriate
- Knee ligament arthrometer exam at 3 months

CRITERIA FOR ADVANCEMENT
- ROM 0 to 130 degrees
- Normal gait pattern
- Demonstrate ability to ascend 8-inch step
- Demonstrate ability to descend a 6-inch step
- Functional progression pending knee ligament arthrometer exam and functional assessment

Postoperative Phase III (Weeks 12 to 20)

GOALS
- Restore full ROM
- Demonstrate ability to descend 8-inch stairs with good leg control without pain
- Improve ADL endurance
- Improve lower extremity flexibility
- Protect patellofemoral joint

PRECAUTIONS
- Avoid descending stairs reciprocally until adequate quadriceps control and lower extremity alignment
- Avoid resistive knee flexion exercises
- Avoid pain with therapeutic exercise and functional activities
- Monitor activity level (prolonged standing/walking)

TREATMENT STRATEGIES
- Leg press/squats (ROM 80- to 0-degree arc)
- AAROM exercises
- Proprioception training: unilateral balance on multiplanar surfaces
  1. Perturbations
- Lunges
- Agility exercises (sport cord)
- Step machine
- Retrograde treadmill running
- Forward running
- Lower extremity PRE and flexibility programs
- Forward Step-Down Test (NeuroCom, Clackamas, OR)
- Active knee extension-PRE (OKC) to ROM 80 to 0 degrees
- NO resistive (OKC) hamstring exercises

CRITERIA FOR ADVANCEMENT
- ROM to WNL
- Demonstrate ability to descend an 8-inch step with good leg control without pain
- Functional progression pending functional assessment
- Improved flexibility to meet demands of running and sport-specific activities

Postoperative Phase IV (Weeks 20 and Beyond)

GOALS
• Hop test ≥85% limb symmetry
• Isokinetic testing ≥85% limb symmetry
• Lack of apprehension with sport-specific movements
• Maximize strength and flexibility to meet demands of individual's sport activity

PRECAUTIONS
• Avoid pain with therapeutic exercise and functional activities
• Protect patellofemoral joint
• Avoid sport activity until adequate strength development and surgeon's clearance

TREATMENT STRATEGIES
• Continue lower extremity strengthening, leg press, squat, OKC extension 0- to 90-degree arc
• Lower extremity flexibility program
• Advance proprioception training
• Advance forward running program
• Advance plyometric program (sport-specific)
• Sport-specific agility activities
• Isokinetic training/testing
• Functional testing
• Knee ligament arthrometer exam at 6 months
• Home therapeutic exercise program: evaluation-based

CRITERIA FOR DISCHARGE
• Hop test ≥85% limb symmetry
• Isokinetic test ≥85% limb symmetry
• Lack of apprehension with sport-specific movements
• Flexibility to accepted levels for sport performance
• Independence with gym program for maintenance and progression of therapeutic exercise program at discharge

Bibliography

Bach, B.R. Jr. Graft Selection for Posterior Cruciate Ligament Surgery. *Oper Tech Sports Med* 1993;1:104-109.

Butler, D.L., Noyes, F.R., Grood, E.S. Ligamentus Restraints to Anterior-Posterior Drawer in the Human Knee. A Biomechanical Study. *J Bone Joint Surg* 1980;62A:259-270.

Clancy, W.G. Jr., Bisson, L.J. Double Tunnel Technique for Reconstruction of the Posterior Cruciate Ligament. *Oper Tech Sports Med* 1999;7:110-117.

Clancy, W.G. Jr Repair and Reconstruction of the Posterior Cruciate Ligament. In Chapman, M.W. (Ed). Operative Orthopaedics. JB Lippincott, Philadelphia, 1988, pp. 1651-1666.

Cooper, D.E., Warren, R.F., Warner, J.P. The PCL and Posterolateral Structures of the Knee: Anatomy, Function, and Patterns of Injury. *Instr Course Lect* 1991;40:249-270.

Cross, M.J., Powell, J.F. Long-term Follow-up of Posterior Cruciate Ligament Rupture: A Study of 116 Cases. *Am J Sports Med* 1984; 12:292-297.

Dejour, H., Walsh, G., Peyrot, J. The Natural History of Rupture of the PCL. *J Orthop Surg* 1988;2:112-120.

Fanelli, G.C. Posterior Cruciate Ligament Injuries in Trauma Patients. *Arthroscopy* 1993;9:291-294.

Fowler, P.J., Messieh, S.S. Isolated Posterior Cruciate Ligament Injuries in Athletes. *Am J Sports Med* 1987;15:553-557.

Girgis, F.G., Marshall, J.L., Al Monajem, A.R. The Cruciate Ligaments of the Knee Joint: Anatomical, Functional and Experimental Analysis. *Clin Orthop* 1975;106:216-231.

Harner, C.D., Höher, J. Evaluation and Treatment of Posterior Cruciate Ligament Injuries. *Am J Sports Med* 1998;26:471-482.

Harner, C.D., Xerogeanes, J.W., Livesay, G.A., Carlin, G.J., Smith, B.A., Kusayama, T., Kashiwaguchi, S., Woo, S.L. The Human Posterior Cruciate Ligament Complex: An Interdisciplinary Study. Ligament Morphology and Biomechanical Evaluation. *Am J Sports Med* 1995;23:736-745.

Kannus, P., Bergfeld, J., Jarvinen, M., Johnson, R.J., Pope, M., Renstrom, P., Yasuda, K. Injuries to the Posterior Cruciate Ligament of the Knee. *Sports Med* 1991;12(2):110-131.

Miyasaka, K.C., Daniel, D.M., Stone, M.L., Hirschman, P. The Incidence of Knee Ligament Injuries in the General Population. *Am J Knee Surg* 1991;4:3-8.

Parolie, J.M., Bergfeld, J.A. Long-term Results of Nonoperative Treatment of Isolated Posterior Cruciate Ligament Injuries in the Athlete. *Am J Sports Med* 1986;14(1):35-38.

Race, A., Amis, A.A. PCL Reconstruction: In Vitro Biomechanical Comparison of "Isometric" Versus Single and Double-bundle "Anatomic" Grafts. *J Bone Joint Surg* 1998;80B:173-179.

Race, A., Amis, A.A. The Mechanical Properties of the Two Bundles of the Human Posterior Cruciate Ligament. *J Biomech* 1994;27:13-24.

Torg, J.S., Barton, T.M. Natural History of the Posterior Cruciate Deficient Knee. *Clin Orthop* 1989;246:208-216.

Van Dommelen, B.A., Fowler, P.J. Anatomy of the Posterior Cruciate Ligament. A Review. *Am J Sports Med* 1989;17:24-29.

CHAPTER 37

Meniscal Repair and Transplantation

John T. Cavanaugh, PT, MEd, ATC

Coleen T. Gately, PT, DPT, MS

Meniscal cartilage plays a significant role in the function and biomechanics of the knee joint. The meniscus functions in load bearing, load transmission, shock absorption, joint stability, joint lubrication, and joint congruity. The meniscus can fail from either mechanical or biochemical (degenerative) causes. The most common mechanism of injury to the menisci involves noncontact forces. Stress across the knee joint from a sudden acceleration or deceleration movement, in conjunction with a change in direction, can trap the menisci between the tibia and femur, resulting in a tear. As a result of these traumas, the patient may present with pain, effusion, locking, and persistent focal joint line tenderness.

If conservative treatment proves to be unsuccessful, surgical intervention is often necessary. Meniscal tear pattern, geometry, site, vascularity, size, stability, tissue viability or quality, as well as associated pathology, are all taken into account when determining whether to resect or repair a meniscal lesion. The literature has demonstrated that removal of the meniscus leads to degenerative changes of the knee joint. Partial meniscectomy when compared with total meniscectomy, reduces the degeneration of articular cartilage. However, results of stresses on the underlying cartilage following partial meniscectomy have been reported to be higher than normal. Therefore, attempts to preserve the injured meniscus are made whenever possible.

The first reported meniscal repair was reported by Annandale in 1885. The goal of a meniscus repair is to allow the torn edges of the meniscus to heal once they have been fixated with sutures. Meniscal repair techniques have evolved from the placement of sutures across the torn meniscus through arthrotomy to using arthroscopy. Published meniscal repair results have supported favorable success at extended follow-up in over 70% to 90% of patients.

As a means to address symptomatic meniscal-deficient patients, the meniscal transplantation procedure was introduced by Milachowski and colleagues in 1984. Ideal candidates for this procedure include patient's whose knees are normally aligned, stable, and demonstrate little degenerative changes. Meniscal transplantation may also be indicated during concomitant anterior cruciate ligament reconstruction, because absence of the meniscus could preclude satisfactory stabilization. Contraindications for meniscal transplantation include advanced articular cartilage wear (especially on the flexion weight-bearing zone of the condyle), axial misalignment, and flattening of the femoral condyle. Reports from 2002 suggest that more than 4000 meniscal transplants have been performed since 1991, with an estimated 800-plus menisci implanted annually. When properly indicated and performed, transplantation leads to good results in over 90% of patients.

Rehabilitation following these procedures are crucial toward the attainment of optimal functional outcome. In this chapter we will discuss the Hospital for Special Surgery's (HSS) clinical guidelines following meniscal repair and transplantation.

Surgical Overview

- The menisci are wedge-shaped crescents of fibrocartilage found between the femur and tibia.
- The menisci allows for a more congruous articulation between the already incongruent femoral condyle and tibial plateau.
- The lateral meniscus is O-shaped, whereas the medial meniscus is C-shaped.
- The lateral meniscus picks up 70% of the load transmitted across the lateral compartment, whereas the medial meniscus and articular cartilage share the load.

- Each meniscus is divided anatomically into horizontal thirds: the posterior horn, mid-body, and anterior horn.
- Menisci are divided into vertical thirds when looking at blood supply. The outer edge of each meniscus has a rich blood supply from the medial and lateral genicular arteries.
  1. Vascularization decreases approaching the inner portion of the meniscus and becomes dependent upon diffusion.
  2. Because of the poor blood supply, tears that approach the inner avascular area have a more difficult time with healing.
  3. Arnoczky and Warren have reported that to allow meniscal tears to heal, the tear needs to be in contact with the peripheral vascular area.
- The surgical management of repairing meniscal tears varies.
  1. In relatively stable tears, the literature has reported the use of rasping and trephination.
  2. Arthroscopic meniscal repair techniques can be divided into three techniques, based upon suture placement. They include an inside-out repair, outside-in repair, and all-inside repair.
- The arthroscopic inside-out surgical technique involves the placement of sutures across the meniscus inside the joint, and the sutures are then tied down outside the joint capsule. This technique has been successful with tears to the middle one-third and, to some degree, tears of the posterior horns.
- The arthroscopic outside-in surgical technique involves the placement of a suture with a Mulberry knot to one side of the meniscal tear inside the joint, and then sutures are tied on the joint capsule. This technique has been advocated in repairing tears to the mid-one-third and anterior horn regions.
- The arthroscopic all-inside surgical technique involves the placement of a suture, screws, and/or darts through an arthroscopic portal to stabilize the tear.
  1. Because it does not make use of any incisions, the all-inside technique is favorable in decreasing the risk of iatrogenic neurovascular damage.

2. This technique has favorable results for posterior horn tears.

- Meniscus allograft transplant (MAT) has evolved into a primarily arthroscopic technique in which a cadaveric meniscus is inserted into a meniscus deficient knee.

    1. The cadaveric meniscus is supplied by a tissue bank. Although there are no set standards, most tissue banks determine implant size through estimates made from radiographs.
    2. Following a diagnostic arthroscopy of the knee, the native meniscus is removed.
    3. Different techniques have evolved in transplanting medial or lateral menisci.

- With a medial meniscus replacement, two bone plugs, one to the anterior horn and another to the posterior horn, are inserted in their respective tibial tunnels while sutures along the rim hold the graft in place.

- With lateral meniscus transplantation, a rectangular bone trough is created between the anterior and posterior lateral meniscal attachment sites. Suture placement holds the meniscus in place.

Rehabilitation Overview

- Rehabilitation programs following meniscal repair and transplantation should reflect an optimal environment for healing.

- Surgical technique, type of repair fixation, location of the repair, concomitant procedures, and surgeon's preference will have a direct influence on weight-bearing status, range of motion (ROM) restrictions, and treatment progressions. Therefore, communication between the surgeon and rehabilitation specialist, particularly in the early protective phases of rehabilitation, is vital.

- Customarily, following meniscal repair and transplantation procedures, immediate ROM is encouraged. Early motion has been shown to minimize the deleterious effects of immobilization, such as articular cartilage degeneration, excessive adverse collagen formation, and pain.

- Weight-bearing following meniscal repair will be typically progressive throughout the early postoperative period.

- Weight-bearing following meniscal transplantation and meniscal repairs involving complex or radial tears will be limited to toe-touch ambulation for the first 4 weeks.
- The involved knee is maintained in full extension, donning a double-upright hinged brace locked at 0 degrees during the designated protection phase, regardless of which meniscal procedure was performed.
- The pre-surgical status of the patient, any associated pathology, and a comprehensive evaluation will each play an important factor in designing an individualized rehabilitation program for each patient.
  1. An elite athlete may progress faster as a result of greater preoperative muscle strength as compared to a nonathlete in weak physical condition.
  2. Patients with degenerative joint disease may need a slower weight-bearing progression.
  3. Patients with patellofemoral disorders may or may not be candidates for certain isotonic or isokinetic knee extension exercises.
- Subjective complaints and physical findings ascertained during evaluations and continual reassessments will direct the rehabilitation program to the proper speed and direction.
- The realistic goals of the patient, surgeon, and rehabilitation specialist should be discussed and defined early in the postoperative course.
  1. The patient should be brought to understand the magnitude of his or her surgery and the timetable for recovery.
  2. Goals should be specific and functional to the individual needs of the patient.
- The patient should be made aware of his or her role in the rehabilitative process. The patient's compliance to activity modifications and home therapeutic exercises is vital for a successful outcome.
- Postoperative guidelines following these procedures abide by a criteria-based progression. ROM and strength requirements are to be met before advancement to subsequent phases.

Meniscal Repair Guidelines Postoperative Phase I (Weeks 0 to 6)

GOALS
- Emphasis on full passive extension
- Control postoperative pain/swelling
- ROM to 90-degree flexion
- Regain quadriceps control
- Independence in home therapeutic exercise program

PRECAUTIONS
- Avoid active knee flexion
- Avoid ambulation without brace locked at 0 degrees before 4 weeks
- Avoid prolonged standing/walking

TREATMENT STRATEGIES
- Towel extensions, prone hangs, and so on
- Quadriceps reeducation (quadriceps sets with electrical muscle stimulator [EMS] or electromyography [EMG])
- Progressive weight-bearing PWB to WBAT with brace locked at 0 degrees with crutches
- Toe-touch weight-bearing for complex or radial tears
- Patellar mobilization
- Active-assisted flexion/extension 90- to 0-degree exercise
- SLRs (all planes)
- Hip PREs
- Proprioception board (bilateral weight-bearing)
- Aquatic therapy-pool ambulation or underwater treadmill (weeks 4 to 6)
- Short crank ergometry (if ROM>85 degrees)
- Leg press (bilateral/60- to 0-degree arc) (if ROM>85 degrees)
- OKC quadriceps isometrics (submaximal/bilateral at 60 degrees) (if ROM>85 degrees)
- Upper extremity cardiovascular exercises as tolerated
- Hamstring and calf stretching
- Cryotherapy
- Emphasize patient compliance to home therapeutic exercise program and weight-bearing and ROM precautions/progression

Continued

Meniscal Repair Guidelines Postoperative Phase I (Weeks 0 to 6)—Cont'd

CRITERIA FOR ADVANCEMENT
- Ability to SLR without quadriceps lag
- ROM 0 to 90 degrees
- Demonstrate ability to unilateral (involved extremity) weight-bear without pain

Meniscal Repair Guidelines Postoperative Phase II (Weeks 6 to 14)

GOALS
- Restore full ROM
- Restore normal gait (non-antalgic)
- Demonstrate ability to ascend and descend 8-inch stairs with good leg control without pain
- Improve ADL endurance
- Improve lower extremity flexibility
- Independence in home therapeutic exercise program

PRECAUTIONS
- Avoid descending stairs reciprocally until adequate quadriceps control and lower extremity alignment
- Avoid pain with therapeutic exercise and functional activities
- Avoid running and sport activity

TREATMENT STRATEGIES
- Progressive weight-bearing/WBAT with crutches/cane (brace opened 0 to 60 degrees), if good quadriceps control (good quadriceps set/ability to SLR without lag or pain)
- Aquatic therapy—pool ambulation or underwater treadmill
- Discontinue crutches/cane when gait is non-antalgic
- Brace changed to surgeon's preference (OTS brace, patellar sleeve, etc.)
- AAROM exercises
- Patellar mobilization
- SLRs (all planes) with weights
- Proximal PREs
- Neuromuscular training (bilateral to unilateral support)

- Balance apparatus, foam surface, perturbations
- Short crank ergometry
- Standard ergometry (if knee ROM > 115 degrees)
- Leg press (bilateral/eccentric/unilateral progression)
- Squat program (PRE) 0 to 60 degrees
- OKC quadriceps isotonics (pain-free arc of motion) (CKC preferred)
- Initiate forward step-up and step-down programs
- StairMaster
- Retrograde treadmill ambulation
- Quadriceps stretching
- Elliptical machine
- Forward Step-Down Test (NeuroCom)
- Upper extremity cardiovascular exercises as tolerated
- Cryotherapy
- Emphasize patient compliance to home therapeutic exercise program

CRITERIA FOR ADVANCEMENT
- ROM to WNL
- Ability to descend 8-inch stairs with good leg control without pain

Meniscal Repair Guidelines Postoperative Phase III (Weeks 14 to 22)

GOALS
- Demonstrate ability to run pain-free
- Maximize strength and flexibility as to meet demands of ADL
- Hop test ≥85% limb symmetry
- Isokinetic test >85% limb symmetry
- Lack of apprehension with sport-specific movements
- Flexibility to accepted levels of sport performance
- Independence with gym program for maintenance and progression of therapeutic exercise program at discharge

PRECAUTIONS
- Avoid pain with therapeutic exercise and functional activities

Continued

Meniscal Repair Guidelines Postoperative Phase III (Weeks 14 to 22)—Cont'd

- Avoid sport activity until adequate strength development and surgeon's clearance

TREATMENT STRATEGIES
- Progress squat program <90-degree flexion
- Lunges
- Retrograde treadmill running
- Start forward running (treadmill) program at 4 months postoperatively if 8-inch step down satisfactory
- Continue lower extremity strengthening and flexibility programs
- Agility program/sport-specific (sports cord)
- Start plyometric program when strength base is sufficient
- Isotonic knee flexion/extension (pain- and crepitus-free arc)
- Isokinetic training (fast to moderate to slow velocities)
- Functional testing (hop test)
- Isokinetic testing
- Home therapeutic exercise program: evaluation-based

CRITERIA FOR ADVANCEMENT
- Symptom-free running and sport-specific agility
- Hop test ≥85% limb symmetry
- Isokinetic test >85% limb symmetry
- Lack of apprehension with sport-specific movements
- Flexibility to accepted levels of sport performance
- Independence with gym program for maintenance and progression of therapeutic exercise program at discharge

Meniscal Transplantation Guidelines Postoperative Phase I (Weeks 0 to 6)

GOALS
- Emphasis on full passive extension
- Control postoperative pain/swelling
- ROM to 90-degree flexion

- Regain quadriceps control
- Independence in home therapeutic exercise program

PRECAUTIONS
- Avoid active knee flexion
- Avoid ambulation without brace locked at 0 degrees before 4 weeks
- Avoid prolonged standing/walking

TREATMENT STRATEGIES
- Towel extensions, prone hangs, and so on
- Quadriceps reeducation (quadriceps sets with EMS or EMG)
- Toe-touch weight-bearing with brace locked at 0 degrees, with crutches for 4 weeks
- Progressive weight-bearing PWB to WBAT, weeks 4 to 6
- Patellar mobilization
- CPM machine
- Active-assisted flexion/extension 90- to 0-degree exercise
- SLRs (all planes)
- Hip PREs
- Proprioception board (bilateral weight-bearing)
- Aquatic therapy—pool ambulation or underwater treadmill (weeks 4 to 6)
- Short crank ergometry (if ROM>85 degrees)
- Leg press (bilateral/60- to 0-degree arc) (if ROM>85 degrees) (weeks 4 to 6)
- OKC quadriceps isometrics (submaximal/bilateral at 60 degrees) (if ROM>85 degrees)
- Upper extremity cardiovascular exercises as tolerated
- Hamstring and calf stretching
- Cryotherapy
- Emphasize patient compliance to home therapeutic exercise program and weight-bearing and ROM precautions/progression

CRITERIA FOR ADVANCEMENT
- Ability to SLR without quadriceps lag
- ROM 0 to 90 degrees
- Demonstrate ability to unilateral (involved extremity) weight-bear without pain

Meniscal Transplantation Guidelines
Postoperative Phase II (Weeks 6 to 14)

GOALS
- Restore full ROM
- Restore normal gait (non-antalgic)
- Demonstrate ability to ascend 8-inch stairs with good leg control without pain
- Improve ADL endurance
- Improve lower extremity flexibility
- Independence in home therapeutic exercise program

PRECAUTIONS
- Avoid descending stairs reciprocally until adequate quadriceps control and lower extremity alignment
- Avoid pain with therapeutic exercise and functional activities
- Avoid running and sport activity

TREATMENT STRATEGIES
- Progressive weight-bearing/WBAT with crutches/cane (brace opened 0 to 60 degrees), of good quadriceps control (good quadriceps set/ability to SLR without lag or pain)
- Aquatic therapy—pool ambulation or underwater treadmill
- D/C crutches/cane when gait is non-antalgic
- Brace changed to surgeon's preference (OTS brace, patellar sleeve, etc.)
- AAROM exercises
- Patellar mobilization
- SLRs (all planes) with weights
- Proximal PREs
- Neuromuscular training (bilateral to unilateral support)
- Balance apparatus, foam surface, perturbations
- Short crank ergometry
- Standard ergometry (if knee ROM > 115 degrees)
- Leg press (bilateral/eccentric/unilateral progression)
- Squat program (PRE) 0 to 45 degrees
- OKC quadriceps isotonics (pain-free arc of motion; CKC preferred)
- Initiate forward step-up program
- StairMaster
- Retrograde treadmill ambulation

- Quadriceps stretching
- Elliptical machine
- Upper extremity cardiovascular exercises as tolerated
- Cryotherapy
- Emphasize patient compliance to home therapeutic exercise program

CRITERIA FOR ADVANCEMENT
- ROM to WNL
- Ability to descend 8-inch stairs with good leg control without pain

Meniscal Transplantation Guidelines Postoperative Phase III (Weeks 14 to 22)

GOALS
- Maximize strength and flexibility as to meet demands of ADL
- Demonstrate ability to descend 8-inch stairs with good leg control without pain
- Isokinetic test >75% limb symmetry
- Independence with gym program for maintenance and progression of therapeutic exercise program at discharge

PRECAUTIONS
- Avoid pain with therapeutic exercise and functional activities
- Avoid sport activity until adequate strength development and surgeon's clearance

TREATMENT STRATEGIES
- Progress squat program <60-degree flexion
- Continue lower extremity strengthening and flexibility programs
- Initiate forward step-down program
- Forward Step-Down Test (NeuroCom)
- Isotonic knee flexion/extension (pain- and crepitus-free arc)
- Isokinetic training (fast to moderate to slow velocities)

Continued

**Meniscal Transplantation
Guidelines Postoperative Phase III
(Weeks 14 to 22)—Cont'd**

- Isokinetic testing
- Home therapeutic exercise program:
  evaluation-based

CRITERIA FOR ADVANCEMENT
- Isokinetic test >75% limb symmetry
- Ability to descend 8-inch stairs with good leg control
  without pain

**Meniscal Transplantation Guidelines
Postoperative Phase IV (Weeks 22 to 30)**

GOALS
- Demonstrate ability to run pain-free
- Maximize strength and flexibility as to meet demands of
  recreational activity
- Isokinetic test >85% limb symmetry
- Lack of apprehension with recreation-type sport
  movements
- Independence with gym program for maintenance and
  progression of therapeutic exercise program at discharge

PRECAUTIONS
- Avoid pain with therapeutic exercise and functional
  activities
- Avoid sport activity until adequate strength development
  and surgeon's clearance

TREATMENT STRATEGIES
- Progress squat program <90-degree flexion
- Retrograde treadmill running
- Start forward running (treadmill) program at 6 months
  postoperatively if 8-inch step-down satisfactory
- Continue lower extremity strengthening and flexibility
  programs
- Isotonic knee extension (pain- and crepitus-free arc)
- Isokinetic training (fast to moderate to slow velocities)
- Isokinetic testing
- Home therapeutic exercise program: evaluation-based

CRITERIA FOR ADVANCEMENT
- Symptom free running (if appropriate)
- Isokinetic test >85% limb symmetry
- Flexibility to accepted levels of recreational activity
- Independence with gym program for maintenance and progression of therapeutic exercise program at discharge

Bibliography

Akeson, W.H., Woo, S.L., Amiel, D., Coutts, R.D., Daniel, D. The Connective Tissue Response to Immobility: Biomechanical Changes in Periarticular Connective Tissue of the Immobilized Rabbit Knee. *Clin Orthop* 1973;93:356-362.

Albrecht-Olsen, P., Kristensen, G., Burgaard, P., Joergensen, U., Toerholem, C. The Arrow Versus Horizontal Suture in Arthroscopic Meniscus Repair. A Prospective Randomized Study with Arthroscopic Evaluation. *Knee Surg Sports Traumatol Arthrosc* 1999;7(5):268-273.

Allen, C.R., Wong, E.K., Livesay, G.A., Sakare, M., Fu, F.H., Woo, S.L. The Importance of the Medial Meniscus in the Anterior-Cruciate Ligament-Deficient Knee. *J Orthop Res* 2000;18(1):109-115.

Allen, P.R., Denham, R.A., Swan, A.V. Late Degenerative Changes after Meniscectomy. Factors Affecting the Knee after Operation. *J Bone Joint Surg Br* 1984;66(5):666-671.

Annandale, T. An Operation for Displaced Semilunar Cartilage. *Br Med J* 1885;1:779.

Arnoczky, S.P., Warren, R.F. Microvasculature of the Human Meniscus. *Am J Sports Med* 1982;10(2):90-95.

Belzer, J., Cannon, W. Meniscal Tears: Treatment in the Stable and Unstable Knee. *J Am Acad Orthop Surg* 1993;1(1):41-47.

Cannon, W.D. Jr., Morgan, C.D. Meniscal Repair. Part II: Arthroscopic Repair Techniques. *J Bone Joint Surg* 1994;76A:294-311.

Cannon, W.D., Vittori, J.M. The Incidence of Healing in an Arthroscopic Meniscal Repairs in ACL-Reconstructed Knees Versus Stable Knees. *Am J Sports Med* 1992;20(2):176-181.

Cavanaugh, J.T. Rehabilitation Following Meniscal Surgery. In Engle, R.P. (Ed). Knee Ligament Rehabilitation. Churchill Livingstone, New York, 1991, pp. 59-69.

Chen, M.I., Branch, T.P., Hutton, W.C. Is It Important to Secure the Horns During Lateral Meniscal Transplantation? A Cadaveric Study. *Arthroscopy* 1996;12(2):174-181.

Cole, B.J., Carter, T.R., Rodeo, S.A. Allograft Meniscal Transplantation: Background, Techniques, and Results. *Instr Course Lect* 2003;52:383-396.

Day, B., Mackenzie, W.G., Shim, S.S., Leung, G. The Vascular and Nerve Supply of the Human Meniscus. *Arthroscopy* 1985;1(1):58-62.

Fairbank, T.J. Knee Joint Changes after Meniscectomy. *J Bone Joint Surg Br* 1948;30B(4):664-670.

Ferkel, R.D., Davis, J.R., Friedman, M.J., Fox, J.M., DelPizzo, W., Snyder, S.J., Berasi, C.C. Arthroscopic Partial Medial Meniscectomy: An Analysis of Unsatisfactory Results. *Arthroscopy* 1985;1(1):44-52.

Gillquist, J., Messner, K. Long-term Results of Meniscal Repair. *Sports Med Arthrosc* 1993;1:159-163.

Henning, C.E. Arthroscopic Repair of Meniscal Tears. *Orthopedics* 1983;6:1130-1132.

Jorgensen, U., Sonne-Holm, S., Lauridsen, F., Rosenklint, A. Long-term Follow-up of Meniscectomy in Athletes. A Prospective Longitudinal Study. *J Bone Joint Surg Br* 1987;69B(1):80-83.

Kurosawa, H., Fukubayashi, T., Nakajima, H. Load-bearing Mode of the Knee Joint: Physical Behavior of the Knee Joint with or without Menisci. *Clin Orthop Relat Res* 1980;149:283-290.

Levy, I.M., Torzilli, P.A., Warren, R.F. The Effect of Medial Meniscectomy on Anterior-Posterior Motion of the Knee. *J Bone Joint Surg Am* 1982;64A(6):883-888.

McGinty, J.B., Geuss, L.F., Marvin, R.A. Partial or Total Meniscectomy. A Comparative Analysis. *J Bone Joint Surg Am* 1977;59:763-766.

Milachowski, K.A., Weismeier, K., Wirth, C.J. Homologous Meniscus Transplantation. Experimental and Clinical Results. *Int Orthop* 1989;13(1):1-11.

Morgan, C.D., Casscells, S.W. Arthroscopic Meniscus Repair: A Safe Approach to the Posterior Horns. *Arthroscopy* 1986;2(1):3-12.

Morgan, C.D. The "All-inside" Meniscus Repair. *Arthroscopy* 1991; 7(1):120-125.

Northmore-Ball, M.D., Dandy, D.J., Jackson, R.W. Arthroscopic Open Partial and Total Meniscectomy. A Comparative Study. *J Bone Joint Surg Br* 1983;65(4):400-404.

Noyes, F.R., Barber-Westin, S.B., Rankin, M.D., Rankin, M. Meniscal Transplantation in Symptomatic Patients Less Than Fifty Years Old. *J Bone Joint Surg* 2004;86A(7):1392-1404.

Noyes, F.R., Mangine, R.E., Barber, S. Early Knee Motion after Open and Arthroscopic ACL Reconstruction. *Am J Sports Med* 1987;15(2):149-160.

Okuda, K., Ochi, M., Shu, N., Uchio, Y. Meniscal Rasping for Repair of Meniscal Tear in the Avascular Zone. *Arthroscopy* 1999;15(3): 281–286.

Pollard, M.E., Kang, Q., Berg, E.E. Radiographic Sizing for Meniscal Transplantation. *Arthroscopy* 1995;11(6):684–687.

Radin, E.L. Factors Influencing the Progression of Osteoarthrosis. In Ewing, J.W (Ed). Articular Cartilage and Knee Joint Function. Raven Press, New York, 1990, pp. 301–309.

Rodeo, S.A. Arthroscopic Meniscal Repair with Use of the Outside-in Technique. *J Bone Joint Surg Am* 2000;82(1):127–141.

Rodeo, S. Meniscal Allografts—Where Do We Stand? *Am J Sports Med* 2001;29(2):246–261.

Salter, R.B., Simmonds, D.F., Malcolm, B.W., Rumble, E.J., MacMichael, D., Clements, N.D. The Biological Effect of Continuous Passive Motion on the Healing of Full-thickness Defects in Articular Cartilage. An Experimental Investigation in the Rabbit. *J Bone Joint Surg* 1980;62A(8):1232–1251.

Scott, G.A., Jolly, B.C., Henning, C.E. Combined Posterior Incision and Arthroscopic Intra-articular Repair of the Meniscus. An Examination of Factors Affecting Healing. *J Bone Joint Surg Am* 1986;68(6): 847–861.

Sgaglione, N.A., Steadman, J.R., Shaffer, B., Miller, M.D., Fu, F.H. Current Concepts in Meniscus Surgery: Resection to Replacement. *Arthroscopy* 2003;19(Suppl 1):161–188.

Shaffer, B., Kennedy, S., Klimkiewicz, J., Yao, L. Preoperative Sizing of Meniscal Allografts in Meniscus Transplantation. *Am J Sports Med* 2000;28(4):524–533.

Sommerlath, K., Gillquist, J. Knee Function after Meniscus Repair and Total Meniscectomy: A 7-year Follow-up Study. *Arthroscopy* 1987; 3(3):166–169.

Stone, K.R., Rosenberg, T. Surgical Technique of Meniscal Replacement Arthroscopy. *J Arthrosc Relat Surg* 1993;9(2): 234–237.

Uchio, Y., Ochi, M., Adachi, N., Kawasaki, K., Iwasa, J. Results of Rasping of Meniscal Tears with and without Anterior Cruciate Ligament Injury as Evaluated by Second-look Arthroscopy. *Arthroscopy* 2003;19(5):463–469.

van Arkel, E.R., deBoer, H.H. Human Meniscal Transplantation. Preliminary Results at 2- to 5-year Follow-up. *J Bone Joint Surg Br* 1995;77(4):589–595.

Walker, P.S., Erkman, M.J. The Role of the Menisci in Force Transmission Across the Knee. *Clin Orthop Relat Res* 1975;109: 184–192.

Wirth, C.J., Peters, G. Meniscus Injuries of the Knee Joint: Pathophysiology and Treatment Principles. In Baillière's Clinical Orthopedics: Baillière Tindall. London, 1997, pp. 123–144.

Zhang, Z., Arnold, J.A., Williams, T., McCann, B. Repair by Trephination and Suturing of Longitudinal Injuries in the Avascular Area of the Meniscus in Goats. *Am J Sports Med* 1995;23(1):35–41.

Chapter 38

Achilles Tendon Repair

Robert A. Maschi, PT, DPT, CSCS

Heather M. Cloutman, PT, MSPT, CSCS

Nicole Fritz, PT, DPT

The incidence of Achilles tendon rupture is increasing in Western society where lifestyles are sedentary and interest in athletic activities has increased. Acute ruptures are commonly associated with white-collar professional men in the third or fourth decades of life who are involved in recreational athletics. The majority of injuries occur during racquet or ball sports, which involve acceleration/deceleration mechanisms, sprint starts and jumping. Traumatic injury is another common cause of acute Achilles tendon rupture, including falling from a height, falling down stairs, or slipping into a hole.

Operative repair of an Achilles tendon rupture combined with early rehabilitation enables the patient to return to preinjury functional level, achieve normal ankle range of motion (ROM), and decrease the risk of rerupture. The Hospital for Special Surgery (HSS) Achilles tendon repair rehabilitation guideline is presented.

Surgical Overview

- Open repair of the Achilles tendon is accomplished by exposing the tendon via an incision on the posterior aspect of the leg.
- The paratenon is opened and the tendon ends are juxtaposed and sutured together. Many different suture techniques can be used, and these vary among surgeons.
- If the tendon ends are frayed where the Achilles has ruptured often a circumferential suture is used as well. The repair can be reinforced with the plantaris tendon grafts.

- The paratenon is closed and then the skin is closed and covered with a sterile dressing.
- A plantar splint is placed at this time to prevent dorsiflexion, which could disrupt the repair. Some surgeons prefer to use a cast or an anterior splint.
- A Cam walker boot can also be used after sutures are removed in 10 to 14 days, which allows for examination of the wound and early mobilization.
- Meticulous soft tissue handling and closure of the paratenon are key elements of the procedure.

Rehabilitation Overview

- The rehabilitation program following Achilles tendon repair begins 2 to 6 weeks postoperatively.
- Special attention must be given by the rehabilitation specialist to protect the repair. For example, it is imperative that passive heel cord stretching is avoided until at least 12 weeks postoperatively. In addition, weight-bearing should be progressed incrementally and guided by communication with the surgeon.
- The clinician must consider the four phases of tendon healing (inflammation, proliferation, remodeling, and maturation) throughout the progression of the postoperative rehabilitation program.
- The tendon is weakest during the first 6 weeks of healing (inflammation and proliferation phases) and then slowly increases in strength over the next 6 weeks to 12 months (remodeling and maturation phases).
- The patient is progressed via criteria-based functional progression.

Postoperative Phase I: Protection and Healing (Weeks 1 to 6)

GOALS
- Protect repair
- Control edema and pain
- Minimize scar formation
- Improve ROM of dorsiflexion to neutral (0 degrees)
- Increase proximal lower extremity musculature 5/5 in all planes

- Progressive weight-bearing–surgeon directed
- Independence in home exercise program

PRECAUTIONS
- Avoid passive heel cord stretching
- Limit active dorsiflexion ROM to neutral (0 degrees) with knee flexed at 90 degrees
- Avoid heat application
- Avoid prolonged dependent position

TREATMENT STRATEGIES
- Progress weight-bearing status in the Cam boot with crutches or cane-surgeon directed
- AROM dorsiflexion/plantar flexion/inversion/eversion
- Scar massage
- Joint mobilizations
- Proximal musculature strengthening
- Modalities
- Cryotherapy

CRITERIA FOR ADVANCEMENT
- Pain and edema controlled
- Weight-bearing status-surgeon directed
- ROM dorsiflexion to neutral (0 degrees)
- Proximal lower extremity muscle strength 5/5

Postoperative Phase II: Early Mobilization (Weeks 6 to 12)

GOALS
- Normalize gait
- Restore full functional ROM necessary for normal gait (15-degree dorsiflexion) and for ascending stairs (25 degrees)
- Normalize dorsiflexion, inversion, and eversion ankle strength 5/5

PRECAUTIONS
- Avoid pain with therapeutic exercise and functional activities
- Avoid passive heel cord stretching

Continued

Postoperative Phase II: Early Mobilization (Weeks 6 to 12)—Cont'd

TREATMENT STRATEGIES
- Gait training WBAT to FWB with/without orthoses or assistive device
  1. d/c crutches when gait is non-antalgic
- Underwater treadmill system for gait training
- Heel lift in shoe to assist nonapprehensive and normalized gait
- AROM dorsiflexion/plantar flexion/inversion/eversion
- Proprioception training: BAPS
- Isometrics/isotonics: inversion/eversion
- Week 6: PREs plantar flexion/dorsiflexion with knee flexed to 90 degrees
- Week 8: PREs plantar flexion/dorsiflexion with knee extended 0 degrees
- Plantar flexor strengthening using a leg press and leg curl machine
- Bike
- Alphabet drawing using multiaxial plate
- Retro treadmill
- Modalities
- Scar massage
- Forward step-up program

CRITERIA FOR ADVANCEMENT
- Normal gait pattern
- Full PROM dorsiflexion, 20 degrees
- Manual muscle test grade of 5/5 for dorsiflexion, inversion, and eversion

Note: PREs for the proximal musculature of the involved extremity are advanced.

Phase III: Early Strengthening (Weeks 12 to 20)

GOALS
- Restore full AROM
- Normalize plantar flexion strength 5/5
- Normalize balance (tested using NeuroCom or Biodex Balance System)
- Return to functional activities without pain
- Ability to descend stairs

PRECAUTIONS
- Avoid pain with therapeutic exercise and functional activities
- Avoid high loading the Achilles tendon (i.e., aggressive stretching in dorsiflexion with body weight or jumping)

TREATMENT STRATEGIES
- Inversion/eversion isotonics/isokinetics
- Bike, StairMaster, VersaClimber
- Proprioception training: Prop board/BAPS/foam rollers/trampoline/NeuroCom
- Aggressive plantar flexion PREs (emphasize eccentric activity)
- Submaximal sport-specific skill development
- Progress proprioception program
- Running in underwater treadmill system
- Progress proximal strengthening of lower extremities (PREs)
- Isokinetic PF/DF
- Flexibility as needed for activity
- Forward step-down program

CRITERIA FOR ADVANCEMENT
- No apprehension with ADL
- Normal flexibility
- Adequate strength base shown by ability to perform 10 unilateral heel raises
- Ability to descend stairs reciprocally
- Symmetrical lower extremity balance

Postoperative Phase IV: Late Strengthening (Weeks 20 to 28)

GOALS
- Demonstrate ability to run forward on a treadmill symptom-free
- Average peak torque of 75% with isokinetic testing
- Maximize strength and flexibility as to meet all demands of ADL
- Return to functional activity without limitation

Continued

Postoperative Phase IV: Late Strengthening (Weeks 20 to 28)—Cont'd

- Higher level dynamic activity with lack of apprehension with sport-specific movements

PRECAUTIONS
- No apprehension or pain with dynamic activity
- Avoid running or sport activity until adequate strength and flexibility is achieved

TREATMENT STRATEGIES
- Start forward treadmill running
- Isokinetic testing and training
- Continue lower extremity strengthening and flexibility program
- Advance proprioception training with perturbation
- Light plyometric training (bilateral jumping activities)
- Continue aggressive plantar flexion PREs (emphasize eccentric activity)
- Submaximal sport-specific skill development drills
- Progress bike, StairMaster, VersaClimber
- Continue to progress proximal strengthening of lower extremities (PREs)

CRITERIA FOR ADVANCEMENT
- Pain-free running
- Average peak torque of isokinetic test=75%
- Normal flexibility
- Normal strength (5/5 throughout ankle)
- Sport-specific drills with no apprehension

Postoperative Phase V: Return to Full Sport (Week 28 to Year 1)

GOALS
- Lack of apprehension with sports activity
- Maximize strength and flexibility to meet demands of individual sport activity
- 85% limb symmetry with vertical jump test
- 85% limb symmetry for average peak isokinetic torque (PF/DF/INV/EV)

PRECAUTIONS
- Avoid pain with therapeutic, functional, and sport activity
- Avoid full sport activity until adequate strength and flexibility

TREATMENT STRATEGIES
- Advanced functional exercises and agility exercises
- Plyometrics
- Sport-specific exercises
- Isokinetic testing
- Functional test assessment, such as vertical jump test

CRITERIA FOR DISCHARGE
- Flexibility and strength to accepted levels for sports performance
- Lack of apprehension with sport-specific movements
- 85% limb symmetry with functional tests
- 85% limb symmetry for average peak isokinetic torque (PF/DF/INV/EV)
- Independent performance of gym/home exercise program

Bibliography

Aoki, M., Ogiwara, N., Ohta, T., Nabeta, Y. Early Motion and Weightbearing After Cross-Stitch Achilles Tendon Repair. *Am J Sports Med* 1998;26(6):794-800.

Bates, A., Hanson, N. The Principles and Properties of Water. In Aquatic Exercise Therapy. WB Saunders, Philadelphia, 1996, pp. 1-320.

Cetti, R., Christensen, S.E., Ejsted, R., Jensen, N.M., Jorgensen, U. Operative Versus Nonoperative Treatment of Achilles Tendon Rupture: A Prospective Randomized Study and Review of the Literature. *Am J Sports Med* 1993;21(6):791-799.

Curwin, S. Tendon Injuries: Pathology and Treatment. In Zachazewski, J.E., Magee, D.J., Quillen, W.S. (Eds). Athletic Injuries and Rehabilitation. WB Saunders, Philadelphia, 1996.

Davies, G. Open Kinetic Chain Assessment and Rehabilitation, Athletic Training. *Sports Health Care Perspect* 1995;1(4):347-370.

Kendall, F., McCreary, E. Muscles Testing and Function, 4th ed., chap 7. Williams & Wilkins, Baltimore, 1993.

Leadbetter, W.B. Cell Matrix Response in Tendon Injury. *Clin Sports Med* 1992;11(3):533.

Maffulli, N. Current Concepts Review: Rupture of the Achilles Tendon. *J Bone Joint Surg* 1999;81:1019–1036.

Maffuli, N., Tallon, C., Wong, J., Lim, K.P., Bleakney, R. Early Weightbearing and Ankle Mobilization after Open Repair of Acute Midsubstance Tears of the Achilles Tendon. *Am J Sports Med* 2003;31(5):692–700.

Mandelbaum, B., Gruber, J., Zachazewski, J. Rehabilitation of the Postsurgical Orthopedic Patient: Achilles Tendon Repair and Rehabilitation. Mosby, St. Louis, 2001.

Mandelbaum, B.R., Myerson, M.S., Forester, R. Achilles Tendon Ruptures. A New Method of Repair, Early Range of Motion, and Functional Rehabilitation. *Am J Sports Med* 1995;23:392–395.

Motta, P., Errichiello, C., Pontini, I. Achilles Tendon Rupture. A New Technique for Easy Surgical Repair and Immediate Movement of the Ankle and Foot. *Am J Sports Med* 1997;25(2):172–176.

Myerson, M.S. Achilles Tendon Ruptures. *Instr Course Lect* 1999;48:219–230.

Nicholas, J.A., Hershman, E.B. The Lower Extremity and Spine in Sports Medicine, 2nd ed. Mosby, St. Louis, 1995.

Norkin, C.C., Levangie, P.K. Joint Structure and Function: A Comprehensive Analysis. FA Davis, Philadelphia, 1992.

Petschnig, R., Baron, R., Albrecht, M. The Relationship Between Isokinetic Quadriceps Strength Tests and Hop Tests for Distance and One-Legged Vertical Jump Test Following ACL Reconstruction. *J Orthop Sports Phys Ther* 1998;28(1):23–31.

Schepsis, A.A., Jones, H., Haas, A.L. Achilles Tendon Disorders in Athletes. *Am J Sports Med* 2002;30(2):287–305.

Soldatis, J.J., Goodfellow, D.B., Wilber, J.H. End-to-end Operative Repair of Achilles Tendon Ruptures. *Am J Sports Med* 1997;24(1):90–95.

Thomas, M., Fiatarone, M., Fielding, R. Leg Power in Young Women: Relationship to Body Composition, Strength, and Function. *Med Sci Sports Exerc* 1996;28(10):1321–1326.

Threlkeld, J., Horn, T.S., Wojtowicz, G.M., Rooney, J.G., Shapiro, R.S. Kinematics, Ground Reaction Force, and Muscle Balance Produced by Backward Running. *J Orthop Sports Phys Ther, American Physical Therapy Association*, 1989.

CHAPTER 39

Lateral Ankle Reconstruction

Jaime Edelstein, PT, MSPT, CSCS

Dennis J. Noonan, ATC, CMT

The lateral ligaments of the ankle are the most commonly injured structures in the body of an athlete. The ligaments involved in this injury are the anterior talofibular ligament (ATFL), calcaneofibular ligament (CFL), and posterior talofibular ligament (PTFL). The etiology of a lateral ankle sprain is related specifically to sports involving running or jumping, such as soccer, basketball, and dance. Eighty percent to 85% of acute ankle sprains are treated successfully with conservative treatment. Research has shown that those who have sustained an ankle sprain are approximately 10% to 20% more susceptible to develop chronic instability, pain on exertion, or recurrent swelling.

Ankle Instability

- Chronic lateral ankle instability is defined as instability and associated symptoms for greater than 6 months. These signs and symptoms are caused by either mechanical or functional instability.
- *Mechanical instability*, referred to as *laxity*, is defined as ankle movement beyond the physiological limit of the ankle's range of motion (ROM).
  1. True mechanical instability may be demonstrated using clinical tests, including the anterior drawer, the talar tilt, or diagnostically using a wide variety of radiographic tests, including stress radiography, magnetic resonance imaging (MRI), computed tomography (CT scan), and bone scan.
  2. The presence of mechanical instability alone does not correlate to a need for surgical repair.

373

- Functional instability, a term first defined by Freeman et al., is a subjective feeling of "giving way" or evidence of recurrent, symptomatic ankle sprains. As well documented, mechanical instability is not a reliable indicator of a functionally unstable ankle.
- Studies have shown that joint position sense and kinesthesia are greatly diminished in individuals with chronic ankle instability (CAI), which, in turn, leads to repetitive lateral ankle sprains. Other proprioceptive deficits may be accountable for these levels of instability.
- Additional contributing factors leading to functional instability include deficits in center of pressure excursion measures, postural stability, ROM, and invertor and evertor muscles strength.
- The focus of conservative rehabilitation for this population has been placed on challenging and regaining postural-control strategies, in addition to strengthening, flexibility, and regaining ROM.
- The 10% to 20% of individuals who have functional instability, with or without true mechanical instability, may require surgical intervention. These individuals have failed conservative treatment with guided physical therapy and are still having subjective complaints and recurrent incidents of instability.
- More than 50 surgical procedures have been described to treat lateral ankle instability. The surgical procedures for treating this pathology may be described as anatomical or nonanatomical.
- The preferred surgical procedure at the Hospital for Special Surgery (HSS) is the modified Broström-Gould Procedure, an anatomical procedure. The rehabilitation guidelines for this procedure are described in this chapter.

Surgical Overview

- The ATFL resists inversion of the talus within the ankle mortis (talar tilt). The CFL acts as a restraint against subtalar inversion and thereby indirectly acts as a restraint for talar tilt. Without these restraints the ankle will be mechanically unstable.

- Anatomical repairs involve the ATFL and the CFL being imbricated and sutured. In cases where the ATFL and CFL tissues are obliterated, ligament augmentation may also be performed, using fascia lata, plantaris tendon, Achilles tendon, or allograft.

- The nonanatomical procedures are checkrein and tenodesis procedures using the peroneus brevis tendon.
  1. Nonanatomical surgical procedures have been developed and modified by multiple surgeons.
  2. All of these physicians developed surgical variations using the peroneus brevis to reconstruct and stabilize the lateral ankle.

- A tenodesis is the procedure of choice when an individual has general ligamentous laxity, has failed a modified Broström-Gould procedure, is an obese individual, or a direct repair is not possible because of chronic, repetitive trauma.

- Because all of these tenodesis procedures somewhat change the biomechanics of the subtalar joint, instability may be a complication for any of the tenodesis surgical procedures. Subjective complaints of instability following anatomical procedure tend to be less prevalent (0% to 3%).

- In 1966, Broström repaired the ATFL and CFL by attenuating and shortening the ATFL and CFL ligaments. This allowed for isometry of the ligaments as well as full ROM at the talocrural and subtalar joints. However, this procedure had a high rate of subtalar instability.

- In 1980, Gould et al. addressed this instability by developing the modified Broström procedure, whereby the extensor retinaculum was sutured to the anterior aspect of the fibula.

- The surgical procedure entails the foot being placed in a vertical or slightly internally rotated position.

- A curvilinear incision is made anteriorly to the distal fibula, stopping at the peroneals. Care must be taken because the sural nerve lies just below this incision over the peroneal tendons.

- The joint capsule is dissected along the anterior border of the lateral malleolus. The ATFL lies within the joint capsule, and the CFL lies deep to the capsule. Once both structures are identified, the repair can be made.

- The final phase is to attach the posterior portion of the extensor retinaculum to the distal fibula via sutures passed through holes in the fibula.
- This type of procedure reinforces the repair as well as limits inversion. This limitation of inversion is considered an acceptable outcome of the procedure given that instability was the initial pathology being corrected.
- The patient is placed in a short leg cast or bivalve cast and is non–weight-bearing following surgery.
- Outcome studies have reported at least an 85% success rate.

Rehabilitation Overview

- Rehabilitation following a modified Broström procedure begins immediately postoperatively with gait training, patient education, and a home exercise program.
- The individual is initially non–weight-bearing following surgery.
- The ankle is in a neutral position in the cast.
- Once active range of motion (AROM) is allowed, special care must be taken in limiting forces into inversion through the earliest phase of the healing process. Excessive tensile forces on the repair could potentially disrupt the repair.
- Formal physical therapy is initiated 6 weeks following surgery.
  1. The patient bears weight as tolerated in an Aircast and uses either a cane or crutches as an assistive device.
  2. Initial rehabilitation will focus on review of the home exercise program and continued patient education and progression of ROM into all planes.
- During the initial physical therapy outpatient evaluation, it is necessary to assess for intrinsic mechanical factors, including hind foot varus or generalized ligamentous laxity, because this will affect postoperative stresses on the repair as well as overall treatment approaches.
- The format for progression in rehabilitation is functionally based.

- It is important to note that most of the research and literature supporting this proposed guideline is relative to functional ankle instability (FAI). Lateral ankle reconstruction and FAI are comparable in their philosophies.
- Proprioceptive training is very important with this population as well as strengthening of the evertors and the invertors.
- Return to full activity or to sport is expected to occur at approximately 3 months. Athletes returning to play will be expected to participate initially with a lace-up ankle brace or taping for 4 to 6 months.
- Objective measures and subjective reports, however, will outweigh a rehabilitation timeline.
- Understanding the goals and abilities of the population being instructed is vital.

Postoperative Phase I (Weeks 6 to 8)

GOALS
- Patient education, wound recognition, infection avoidance
- Edema control
- Regaining ROM, progressing motion into inversion and plantar flexion. Achieve 75% functional ROM
- Prevent deconditioning
- Pain reduction
- Reduce scar adhesions/myofascial restriction
- Normalized gait without assistive device on level surfaces

PRECAUTIONS
- Avoid standing or walking for extensive periods of time
- Excessive tensile force into plantar flexion or inversion. No active assist or passive stretching into these planes of motion

TREATMENT STRATEGIES
- Edema control: cryotherapy, contrast baths, elevation, IFC electrical stimulation, retrograde massage
- ROM:
  1. AROM into eversion (EV), plantar flexion (PF), inversion (INV)
     - Straight plane movements, circles, alphabets A to Z
  2. Sitting: BAPS board, rocker board, foam roll

Continued

Postoperative Phase I (Weeks 6 to 8)—Cont'd

- Flexibility: gastrocnemius and soleus
  1. Towel/strap stretch, manual stretch by therapist
- Cross training: pool, UBE, core stabilization
- Gait training
  1. Use mirror for feedback, assistive device as needed
  2. Pool/AquaCiser
- Strengthening:
  1. Foot intrinsics: towel grab, marble pick-up
  2. Isometrics: evertors, invertors, dorsiflexion, and plantar flexors
  3. PREs: elastic band, ankle weights, manual resistance
  4. Proximal strengthening: open chain hip, light leg press/ball squats
- Mobilization: soft tissue
  1. Scar
  2. Plantar fascia, lumbricals
- Proprioception: bilateral
  1. Rocker board, proprioception board, Biodex Balance System

CRITERIA FOR ADVANCEMENT
- Normalized gait, pain-free without assistive device
- Pain-free eversion with 4/5 strength throughout full ROM
- ROM: PF 15 degrees

Postoperative Phase II (Weeks 8 to 12)

GOALS
- Restore full ROM
- Patient independent in donning brace
- No edema post-activity
- Normalized, non-antalgic gait on stairs and inconsistent surfaces
- Maintain full body conditioning
- Unilateral calf raise 10 repetitions (5/5 strength)
- Initiate plyometrics
- Initiate jogging to running

PRECAUTIONS
- Patient education to continue activity modification

TREATMENT STRATEGIES
- Protection: Aircast, semi-rigid support
- Edema control: cryotherapy
- ROM: full ROM (by latest 12 weeks); focus on multiplanar movements
  1. Standing/weight-bearing BAPS board
  2. Mobilizations: joint mobilizations, Mulligan techniques
- Flexibility:
  1. Standing gastrocnemius and soleus stretching
  2. Soft tissue mobilization and myofascial release (MFR) to posterior contractile tissues and fascia
     - Gastrocnemius, soleus, tibialis posterior
- Proprioception:
  1. Unilateral standing: eyes open, eyes closed
  2. Dynamic neuromuscular training with Biodex Balance Master system
  3. Unilateral stance on proprioception board, rocker/wobble board, foam block
  4. Add perturbation or other modes of dynamic stability/multitasking
     - Ball toss, reaching
- Strengthening: focus on invertors and evertors as well as all muscle groups that support the ankle
  1. Rhythmic stabilization
  2. Concentric and eccentric
  3. Open chain
     - Thera-Band, manual resistance, isokinetics training
  4. Closed chain
     - Side step with elastic band, contralateral elastic band activity (KE and HE), leg press, step up/step down, sports cord (retro, side to side, carioca)
  5. Muscle endurance: StairMaster, Elliptical
- Plyometrics
  1. Bilateral jumps
  2. Unilateral jumps
- Treadmill
- Cardiovascular: Elliptical, StairMaster, VersaClimber

CRITERIA FOR ADVANCEMENT
- Full ROM
- No residual edema after activity
- No pain after activity
- Non-antalgic, no apprehension with treadmill jog

Postoperative Phase III (Weeks 12 to 16)

GOALS
- Running to sprinting
- Multiplane activities
- Regain full cardiovascular and muscular endurance
- Strength ≥85% limb symmetry through isokinetic testing
- No apprehension with high level activity, direction change
- Functional testing: 85% limb symmetry
- Skill progression, no pain, no apprehension
- Return to full sport, high level activity

PRECAUTIONS
- Continue to wear ankle brace during sports for 6 months
- Apprehension or pain with return to sport
- Volume awareness with high intensity activities and drills

TREATMENT STRATEGIES
- Protection: lace-up ankle brace for activities
- Strengthening
  1. Testing: isokinetic, dynamometry, functional testing
  2. Increase workload, resistance, and intensity in PREs
- Endurance
  1. Jumping rope: bilateral skip, alternating skip, then unilateral skip
  2. Isokinetics
- Proprioception
  1. Single-leg stance on change of surfaces (most stable to least stable)
  2. Add perturbation or other modes of dynamic stability/ multitasking, visual input changes
  3. Ball toss, reaching, walking, jogging with variation in speed of movement and intensity of perturbation
  4. Introduction of sport-specific skills
- Plyometrics: advanced
  1. Depth pumps, jumps in series, dot drills
- Return to sport functional progression and testing

SPORT-SPECIFIC ACTIVITIES
- Single skill activities (e.g., shooting baskets from stationary stance)
- Add multitasking skills (e.g., dribble and shot drills; running, throwing, and catching ball)
  1. Progress from linear movement to change of direction
- Add defensive player/coach to drill

- Practice drills with team
- Scrimmage with team
- Return to play

CRITERIA FOR DISCHARGE
- Regain full cardiovascular and muscular endurance
- Strength ≥85% limb symmetry through isokinetic testing
- No apprehension with high level activity, direction change
- Functional testing: 85% limb symmetry
- Skill progression, no pain, no apprehension
- return to full sport, high level activity

Bibliography

Baumhauer, J.F., O'Brien, T. Surgical Considerations in the Treatment of Ankle Instability. *J Athl Train* 2002;37(4):458-462.

Bernier, J.N., Perrin, D.H. Effect of Coordination Training on Proprioception of the Functionally Unstable Ankle. *J Orthop Sports Phys Ther* 1998;27(4):264-275.

Broström, L. Sprained Ankles. *Acta Orthop Scand* 1966;132(6): 551-565.

Clanton, T.O. Lateral Ankle Sprains. In Coughlin, M.J., Mann, R.A. (Eds). Surgery of the Foot and Ankle, 7th ed., vol 2. Mosby, St. Louis, 1999, pp. 1191-1210.

Freeman, M.A., Dean, M.R., Hanham, I.W. The Etiology and Prevention of Functional Instability of the Foot. *J Bone Joint Surg Br* 1965;47:678-685.

Garrick, J.G. The Frequency of Injury, Mechanism of Injury, and Epidemiology of Ankle Sprains. *Am J Sports Med* 1977;5(6): 241-242.

Girard, P., Anderson, R.B., Davies, W.H., Isear, J.A., Kiebzak, G.M. Clinical Evaluation of the Modified Broström-Evans Procedure to Restore Ankle Stability. *Foot Ankle Int* 1999;20(4):246-252.

Gould, N., Seligson, D., Gassman, J. Early and Late Repair of Lateral Ligament of the Ankle. *Foot Ankle* 1980;1(2):84-89.

Hamilton, W.G. Ankle Instability Repair: The Broström-Gould Procedure. In Johnson, K.A. (Ed). The Foot and Ankle. Raven Press, Ltd., New York, 1994, pp. 437-446.

Hamilton, W.G., Thompson, F.M., Snow, S.W. The Modified Brostrom Procedure for Lateral Ankle Instability. *Foot Ankle* 1993; 14(1):1-7.

Hollis, J.M., Blasier, R.D., Flahiff, C.M., Hofmann, O.E. Biomechanical Comparison of Reconstruction Techniques in Simulated Lateral Ankle Ligament Injury. *Am J Sports Med* 1995;23(6):678-682.

Karlsson, J., Eriksson, B.I., Bergsten, T., Rudholm, O., Sward, L. Comparison of Two Anatomic Reconstructions for Chronic Lateral Instability of the Ankle Joint. *Am J Sports Med* 1997;25(1):48-53.

Karlsson, J., Lansinger, O. Lateral Instability of the Ankle Joint. Nonsurgical Treatment Is the First Choice, 20% Need Ligament Surgery. *Lakartidnengen* 1991;88:1399-1402.

Konradsen, L., Holmer, P., Sondergaard, L. Early Mobilizing Treatment for Grade III Ankle Ligament Injuries. *Foot Ankle* 1991;12(2):69-73.

Louwerens, J.W., Snijders, C.J. Lateral Ankle Instability: An Overview. In Ranawat, C.S., Positano, R.G. (Eds). Disorders of the Heel, Rearfoot, and Ankle, chap 24. Churchill Livingstone, New York, 1999, pp. 341-353.

Messer, T.M., Cummins, C.A., Ahn, J., Kelikian, A.S. Outcome of the Modified Brostrom Procedure for Chronic Lateral Ankle Instability Using Suture Anchors. *Foot Ankle Int* 2000;21(12):996-1003.

Riemann, B.L., Caggiano, N.A., Lephart, S.M. Examination of Clinical Method of Assessing Postural Control During a Functional Performance Task. *J Sports Rehabil* 1999;8:171-183.

Riemann, B.L. Is There a Link Between Chronic Ankle Instability and Postural Instability? *J Athl Train* 2002;37(4):386-393.

Rosenbaum, D., Engelhardt, M., Becker, H.P., Claes, L., Gerngro, H. Clinical and Functional Outcome after Anatomic and Nonanatomic Ankle Ligament Reconstruction: Evans Tenodesis Versus Periosteal Flap. *Foot Ankle Int* 1999;20(10):636-639.

Ryan, L. Mechanical Stability, Muscle Strength and Proprioception in the Functionally Unstable Ankle. *Aust J Physiother* 1994;40(1): 41-47.

Sammarco, G.J., Idusuyi, O.B. Reconstruction of the Lateral Ankle Ligaments Using a Split Peroneus Brevis Tendon Graft. *Foot Ankle Int* 1999;20(2):97-103.

Sammarco, V.J. Complications of Lateral Ankle Ligament Reconstruction. *Clin Orthop Relat Res* 2001;391:123-132.

Schmidt, R., Cordier, E., Bertsch, C., Eils, E., Neller, S., Benesch, S., Herbst, A., Rosenbaum, D., Claes, L. Reconstruction of the Lateral Ligaments: Do the Anatomical Procedures Restore Physiologic Ankle Kinematics? *Foot Ankle Int* 2004;25(1):31-36.

Tropp, H. Commentary: Functional Ankle Instability Revisited. *J Athl Train* 2002;37:512-515.

Tropp, H. Pronator Muscle Weakness in Functional Instability of the Ankle Joint. *Int J Sports Med* 1986;7:291-294.

CHAPTER 40

Rotator Cuff Repair: Arthroscopic and Open

Robert A. Maschi, PT, DPT, CSCS

Greg Fives, PT, MSPT, SCS

Rotator cuff pathology is a significant cause of pain and disability in the general population. Rotator cuff tears may occur as the result of trauma, degeneration secondary to repetitive microtrauma, or a combination of both. Rotator cuff repair is a common intervention used by surgeons to improve the function and pain level in this population.

Factors, such as choice of technique, size and location of the tear, and quality of the tissue involved, will influence the timing of therapeutic interventions and the progression of rehabilitation. The Hospital for Special Surgery (HSS) postoperative guidelines and approach to rehabilitation following arthroscopic rotator cuff repair is presented in this chapter.

Surgical Overview

- The muscles of the rotator cuff consist of the subscapularis, supraspinatus, infraspinatus, and teres minor.
- All of the tendons of the cuff blend with and reinforce the glenohumeral joint capsule.
- The primary function of the rotator cuff is to balance the force couples about the glenohumeral joint during active elevation of the upper extremity. With this in mind, the primary goal of rotator cuff repair surgery is to restore, as closely as possible, the anatomical cuff configuration and these biomechanical force couples.
- In 1911, Codman first described open surgical repair of the supraspinatus. Since then, rotator cuff repair techniques have evolved significantly, and the introduction of shoulder arthroscopy in 1980 dramatically changed the way rotator cuff repairs are performed.

- Surgical techniques progressed from open to arthroscopic-assisted mini-open repair techniques during the early to mid-1990s.
- The trend now seems to be the progression to an all-arthroscopic surgical technique.
  1. The advantages associated with an all-arthroscopic rotator cuff repair are deltoid preservation; smaller skin incisions; better visualization and evaluation of the glenohumeral joint and rotator cuff defect; improved ability to mobilize and release the rotator cuff; decreased post-operative pain and stiffness; and improved rehabilitation potential.
  2. Some disadvantages include bone-tendon fixation and the technical difficulty of performing the procedure.
- Overall, the results of arthroscopic repairs appear to be very promising. Wolf et al. showed good to excellent results in 94% of patients who underwent arthroscopic rotator cuff repair.
- Surgery initially involves positioning the patient in the lateral decubitus or upright beach chair position.
  1. Bony landmarks are identified and marked, and the arthroscope is placed into the joint space via posterior, anterior, and lateral portals.
  2. The glenohumeral joint is then inspected via the arthroscope to help identify possible concomitant intra-articular pathologies.
  3. The tear is located and evaluated in regard to its size and shape.
  4. The amount of retraction of the rotator cuff is assessed, as is cuff mobility, using grasper hooks.
  5. If present, adhesions are released to improve cuff mobility.
  6. Excursion of the cuff is determined to identify the exact area of bony preparation and the anatomical "footprint" of the cuff.
  7. The torn tendon edges are débrided of devascularized tissue, and sutures are placed through the torn edges.
  8. The cuff is fixated with anchors placed into the tuberosity, if an anatomical repair is possible.

9. Acromioplasty and/or subacromial decompression may not be needed at the time of rotator cuff repair if the acromion does not compromise the subacromial space and/or if the cuff tear is secondary to trauma or intrinsic tendinopathy caused by eccentric tendon overload.

10. Patients are placed in a postoperative sling or abduction brace to immobilize and protect the repair and discharged home on the day of surgery.

Rehabilitation Overview

- The rehabilitation program following rotator cuff repair must take into account the healing time of surgically repaired tissue.

- The program should balance the aspects of tissue healing and appropriate interventions to restore range of motion (ROM), strength, and function.

- Factors that influence the rate at which a patient can be progressed through the program include surgical technique, quality of the tissue repaired, size of the tear, and location of the tear.

- Good tissue quality will allow a secure repair, which may allow for a faster rehabilitation than a more tenuous repair of poorer quality tissue. Tissue quality can be influenced by conditions, such as rheumatoid arthritis, diabetes, and by the chronicity of the tear, previous surgery, repeated injections, or chronic steroid use. These can increase the risk of suture pull-out.

- Functional outcome is also directly related to the size of the tear.

  1. Tear size, not age, is more of a factor in predicting a successful outcome after rotator cuff repair.

  2. Larger tears involve more tissue and are often retracted, which requires greater mobilization of the tissue to achieve closure. Therefore, in larger tears tissue trauma is greater, which requires a more conservative postoperative rehabilitation course.

- The location of the tear will also affect interventions.

  1. For example, a small tear of the supraspinatus may allow for early activation of the internal and external rotators,

whereas a tear extending into the infraspinatus and teres minor or the subscapularis will delay strengthening of the corresponding musculature.

2. The therapist must take into account what structures are involved to avoid disruption of healing tissues in the early phases of rehabilitation. Communication with the referring surgeon is essential to determine this information.

3. One must keep in mind that the information in this chapter should serve as a guideline only and that progression through the rehabilitative course will vary, depending on all points previously mentioned.

Postoperative Phase I: Maximum Protection (Weeks 0 to 3)

GOALS

- Protect surgical repair
- Decrease pain/inflammation
- Gradually increase shoulder ROM (surgeon directed) external rotation (ER) to 45 degrees, internal rotation (IR) to 45 degrees, and forward flexion (FF) to 120 degrees
- Improve proximal (scapula) and distal strength and mobility
- Independence in an HEP

PRECAUTIONS

- Maintain sling immobilization when not performing exercises
- NO active movements at the operated shoulder joint other than gentle self-care activity below shoulder level
- Avoid exceeding ROM limitations set by surgeon
- Avoid pain with ROM and isometric exercises

TREATMENT STRATEGIES

- Sling immobilization (surgeon directed)
- Patient education: sleeping postures, activity modification
- Cryotherapy (Cryo/cuff, gel packs, ice)
- Pendulum exercises
- AAROM/PROM exercises
  1. PROM by the rehabilitation specialist
  2. AAROM forward flexion in supine with contralateral upper extremity

   3. Supine wand ER/IR in scapular plane
   4. Continuous passive motion (CPM) for ER if needed
- Active range of motion (AROM) exercises
   1. Elbow/forearm/wrist/hand
- Scapula stabilization exercises-side-lying (progress to manual resistance)
- Submaximal deltoid isometrics in neutral as ROM improves (short lever arm)
- Progress and update HEP

CRITERIA FOR ADVANCEMENT
- Normal scapular mobility
- Full AROM distal to shoulder
- Shoulder ROM to within surgeon's set goals

Postoperative Phase II: Moderate Protection (Weeks 3 to 7)

GOALS
- Protect surgical repair
- Decrease pain/inflammation
- Improve ROM 80% to 100% forward flexion and external rotation
- Improve proximal scapula strength and stability
- Improve scapulohumeral rhythm and neuromuscular control
- Decrease rotator cuff inhibition

PRECAUTIONS
- Avoid pain with ADL
- Avoid active elevation of arm
- No maximal cuff activation
- Avoid pain with ROM/therapeutic exercise
- Avoid exceeding ROM limitations

TREATMENT STRATEGIES
- Continue exercises in phase I, progressing ROM as tolerated
- Discontinue sling (surgeon directed)
- AAROM exercises
   1. Supine forward flexion with wand (scapula plane)
   2. Continue wand ER/IR

Continued

Postoperative Phase II: Moderate Protection (Weeks 3 to 7)—Cont'd

   3. Joint mobilization techniques
   4. Initiate pulleys as ROM and upper extremity control improves
   5. Airdyne ergometer
   6. Initiate hydrotherapy (pool) program
- Physio ball scapular stabilization (below horizontal)
- Isometric exercises
   1. ER/IR (submaximal) at modified neutral
   2. Progress deltoid isometrics to long lever arm in neutral
- Isotonic exercises
- Scapula, elbow
- Begin humeral head stabilization exercises as ROM improves (>90 degrees)
- Modalities as needed
- Modify HEP

CRITERIA FOR ADVANCEMENT
- Ability to activate cuff and deltoid without pain
- Tolerates arm out of sling
- ROM 80% or greater for forward flexion and external rotation

Postoperative Phase III: Early Strengthening (Weeks 7 to 13)

GOALS
- Eliminate/minimize pain and inflammation
- Restore full PROM
- Improve strength/flexibility
- Restore normal scapulohumeral rhythm below 90-degree elevation
- Gradual return to light ADL below 90-degree elevation

PRECAUTIONS
- Monitor activity level
- Limit overhead activity
- Avoid shoulder "shrug" with activity and exercise
- Patient to avoid jerking movements and lifting heavy objects

TREATMENT STRATEGIES
- Activity modification, continue cryotherapy PRN
- Continue wand exercises for external/internal rotation and flexion
- Continue joint mobilization techniques—progress to grades III and IV
- Flexibility exercises, horizontal adduction (posterior capsule stretching)
- Progress to functional ROM exercises (IR behind back, towel pass)
- Periscapular isotonic strengthening
  1. Scapular protraction
  2. Progress to scapular retraction exercises
  3. Shoulder extension with elastic bands
  4. Dumbbell rowing
- Rotator cuff isotonic strengthening exercises
  1. AROM, side-lying ER
  2. ER/IR at modified neutral with elastic bands, if sufficient scapular strength base developed
- Functional strengthening exercises
  1. AROM supine forward flexion (scapular plane)
  2. Progress to standing forward flexion
- Progress to rhythmic stabilization exercises
- Progress to closed-chain exercises
- Upper body ergometer (UBE) as ROM and strength improve

CRITERIA FOR ADVANCEMENT
- Minimal pain and/or inflammation
- Full PROM
- Improved rotator cuff and scapular strength
- Normal scapulohumeral rhythm with shoulder elevation below 90 degrees
- Independence with current HEP

Postoperative Phase IV: Late Strengthening (Weeks 14 to 19)

GOALS
- Improve strength to 5/5 for scapula and shoulder musculature

Continued

Postoperative Phase IV: Late Strengthening (Weeks 14 to 19)—Cont'd

- Improve neuromuscular control
- Normalize scapulohumeral rhythm throughout the full ROM

PRECAUTIONS
- Progress to overhead activity only when proper proximal stability is attained

TREATMENT STRATEGIES
- Continue to progress isotonic strengthening for periscapular and rotator cuff musculature
  1. Latissimus pull-down (LPD)
  2. Row machine
  3. Chest press
- Continue flexibility-side-lying posterior capsule stretch
- Progress scapular stabilization program
- Initiate isokinetic strengthening (IR/ER) in scapular plane
- Initiate plyometric exercises below horizontal, if sufficient strength base (surgeon directed)

CRITERIA FOR ADVANCEMENT
- Normal scapulohumeral rhythm throughout the full ROM
- Normal strength 5/5 manual muscle test (MMT) of scapular and humeral muscles

Postoperative Phase V: Return to Sport (Weeks 20 to 24)

GOALS
- Maximize flexibility, strength, and neuromuscular control to meet demands of sport, return to work, recreational, and daily activity
- Isokinetic testing: 85% limb symmetry
- Independent in home and gym therapeutic exercise programs for maintenance and progression of functional level at discharge

PRECAUTIONS
- Avoid pain with therapeutic exercises and activity
- Avoid sport activity until adequate strength, flexibility, and neuromuscular control

- Surgeon's clearance needed for sport activity

TREATMENT STRATEGIES
- Continue to progress isotonic strengthening for periscapular and rotator cuff musculature
- Isokinetic training and testing for external and internal rotators
- Continue flexibility and stabilization programs
- Individualize program to meet demands of sport-specific requirements
- Plyometrics (above horizontal)
- Interval training program for pitchers and overhead athletes
- Periodization training

CRITERIA FOR DISCHARGE
- Isokinetic testing close to normal ER/IR ratios (66%), 85% symmetry
- Independence with home/gym program at discharge for maintenance and progression of flexibility, strength, and neuromuscular control

Bibliography

Baker, C.L., Whaley, A.L., Baker, M. Arthroscopic Rotator Cuff Tear Repair. *J Surg Orthop Adv* 2003;12(4):175–190.

Burkhart, S.S., Danaceau, S.M., Pearce, C.E. Jr. Arthroscopic Rotator Cuff Repair: Analysis of Results by Tear Size and by Repair Technique-margin Convergence Versus Direct Tendon-to-bone Repair. *Arthroscopy* 2001;17:905–912.

Codman, E.A. Complete Rupture of the Supraspinatus Tendon. Operative Treatment with Report of Two Successful Cases. *Boston Med Surg J* 1911;164:708–710.

Debeyre, J., Patte, D., Elmelik, E. Repair of Ruptures of the Rotator Cuff of the Shoulder with a Note on Advancement of the Supraspinatus Muscle. *J Bone Joint Surg* 1965;47B:36–42.

Galatz, L.M., Ball, C.M., Teefey, S.A., Middleton, W.D., Yamaguchi, K. The Outcome and Repair Integrity of Completely Arthroscopically Repaired Large and Massive Rotator Cuff Tears. *J Bone Joint Surg Am* 2004;86A(2):219.

Gartsman, G.M. All Arthroscopic Rotator Cuff Repairs. *Orthop Clin North Am* 2001;32(3):501–510.

Gartsman, G.M., Khan, M., Hammerman, S.M. Arthroscopic Repair of Full-thickness Tears of the Rotator Cuff. *J Bone Joint Surg Am* 1998;80:832–840.

Goldberg, B.A., Lippitt, S.B., Matsen, F.A. III. Improvement in Comfort and Function after Cuff Repair Without Acromioplasty. *Clin Orthop* 2001;390:142–150.

Gore, D.R., Murray, M.P., Sepic, S.B., Gardner, G.M. Shoulder Muscle Strength and Range of Motion Following Surgical Repair of Full Thickness Rotator Cuff Tears. *J Bone Joint Surg Am* 1986; 69: 266–272.

Grondel, R.J., Savoie, F.H. III, Field, L.D. Rotator Cuff Repairs in Patients 62 Years of Age or Older. *J Shoulder Elbow Surg* 2001; 10:97–99.

Lo, I.K., Burkhart, S.S. Current Concepts in Arthroscopic Rotator Cuff Repair. *Am J Sports Med* 2003;31(2):308–324.

Post, M., Sliver, R., Singh, M. Rotator Cuff Tears: Diagnosis and Treatment. *Clin Orthop* 1983;173:78–91.

Severud, E.L., Ruotolo, C., Abbott, D.D., Nottage, W.M. All-Arthroscopic Versus Mini-open Rotator Cuff Repair: A Long-term Retrospective Outcome Comparison. *Arthroscopy* 2003;19:234–238.

Tauro, J.C. Arthroscopic Rotator Cuff Repair: Analysis of Technique and Results at 2- and 3-year Follow-up. *Arthroscopy* 1998;14:45–51.

Wahl, C.J., Wickiewicz, T.L. Surgical Treatment of Rotator Cuff Tears. *Curr Opin Orthop* 2002;13(4):281–287.

Watson, M. Major Ruptures of the Rotator Cuff: The Result of Surgical Repair in 89 Patients. *J Bone Joint Surg Br* 1985;67:618–624.

Wilk, K.E., Crockett, H.C., Andrews, J.R. Rehabilitation after Rotator Cuff Surgery. *J Shoulder Elbow Surg* 2000;1:1–18.

Wolf, E.M., Pennington, W.T., Agrawal, V. Arthroscopic Rotator Cuff Repair: 4- to 10-year Results. *Arthroscopy* 2004;20(1):5–12.

Yamaguchi, K., Levine, W.N., Marra, G., Galatz, L.M., Klepps, S., Flatow, E.L. Transitioning to Arthroscopic Rotator Cuff Repair: The Pros and Cons. *Instr Course Lect* 2003;52:81–92.

Yel, M., Shankwiler, J.A., Noonan, J.E. Jr., Burkhead, W.Z. Jr. Results of Decompression and Rotator Cuff Repair in Patients 65 Years Old and Older: 6- to 14-year Follow-up. *Am J Orthop* 2001; 30:347–352.

CHAPTER 41

Subacromial Decompression

Lee Rosenzweig, PT, DPT, CHT

Adam Pratomo, PT, MSPT

Impingement of the rotator cuff tendons and bursae in the subacromial space is the most common cause of shoulder pathology. The pathophysiology of the impingement process involves repetitive encroachment and subsequent micro-trauma to these structures as a result of narrowing of the space between the humeral head and acromion. Neer first described the pathology of shoulder impingement syndrome in 1972.

Neer performed the first open anterior acromioplasty, which was the standard surgical procedure for stages II and III impingement lesions through the 1980s. During this time, Ellman began to perform an arthroscopic technique for sub-acromial decompression (SAD), and this type of procedure has now become widely accepted. The objectives of arthro-scopic SAD are the same as those for open decompression: removal of the structures that are creating impingement within the confines of the subacromial space.

SAD is typically recommended to patients who have failed a 6- to 12-month course of rehabilitation. The success rate of patients who have undergone arthroscopic SAD has been reported to be from 43% to 90%. The chapter will present the Hospital for Special Surgery's (HSS) surgical approach and treatment guidelines for managing patients who have undergone SAD.

Surgical Overview

- Anatomically, the subacromial space is considered an inter-stitial pseudo-articulation among the proximal humerus, cora-cromial arch, acromioclavicular joint, superficial surface of the rotator cuff, and the subacromial and subdeltoid bursa.

- The acromioclavicular joint lies in the anteromedial most aspect, and its anterior wall is composed of the coracoacromial ligament going from the anterior aspect of the acromion to the coracoid process.
- The normal subacromial space is 7 to 14 mm, and narrowing of this space has been associated with rotator cuff pathology.
- The indications for surgical management of impingement are pain or weakness that interferes with work, sports, or activities of daily living (ADL).
- The first reported arthroscopic SAD was performed by Ellman in 1983.
  1. In the procedure, a mechanical suction shaver is used to initially perform a bursectomy to establish visualization within the subacromial space.
  2. The coracoacromial ligament is released with a surgical electrode, and electrocautery is used to release adhesions.
  3. Osteophytes along the undersurface of the acromioclavicular joint are removed with a motorized burr.
- Proper decompression includes (1) extensive complete subacromial bursectomy, (2) coracoacromial ligament resection, (3) resection of the undersurface of the anterior acromion, and (4) removal of impinging acromioclavicular joint osteophytes.

Rehabilitation Overview

- Rehabilitation begins immediately after surgery, and the patient is typically released from the hospital on the same day.
- A sling is used based on patient comfort for the first 2 to 7 days, but early mobilization is encouraged.
- Treatment goals are to restore full ROM, strength, flexibility, neuromuscular control, and return to previous level of function.
- The patient is instructed in a series of range of motion (ROM) exercises to prevent stiffness and promote mobility.

- Patients are advanced when they meet the goals and criteria defined in each phase of rehabilitation. Individual progression is also based on the level of pain during activity.
- Exercise should emphasize forward flexion, internal/external rotation, posterior capsule flexibility, and scapular stability.
- ROM exercises should be performed daily until full range is achieved.
- As ROM improves, strengthening exercises can be incorporated, with an emphasis on muscular balance of the scapulohumeral and scapulothoracic muscles.
- The rehabilitation specialist must carefully assess flexibility, scapulohumeral rhythm, and posture.
- Poor posture during exercise can affect the congruency of the shoulder joint and place the musculature in a poor mechanical position. Correct positioning during exercise will permit the glenohumeral muscles to work within the ideal length-tension relationship.
- Proper scapulothoracic function is also important to allow a stable base for glenohumeral rotation.
    1. The scapular muscles must work in unison to maximize congruency between the humeral head and the glenoid during movement.
    2. Once sufficient scapular stability exists, rotator cuff strengthening is incorporated.
- Impingement commonly occurs when rotator cuff strength is insufficient to stabilize the humeral head during elevation, causing insufficient space for the rotator cuff tendons.
- Superior translation of the humeral head of up to 1.5 mm occurs when the arm reaches 120 degrees of elevation. Abduction with insufficient rotator cuff strength can also result in sharp increases in this superior translation.
- All exercises should be initially kept below the horizontal until sufficient rotator cuff and scapular strength are established to prevent impingement.
- Patients progress to overhead activity when they demonstrate pain-free ROM in conjunction with adequate strength.

- Appropriate patients progress to sport-specific activities, depending on the requirements of the sport.
- It is important to emphasize activity modification throughout the course of rehabilitation to avoid causing inflammation and delayed recovery.

Postoperative Rehabilitation Phase I (Days 0 to 14)

GOALS
- Control postoperative pain and swelling
- Forward flexion ROM to 120 degrees
- External rotation to 60 degrees
- Independent with home exercise program
- Independent with light ADL, dressing
- Precautions:
  1. Pain with exercises
  2. Overhead activity
  3. Carrying heavy objects

TREATMENT STRATEGIES
- Instruction in home exercise program
- Codman's/pendulums
- Supine forward flexion AAROM, AROM
- Cane external rotation with a towel under the elbow (scapular plane)
- Scapular mobilization in side-lying
- Scapular AROM in side-lying (retraction, protraction, elevation, depression)
- Manually resisted scapular strengthening in side-lying
- Standing scapular retraction with elastic bands
- Deltoid and rotator cuff isometrics
- Distal strengthening (wrist and elbow)
- Modalities (TENS, cryotherapy)

CRITERIA FOR ADVANCEMENT
- Forward flexion ROM, 120 degrees
- External rotation to 60 degrees
- Independent with home exercise program
- Controlled pain

Postoperative Rehabilitation Phase II (Weeks 2 to 6)

GOALS
- Full ROM
- Strength 4/5 throughout the involved upper extremity
- Independent with light ADL (appropriate for preoperative functional level)
- Independent home exercise program
- Normal scapulohumeral rhythm <90 degrees elevation

PRECAUTIONS
- Avoid overhead reaching until appropriate ROM and strength have been achieved
- Avoid painful ROM

TREATMENT STRATEGIES
- ROM (active and passive)
- Pulleys
- Capsular stretching and joint mobilization
- Hydrotherapy
- Progress deltoid strengthening
- Progress rotator cuff strengthening
- Advance scapular strengthening below the horizontal
- Progressive resistance equipment (i.e., row, chest press, latissimus pull-down)
- Upper body ergometry
- Modalities as needed
- Progress to home exercise program

CRITERIA FOR ADVANCEMENT
- Minimal level of pain and swelling
- Full ROM
- Strength 4/5 throughout involved upper extremity
- Normal scapulohumeral rhythm <90 degrees elevation

Postoperative Rehabilitation Phase III (Weeks 6 to 10)

GOALS
- Full ROM
- Normal strength (5/5)

Continued

Postoperative Rehabilitation Phase III (Weeks 6 to 10)—Cont'd

- Improved flexibility (surgical side equal to contralateral side)
- Normal scapulohumeral rhythm throughout ROM

PRECAUTIONS
- Avoidance of pain with therapeutic exercises and functional ADL
- Avoidance of sport activities until adequate flexibility and strength have been established

TREATMENT STRATEGIES
- Continue aggressive ROM activities
- Flexibility exercises
- Aggressive joint mobilization, capsular stretching
- Aggressive scapular strengthening
- Advanced rotator cuff strengthening
- Proprioceptive neuromuscular facilitation diagonal patterns (especially D2 flexion and extension, if appropriate)
- Advanced rotator cuff strengthening (elevated position, if appropriate)
- Rhythmic stabilization exercises
- Modalities as needed
- Modify and advance home exercise program as appropriate

CRITERIA FOR ADVANCEMENT
- Full PROM
- Strength 5/5 throughout upper extremity
- Good flexibility
- Normal scapulohumeral throughout ROM
- Pain-free AROM

Postoperative Rehabilitation Phase IV (Weeks 10 to 14)

GOALS
- Isokinetic testing to be <85% of the contralateral side (internal/external rotation)
- Pain-free during all sport-specific drills

- Functional strength, flexibility, and endurance to meet the demands of the individual's sport

PRECAUTIONS
- Avoidance of pain with therapeutic exercises and functional ADL
- Avoidance of sport activities until adequate flexibility and strength have been established

TREATMENT STRATEGIES
- Full upper extremity strengthening program
- Sport-specific plyometrics
- Isokinetic training and testing
- Advanced neuromuscular training
- Begin sport-specific drills/interval throwing program (surgeon-directed)

CRITERIA FOR DISCHARGE/RETURN TO SPORT
- Patient has met strength, flexibility, and endurance goals specific to his or her sport
- Isokinetic testing to be >85% of the contralateral side (internal/external rotation), pain-free during all sport-specific drills

Bibliography

Beach, W., Caspari, R. Arthroscopic Management of Rotator Cuff Disease. *Arthroscopy* 1993;16:1007-1016.

Bigliani, L.U., Morrison, D.S. Subacromial Impingement Syndrome. In Dee, R., Mango, E., Hurst, L.C. (Eds). Principles of Orthopedic Practice. McGraw-Hill, New York, 1989, p. 627.

Brox, J., Gjengedal, E., Uppheim, G., Bohmer, A.S., Brevik, J.I., Ljunggren, A.E., Staff, P.H. Arthroscopic Surgery Versus Supervised Exercises in Patients with Rotator Cuff Disease (Stage II Impingement Syndrome): A Prospective, Randomized, Controlled Study in 125 Patients with a $2^1/_2$ Year Follow-up. *J Shoulder Elbow Surg* 1999;8:102-111.

Bunker, T.D. Impingement: Needle, Scope or Scalpel? In Bunker, T.D., Schranz, P.J. (Eds). Clinical Challenges in Orthopedics: The Shoulder. Mosby, St. Louis, 1998, p. 62.

Burkhart, S. Arthroscopic Debridement and Decompression for Selected Rotator Cuff Tears. *Orthop Clin North Am* 1993;24: 111-124.

Ellman, H. Arthroscopic Subacromial Decompression: Analysis of One-to Three-year Results. *Arthroscopy* 1987;3:173-181.

Ellman, H. Arthroscopic Subacromial Decompression. *Orthop Trans* 1985;9:48.

Esch, J. Arthroscopic Subacromial Decompression and Postoperative Management. *Orthop Clin North Am* 1993;24:161-171.

Gartsman, G.M. Arthroscopy for Shoulder Stiffness. In Miller, M.D., Cole, B.D. (Eds). Textbook of Arthroscopy. WB Saunders, Philadelphia, 2004, p. 173.

Gleyze, P., Thomas, T., Gazielly, D.F., Bruyere, G., Kelberine, F., Kempf, J.F., Levigne, C., Marcillou, P., Nerot, G. Compared Results of the Different Treatments in Partial-thickness Bursal Side Tears of the Rotator Cuff. A Multi-center Study of 48 Shoulders. In Gazielly, D.F., Gleyze, P., Thomas, T. (Eds). The Cuff. Elsevier, Paris, France, 1997, pp. 257-259.

Hawkins, R.J., Abrams, J.S., Brock, R.M., Hobeika, P. Acromioplasty for Impingement with an Intact Rotator Cuff. *J Bone Joint Surg Br* 1988;70:795-797.

Kapanji, I.A. The Physiology of the Joints-Upper Limb, vol 1. Churchill Livingstone, New York, 1970.

Kibler, W.B. Role of the Scapula in the Overhead Throwing Motion. *Contemp Orthop* 1991;22:525-533.

Kibler, W.B. The Role of the Scapula in Athletic Shoulder Function. *Am J Sports Med* 1998;26:325-336.

Lucas, D. Biomechanics of the Shoulder Joint. *Arch Surg* 1973;107:425.

Ludewig, P.M. Alterations in Shoulder Kinematics and Associated Muscle Activity in People with Symptoms of Shoulder Impingement. *Phys Ther* 2000;80:276-291.

Matsen, F.A., Arntz, C. Subacromial Decompression. In Rockwood, C.A., Matsen, F.A. (Eds). The Shoulder. WB Saunders, Philadelphia, 1998, pp. 795-833.

McShane, R.B., Leinberry, C.F., Fenlin, J.M. Conservative Open Anterior Acromioplasty. *Clin Orthop Relat Res* 1987;223:137-144.

Neer, C.S.III. Anterior Acromioplasty for the Chronic Impingement Syndrome in the Shoulder: A Preliminary Report. *J Bone Joint Surg Am* 1972;54:41-50.

Neer, C.S. Anterior Acromioplasty for Chronic Impingement Syndrome in the Shoulder. *J Bone Joint Surg* 1972;54A:41-50.

Neer, C.S. Impingement Lesions. *Clin Orthop Relat Res* 1983; 173: 70-77.

Olsewski, J., Depew, A. Arthroscopic Subacromial Decompression and Rotator Cuff Debridement for Stage II and Stage III Impingement. *Arthroscopy* 1994;10:61-68.

Paulos, L., Franklin, J. Arthroscopic Shoulder Decompression Development and Application. *Am J Sports Med* 1990;18:235-244.

Ryu, R.K. Arthroscopic Subacromial Decompression: A Clinical Review. *Arthroscopy* 1992;8:141-147.

Sharkey, N.A. The Rotator Cuff Opposes Superior Translation of the Humeral Head. *Am J Sports Med* 1995;23:270-275.

Snyder, S.J., Pachelli, A.F., Del Pizzo, W., Friedman, M.J., Ferkel, R.D., Pattee, G. Partial Thickness Rotator Cuff Tears: Results of Arthroscopic Treatment. *Arthroscopy* 1991;7:1-7.

Speer, K.P., Lohnes, J., Garrett, W.E. Jr Arthroscopic Subacromial Decompression: Results in Advanced Impingement Syndrome. *Arthroscopy* 1991;7:291-296.

Wahl, C.J., Warren, R.F., Altchek, D.W. Shoulder Arthroscopy. In Rockwood, C.A., Matsen, F.A., Wirth, M.A., Lippitt, S.B. (Eds). The Shoulder. WB Saunders, Philadelphia, 2004, pp. 283-354.

Weiner, D.S. Superior Migration of the Humeral Head: A Radiological Aid in the Diagnosis of Tears of the Rotator Cuff. *J Bone Joint Surg* 1970;52B:524.

Yamaguchi, K., Flatlow, E. Arthroscopic Evaluation and Treatment of the Rotator Cuff. *Orthop Clin North Am* 1995;26:643-659.

Anterior Stabilization Surgery

Michael Levinson, PT, CSCS

The etiology of anterior shoulder instability can be either the result of a traumatic, acute episode resulting in a dislocation that may have to be reduced by a physician or a chronic condition. The recurrence rate for anterior dislocations is extremely high, especially in the younger, active population.

The mechanism of injury for a traumatic anterior instability is usually some combination of shoulder external rotation, abduction, and extension. Common mechanisms include falling on an outstretched hand or planting a ski pole and falling forward. Instability can also be chronic, resulting from repetitive activities that can cause excessive laxity of the shoulder capsule and/or tearing of the labrum or individual general systemic laxity. Often the result of anterior shoulder instability is a "Bankart lesion," which is defined as an avulsion of the anteroinferior glenoid labrum. Labral pathology and shoulder instability can be treated conservatively but often requires surgical intervention. This chapter will discuss the Hospital for Special Surgery (HSS) guidelines to rehabilitation following anterior shoulder stabilization.

Surgical Overview

- The labrum is a fibrocartilaginous structure that is attached to the glenoid rim. There is a great deal of anatomical variation.
  1. The glenohumeral ligaments attach to the labrum.
  2. The labrum contributes to glenohumeral stability by increasing the surface contact area for the humeral head and provides resistance to humeral head translation.
- An anterior stabilization may be performed open or arthroscopically.

- Patients with extreme laxity or who have multidirectional instability may need an open procedure.
  1. The most common open procedure performed is done by transecting a portion of the subscapularis muscle.
  2. The torn labrum is then repaired, and the capsule is tightened by making a cut through it and overlapping the margins of the cut.
- In contrast to more traditional open procedures, which have greater morbidity, anterior stabilizations can now be performed arthroscopically.
  1. The arthroscopic procedure reduces the morbidity and risk of loss to range of motion (ROM).
  2. A Bankart lesion is commonly repaired with transglenoid suture anchors.
  3. In addition, any excess laxity in the capsule can be reduced by a similar procedure.
  4. The degree to which the capsule is shifted is based upon the patient's examination under anesthesia.
  5. Following the procedure, the patient's shoulder is placed in an immobilizer in adduction and internal rotation.

Rehabilitation Overview

- The rehabilitation program following an anterior stabilization generally begins 1 to 3 weeks postsurgery.
- The goals are to restore normal strength, ROM, flexibility, and proprioception because loss of proprioception has been demonstrated with shoulder instability.
- The patient constantly wears the immobilizer, except when performing exercises or bathing.
- The program emphasizes early, controlled motion to prevent contractures and avoid excessive passive stretching later in the program.
- External rotation and extension of the shoulder are progressed slowly to protect the repair of the labrum and avoid excessive stretching of the anterior capsule.
  1. Historically, there have been significant failure rates among arthroscopic procedures.
  2. ROM progression following the arthroscopic procedure is slower than the open procedure secondary to the lesser fixation.

- Throughout the program a full upper extremity strengthening program will be progressed functionally to prepare the patient for return to activity.
- The program is based on the patient returning to sport-specific activities no earlier than 3 months post-surgery.
- Overhead activities are progressed last.
- Patient education is critical to avoid reinjury. Patients should understand the precautions associated with this surgery.

Postoperative Phase I (Weeks 1 to 3)

GOALS
- Promote healing: reduce pain, inflammation, and swelling
- Forward flexion to 90 degrees
- Arthroscopic: external rotation to neutral; open: 30 degrees
- Independent home exercise program

PRECAUTIONS
- Immobilizer at all times when not exercising
- External rotation and extension limited to neutral (30 degrees for open)

TREATMENT STRATEGIES
- Immobilizer
- Elbow/wrist active range of motion (AROM)
- Gripping exercises
- Scapular isometrics
- Pain-free, submaximal deltoid isometrics
- Active-assisted range of motion (AAROM): forward flexion (scapular plane)
- AAROM: external rotation to neutral
- Home exercise program
- Modalities as needed

CRITERIA FOR ADVANCEMENT
- External rotation to neutral (30 degrees for open)
- Forward flexion to 90 degrees
- Minimal pain or inflammation

Postoperative Phase II (Weeks 3 to 6)

GOALS
- Continue to promote healing
- Arthroscopic: external rotation to 45 degrees; forward flexion to 120 degrees
- Open: external rotation to 60 degrees; forward flexion to 145 degrees
- Begin to restore scapula and rotator cuff strength

PRECAUTIONS
- Limit external rotation to 45 degrees (arthroscopic)
- Avoid excessive stretch to anterior capsule
- Avoid rotator cuff inflammation

TREATMENT STRATEGIES
- Discontinue immobilizer (surgeon directed)
- Continue AAROM, forward flexion: wand exercises, pulleys
- Continue AAROM, external rotation: wand exercises
- Hydrotherapy (if required)
- Manual scapula side-lying stabilization exercises
- Physio ball scapular stabilization exercises
- Internal/external rotation isometrics in modified neutral (submaximal, pain-free)
- Modalities as needed
- Modify home exercise program

CRITERIA FOR ADVANCEMENT
- Minimal pain and inflammation
- Arthroscopic: external rotation to 45 degrees; forward flexion to 120 degrees
- Open: external rotation to 60 degrees; forward flexion to 145 degrees
- Internal rotation/external rotation strength 4/5

Postoperative Phase III (Weeks 6 to 12)

GOALS
- Restore full shoulder ROM
- Restore normal scapulohumeral rhythm
- Upper extremity strength 5/5

Continued

Postoperative Phase III (Weeks 6 to 12)— Cont'd

- Restore normal flexibility
- Begin to restore upper extremity endurance
- Isokinetic internal/external rotation strength 85% of unaffected side

PRECAUTIONS
- Avoid rotator cuff inflammation
- Continue to protect anterior capsule
- Avoid excessive passive stretching

TREATMENT STRATEGIES
- Continue AAROM for forward flexion and external rotation to tolerance
- Begin AAROM for internal rotation
- Progress scapular strengthening (include closed chain exercises)
- Begin isotonic internal rotation/external rotation strengthening in modified neutral (pain-free)
- Begin latissimus strengthening (progress as tolerated)
- Begin scapular plane elevation (emphasis on correct scapulohumeral rhythm)
- Begin upper body ergometry to restore endurance
- Begin humeral head stabilization exercises (if adequate strength and ROM)
- Begin PNF patterns if internal/external rotation strength is 5/5
- Begin general upper extremity flexibility exercises
- Isokinetic training and testing
- Modalities as needed
- Modify home exercise program

CRITERIA FOR ADVANCEMENT
- Normal scapulohumeral rhythm
- Minimal pain and inflammation
- Internal/external rotation strength 5/5
- Full upper extremity ROM
- Isokinetic internal rotation strength 85% of unaffected side

**Postoperative Phase IV
(Weeks 12 to 18)**

GOALS
- Restore normal neuromuscular function
- Maintain strength and flexibility
- Isokinetic internal/external rotation strength at least equal to the unaffected side
- >66% isokinetic external rotation/internal rotation strength ratio
- Prevent reinjury

PRECAUTIONS
- Pain-free plyometrics
- Significant pain with a specific activity
- Feeling of instability

TREATMENT STRATEGIES
- Continue full upper extremity strengthening program
- Advance internal rotation/external rotation strengthening to 90/90 position if required
- Continue upper extremity flexibility exercises
- Isokinetic strengthening and testing
- Activity-specific plyometrics program
- Address trunk and lower extremity demands
- Continue endurance training
- Begin sport or activity-related program
- Modify home exercise program

CRITERIA FOR DISCHARGE
- Pain-free sport or activity-specific program
- Isokinetic internal/external rotation strength to at least equal to unaffected side
- >66% isokinetic external rotation/internal rotation strength ratio
- Independent home exercise program
- Independent sport or activity-specific program

Bibliography

Arciero, R.A., Taylor, D., Snyder, R.J., Uhorchak, J.M. Arthroscopic Bioabsorbable Tack Stabilization of Initial Anterior Dislocations: A Preliminary Report. *Arthroscopy* 1995;11:410–417.

Bacilla, P., Field, L.D., Savoie, F.H. Arthroscopic Bankart Repair in a High Demand Population. *Arthroscopy* 1997;13:51-60.

Bankart, A. The Pathology and Treatment of Recurrent Dislocation of the Shoulder Joint. *Br J Surg* 1938;26:23.

Burger, R.S., Shengel, D., Bonatus, T., Lewis, J. Arthroscopic Staple Capsulorrhaphy for Recurrent Shoulder Instability. *Orthop Trans* 1990;14:596-597.

Coughlin, L., Rubinovich, M., Johansson, A. Arthroscopic Staple Capsulorrhaphy for Anterior Shoulder Instability. *Am J Sports Med* 1992;20:253-256.

Hovelius, L. Anterior Dislocation of the Shoulder in Teenagers and Young Adults. *J Bone Joint Surg* 1987;69:393.

Hovelius, L. Recurrences after Initial Dislocation of the Shoulder. *J Bone Joint Surg* 1983;65:343-349.

Hovelius, L. Shoulder Dislocation in Swedish Hockey Players. *Am J Sports Med* 1978;6:373-377.

Lephart, S., Warner, J.P., Borsa, P.A., Fu, F.H. Proprioception of the Shoulder Joint in Healthy, Unstable and Surgically Repaired Shoulders. *J Shoulder Elbow Surg* 1994;3:371-380.

Levine, W.M. The Pathophysiology of Shoulder Instability. *Am J Sports Med* 2000;28:910-917.

Rowe, C.R. Acute and Recurrent Anterior Dislocation of the Shoulder. *Orthop Clin North Am* 1980;11:252-269.

Smith, R.H., Brunolti, J. Shoulder Kinesthesia after Anterior Glenohumeral Joint Dislocation. *Phys Ther* 1989;69:106-112.

Zuckerman, J.D., Gallagher, M.D., Cuomo, F., Rokito, A. The Effect of Instability and Subsequent Anterior Shoulder Repair on Proprioceptive Ability. *J Shoulder Elbow Surg* 1997;6:180-186.

CHAPTER 43

Posterior Stabilization Surgery

Michael Levinson, PT, CSCS

Posterior shoulder instability is much less common than anterior instability. Incidence has been reported at 2% to 4% of all shoulder instability patients. It has also been suggested that posterior instability may be related to multidirectional instability. Pathological posterior translation of the humeral head may result in pain, instability, or detachment of the posterior and inferior capsulolabral complex.

The mechanism of injury varies; however, traumatic, acute dislocations are rare and usually result from a high energy posterior force to an outstretched arm or from a seizure. More commonly, injury results from recurrent subluxations that occur with the shoulder in a forward flexed, adducted, and internally rotated position. Contact athletes, such as football linemen, who are subjected to posteriorly directed forces in this position, are often injured in this manner. In addition, activities such as bench pressing may exacerbate these symptoms. Injury may also occur nontraumatically in overhead athletes, such as baseball pitchers or tennis players during the "follow through" phase of throwing, when the shoulder is horizontally adducted and internally rotated. Labral pathology and shoulder instability can be treated conservatively but often requires surgical intervention. In this chapter, the Hospital for Special Surgery (HSS) rehabilitation guideline following posterior shoulder stabilization is presented.

Surgical Overview

- The labrum is a fibrocartilaginous structure that, along with the glenohumeral ligaments, attaches to the glenoid. It contributes to glenohumeral stability by increasing the contact area for the humeral head and provides resistance to humeral head translation.

- The posterior capsulolabral complex is often detached with posterior instability.
- At HSS, the posterior stabilization is done exclusively arthroscopically.
  1. An examination under anesthesia is performed to accurately determine the amount of capsular laxity.
  2. The posterior capsulolabral complex is then reattached to the glenoid labrum through an arthroscope, using either suture anchors or biodegradable tacks.
  3. At this time, any capsular redundancy is eliminated by placation and applying tension to the sutures.
- Following surgery, the patient is immobilized for approximately 4 weeks and positioned in the scapular plane in neutral rotation.

Rehabilitation Overview

- The rehabilitation program following a posterior stabilization generally begins 2 to 4 weeks postsurgery.
- The goals are to restore normal strength, ROM, flexibility, and proprioception.
- The patient is protected with an immobilizer during the early phase of the program.
- The program emphasizes early, controlled motion so as to avoid contracture and need for excessive passive stretching later in the program.
- Internal rotation and horizontal adduction are avoided during the early phases of the program and then progressed cautiously so as to avoid excessive stress to the posterior capsule.
- The reduced morbidity of the arthroscopic procedure should reduce the risk of range of motion (ROM) loss.
- Throughout the program a full upper extremity strengthening program will be progressed appropriately to prepare the patient for return to functional activity. However, particular emphasis will be placed on the posterior glenohumeral and scapular musculature to further assist in protecting the posterior capsulolabral complex.

- The program is based on the patient returning to sport-specific activities no earlier than 16 weeks post-surgery, with contact sports and overhead activities progressed last
- Patient education is critical to avoiding reinjury and adversely affecting the surgical procedure.

Postoperative Phase I (Weeks 2 to 4)

GOALS
- Promote healing: reduce pain, inflammation, and swelling
- Restore ROM: forward flexion to 90 degrees, external rotation to 30 degrees
- Begin to regain humeral head and scapular control
- Independent home exercise program

PRECAUTIONS
- Immobilizer at all times when not exercising
- Internal rotation and horizontal adduction limited to neutral

TREATMENT STRATEGIES
- Immobilizer
- Elbow/wrist active range of motion (AROM)
- Gripping exercises
- Scapular isometrics
- AAROM for forward flexion
- AAROM for external rotation
- Manual side-lying, scapular stabilization exercises
- Pain-free, submaximal deltoid isometrics (3 to 4 weeks)
- Pain-free, submaximal internal/external rotation isometrics (3 to 4 weeks)
- Modalities as needed
- Home exercise program

CRITERIA FOR ADVANCEMENT
- External rotation to 30 degrees
- Minimal pain or inflammation

Postoperative Phase II (Weeks 4 to 6)

GOALS
- Continue to promote healing
- Forward flexion to 90 degrees

Continued

Postoperative Phase II (Weeks 4 to 6)—Cont'd

- Internal rotation to 45 degrees
- Begin to restore strength internal/external rotation to 4/5

PRECAUTIONS
- Internal rotation limited to 45 degrees
- Horizontal adduction limited to neutral
- Protect posterior capsule
- Avoid rotator cuff inflammation

TREATMENT STRATEGIES
- Discontinue immobilizer
- Continue AAROM for external rotation
- Continue AAROM for forward flexion
- Hydrotherapy
- Continue deltoid and internal/external rotation isometrics
- Progress scapular strengthening protecting posterior capsule (modify closed chain exercises)
- Modalities as needed
- Modify home exercise program

CRITERIA FOR ADVANCEMENT
- Minimal pain and inflammation
- Forward flexion to 90 degrees
- Internal/external rotation strength 4/5

Postoperative Phase III (Weeks 6 to 12)

GOALS
- Restore full ROM
- Upper extremity strength 5/5
- Restore normal scapulohumeral rhythm throughout ROM
- Restore normal upper extremity flexibility
- Isokinetic internal/external rotation, strength 85% of unaffected side

PRECAUTIONS
- Avoid rotator cuff inflammation
- Continue to protect posterior capsule
- Avoid excessive passive stretching

TREATMENT STRATEGIES
- Continue AAROM for external rotation and forward flexion
- Begin AAROM for internal rotation
- Continue progressive scapular strengthening program, protecting posterior capsule (avoid or modify closed chain exercises)
- Begin internal/external rotation isotonics in modified neutral
- Begin latissimus strengthening
- Begin scapular plane elevation, if scapula and cuff strength is adequate
- Begin humeral head stabilization exercises, if strength is adequate
- Begin PNF patterns, if internal/external rotation is 5/5
- Begin upper extremity flexibility exercises
- Begin upper body ergometry
- Isokinetic training and testing
- Modalities as needed
- Modify home exercise program

CRITERIA FOR ADVANCEMENT
- Pain-free
- Full shoulder ROM
- Normal glenohumeral rhythm
- Normal upper extremity flexibility
- Upper extremity strength 5/5
- Isokinetic internal/external rotation, strength 85% of unaffected side

Postoperative Phase IV (Weeks 12 to 18)

GOALS
- Restore normal neuromuscular function
- Prevent reinjury
- Maintain strength and flexibility
- Isokinetic internal/external rotation strength at least equal to unaffected side
- >66% isokinetic internal/external rotation ratio

Continued

Postoperative Phase IV (Weeks 12 to 18)—Cont'd

PRECAUTIONS
- Plyometrics should be pain-free
- Significant pain with specific activity
- Feeling of instability
- Avoid loss of strength and instability
- Avoid overtraining

TREATMENT STRATEGIES
- Continue full upper extremity strengthening (emphasize eccentrics)
- Continue upper extremity flexibility exercises
- Advance internal/external rotation strengthening to the 90/90 position (if required)
- Isokinetic training and testing
- Continue endurance training
- Begin activity-specific plyometric program
- Address trunk and lower extremities as required
- Begin sport or activity-specific program
- Modify home exercise program
- Modalities as needed

CRITERIA FOR DISCHARGE
- Isokinetic internal/external rotation strength at least equal to unaffected side
- Pain-free
- Independent home exercise program
- Independent sport or activity-specific program

Bibliography

Arciero, R.A., Mazzocca, A.D. Traumatic Posterior Shoulder Subluxation with Labral Injury: Suture Anchor Technique. *Tech Shoulder Elbow Surg* 2004;5:13-24.

Boyd, H.B., Sisk, T.D. Recurrent Posterior Dislocation of the Shoulder. *J Bone Joint Surg* 1972;54A:779-785.

Levine, W.N., Flatow, E.L. The Pathophysiology of Shoulder Instability. *Am J Sports Med* 2000;28:910-917.

Mair, S.D., Zarzour, R., Speer, K.P. Posterior Labral Injury in Contact Athletes. *Am J Sports Med* 1998;26:753-758.

Perry, J. Anatomy and Biomechanics of the Shoulder in Throwing, Swimming, Gymnastics and Tennis. *Clin Sports Med* 1983;2: 247-254.

Schwartz, E., Warren, R.F., O'Brien, S.J. Posterior Shoulder Instability. *Clin Orthop* 1987;18:409-419.

Williams, R.J., Strickland, S., Cohen, M., Altchek, D.W., Warren, R.F. Arthroscopic Repair for Traumatic Posterior Shoulder Instability. *Am J Sports Med* 2003;31:203-209.

CHAPTER 44

Superior Labrum Anterior to Posterior (SLAP) Repair

Michael Levinson, PT, CSCS

Superior labral lesions were first described by Snyder et al. and termed *superior labrum anterior to posterior* (SLAP) lesions. They defined a SLAP lesion as a labral detachment, which originated posteriorly to the long head of the biceps tendon insertion and extended anteriorly. The lesions were classified into four types, according to their arthroscopic appearance.

The mechanism of injury of a SLAP lesion is unclear. It has been described by Andrews et al. as a chronic traction injury of the biceps on the superior labrum in overhead athletes because stimulation of the biceps has been demonstrated to pull the labrum off the superior glenoid. Conversely, Snyder et al. describes an axial compression force from a fall on an outstretched arm.

Pain is the most common complaint; however, some patients may complain of "catching" or "locking." SLAP lesions can be treated conservatively; however, in cases in which the labrum is detached, especially in the athletic population, surgical intervention is required. Complete SLAP lesions have been shown to result in significant increases in anterior and inferior humeral head translation.

Surgical Overview

- The labrum is a fibrocartilaginous structure that surrounds the glenoid. It contributes to glenohumeral stability by increasing the contact area for the humeral head and provides resistance to humeral head translation.
- The superior labrum is loosely attached to the glenoid rim and may overlap the glenoid surface. The superior labrum also inserts into the long head of the biceps.

- The biceps has also been shown to contribute to the stability of the glenohumeral joint.
- Pathology resulting from the previously described mechanism of injury can include labral fraying, detachment of the labrum, the labrum being displaced into the joint, and partial rupture of the biceps.
- Surgical intervention for SLAP lesions is dictated by the extent of the injury.
  1. In cases in which the biceps attachment is intact, the frayed labrum may simply be debrided.
  2. For cases in which the labrum is detached from the glenoid and the long head of the biceps is unstable, a repair is often necessary.
     - Currently, this procedure can be done arthroscopically.
     - The labrum and the long head of the biceps are reattached, using either suture anchors or bioabsorbable tissue tacks.
     - The patient is then immobilized in a sling until rehabilitation begins.

Rehabilitation Overview

- The rehabilitation program following a SLAP repair generally begins 1 to 3 weeks post-surgery.
- The goals of rehabilitation are to restore normal strength, ROM, flexibility, and normal neuromuscular function.
- The patient constantly wears the immobilizer, except when performing exercises or bathing.
- Early, controlled range of motion (ROM) is allowed to optimize healing and avoid excessive passive stretching later in the program.
- Throughout the program, the patient is progressed slowly into abduction and external rotation so as to avoid excessive stretch to the labrum and traction to the long head of the biceps.
- The reduced morbidity associated with new, improved surgical techniques will reduce the incidence of motion loss.
- The rate of progression is determined by the functional demands of the patient. Patients who require a great deal of external rotation, such as overhead athletes, will be progressed more aggressively.

- Throughout rehabilitation, a full upper extremity strengthening program will be progressed functionally and independently to prepare the patient for return to activity.
- Biceps strengthening is progressed very slowly because biceps activity can cause traction to the labrum and thus jeopardize the repair.
- The program is based on the patient returning to sport-specific activities no earlier than 3 to 4 months post-surgery.

Postoperative Phase I (Weeks 1 to 4)

GOALS
- Promote healing: reduce pain and inflammation
- Forward flexion to 90 degrees
- External rotation to neutral
- Independent home exercise program

PRECAUTIONS
- Immobilizer at all times, except when exercising or bathing
- External rotation and extension limited to neutral

TREATMENT STRATEGIES
- Immobilizer
- Gripping exercises
- Active range of motion (AROM): wrist/elbow (supported to avoid biceps stress)
- Scapular "pinches"
- Pain-free, submaximal deltoid isometrics
- Active-assisted range of motion (AAROM): forward flexion (scapular plane)
- AAROM: external rotation to neutral
- Modalities as needed
- Home exercise program

CRITERIA FOR ADVANCEMENT
- External rotation to neutral
- Forward flexion to 90 degrees
- Minimal pain or inflammation

Postoperative Phase II (Weeks 4 to 8)

GOALS
- Continue to promote healing
- Forward flexion to 145 degrees
- External rotation to 60 degrees
- Begin to restore scapular and upper extremity strength
- Restore normal scapulohumeral rhythm

PRECAUTIONS
- Limit external rotation to 30 degrees until 6 weeks
- Avoid excessive stretch to the labrum and biceps
- Avoid rotator cuff inflammation

TREATMENT STRATEGIES
- Discontinue immobilizer (surgeon directed)
- Continue AAROM forward flexion: wand exercises, pulleys
- Continue AAROM external rotation: limited to 30 degrees until 6 weeks
- Hydrotherapy as required
- Manual scapular side-lying stabilization exercises
- Physio ball stabilization exercises
- Internal/external rotation isometrics (submaximal, pain-free)
- Progress scapular strengthening in protective arcs
- Isotonic internal/external rotation strengthening at 6 weeks
- Scapular plane elevation (emphasis on scapulohumeral elevation)
- Begin latissimus strengthening, limited to 90 degrees forward flexion
- Begin humeral head stabilization exercises
- Modalities as needed
- Modify home exercise program

CRITERIA FOR ADVANCEMENT
- Forward flexion to 145 degrees
- External rotation to 60 degrees
- Normal scapulohumeral rhythm
- Minimal pain and inflammation
- Internal/external rotation strength 5/5

Postoperative Phase III (Weeks 8 to 14)

GOALS
- Restore full shoulder ROM
- Restore normal scapulohumeral rhythm
- Isokinetic internal/external rotation: strength 85% of uninvolved side
- Restore normal flexibility

PRECAUTIONS
- Avoid rotator cuff inflammation
- Avoid excessive passive stretching

TREATMENT STRATEGIES
- Continue AAROM for forward flexion and external rotation
- AAROM for internal rotation
- Aggressive scapular and latissimus strengthening
- Begin biceps strengthening
- Begin PNF patterns if internal/external rotation strength is 5/5
- Progress humeral head stabilization exercises
- Progress internal/external rotation to 90/90 position if required
- General upper extremity flexibility exercises
- Upper body ergometry
- Isokinetic training and testing
- Modalities as needed
- Modify home exercise program

CRITERIA FOR ADVANCEMENT
- Normal scapulohumeral rhythm
- Minimal pain and inflammation
- Full upper extremity ROM
- Isokinetic internal/external rotation strength 85% of uninvolved side

Postoperative Phase IV (Weeks 14 to 18)

GOALS
- Restore normal neuromuscular function
- Isokinetic internal/external rotation strength equal to unaffected side

- Maintain strength and flexibility
- Prevent reinjury

PRECAUTIONS
- Pain-free plyometrics
- Significant pain with specific activity
- Feeling of instability

TREATMENT STRATEGIES
- Continue full upper extremity strengthening program
- Continue upper extremity flexibility exercises
- Activity-specific plyometrics program
- Address trunk and lower extremity demands
- Continue endurance training
- Begin sport or activity-related program
- Modify home exercise program

CRITERIA FOR DISCHARGE
- Isokinetic internal/external rotation strength equal to uninvolved side
- Independent home exercise program
- Independent, pain-free sport or activity-specific program

Bibliography

Andrews, J.R., Carson, W.G., Mcleod, W.D. Glenoid Labrum Tears Related to the Long Head of the Biceps. *Am J Sports Med* 1985; 13:337-341.

Cooper, D.E., Arnoczky, S.P., O'Brien, S.J., Warren, R.F., DiCarlo, E., Allen, A.A. Anatomy, Histology and Vascularity of the Glenoid Labrum. An Anatomical Study. *J Bone Joint Surg* 1992;74:46-52.

DiRaimondo, C.A., Alexander, J.W., Noble, P.C. A Biomechanical Comparison of Repair Techniques for Type II SLAP Lesions. *Am J Sports Med* 2004;32:727-733.

Itoi, E., Kuechle, D.K., Newman, S.R., Morrey, B.F., An, K.N. The Stabilizing Function of the Biceps in Stable and Unstable Shoulders. *J Bone Joint Surg* 1993;75:546-550.

Itoi, E., Motzkin, N.E., Morrey, B.F., An, K.N. Stabilizing Function of the Long Head of the Biceps in Stable and Unstable Shoulders. *J Shoulder Elbow Surg* 1994;3:135-142.

Levine, W.N., Flatow, E.L. The Pathophysiology of Shoulder Instability. *Am J Sports Med* 2000;28:910-917.

McGlynn, F.J., Caspari, R.B. Arthroscopic Findings in the Subluxating Shoulder. *Clin Orthop* 1984;183:173-178.

Mileski, R.A., Snyder, S.J. Superior Labral Lesions in the Shoulder: Pathoanatomy and Surgical Management. *J Am Acad Orthop Surg* 1998;6:121-131.

Pagnani, M.J., Deng, X.H., Warren, R.F. Effect of Lesions of the Superior Portion of the Glenoid Labrum on Glenohumeral Translation. *J Bone Joint Surg* 1995;77:1003-1010.

Rodosky, M.W., Harner, C.D., Fu, F.H. The Role of the Long Head of the Biceps Muscle and Superior Glenoid Labrum in Anterior Instability of the Shoulder. *Am J Sports Med* 1994;22:121-130.

Snyder, S.J., Banas, M.P., Karzel, R.P. An Analysis of 140 Injuries to the Superior Glenoid Labrum. *J Shoulder Elbow Surg* 1995;4:243-248.

Snyder, S.J., Karzel, R.P., Del Pizzo, W., Ferkel, R., Friedman, M. SLAP Lesions of the Shoulder. *Arthroscopy* 1990;6:274-279.

CHAPTER 45

Ulnar Collateral Ligament Reconstruction

Michael Levinson, PT, CSCS

Injury of the ulnar collateral ligament (UCL) is almost exclusively limited to the competitive throwing population. More specifically, it is most common in baseball players. The UCL of the elbow has been shown to contribute 54% of the resistance to valgus stress while throwing. Injury is a result of the extreme valgus forces placed on the elbow, especially during pitching. Tearing of the UCL can result in pain and instability. Conservative treatment has not been seen to be successful for this injury, especially with pitchers. Continued pitching with this injury can lead to arthritic changes.

To restore stability, a reconstruction is often indicated. The most common graft choice for the reconstruction is the palmaris longus tendon. In the absence of this muscle, the graft is generally taken from the patient's gracilis. Graft choice does not affect the Hospital for Special Surgery (HSS) guideline. The HSS UCL reconstruction guideline is based on the "docking technique" described by Altchek et al.

Surgical Overview

- A UCL reconstruction, using a palmaris longus tendon graft, is performed using a combination of open and arthroscopic surgery.
- Most commonly, the graft is harvested from the ipsilateral palmaris longus tendon.
- Exposure is created by splitting the flexor carpi ulnaris muscle.
- Bone tunnels are created in the humerus and ulna.
- The graft is "docked" securely into the tunnels, using sutures.

- The elbow is then taken through a full range of motion (ROM) to determine final graft tension and placed in a splint at 60-degree flexion.

Rehabilitation Overview

- The rehabilitation program following UCL reconstruction begins immediately after surgery, with the patient instructed in a home exercise program.
- Formal physical therapy usually does not begin until approximately 4 to 6 weeks post-surgery.
- Care must be taken to protect the graft throughout the progression of the rehabilitation program.
- The program emphasizes early, controlled motion so as to avoid any excessive passive stretching later in the program. This will allow the graft to remain as tight as possible until the patient is allowed to return to activity.
- The program also limits excessive stress to the wrist and elbow during the early phases to allow optimal soft tissue healing.
- Shoulder and scapular strengthening are a key component of the program.
- Following kinetic chain principles, improved proximal strength and efficiency should reduce stress on the elbow.
- The program is based on the patient beginning an interval throwing program at 4 months post-surgery and a hitting program at 5 months.

Postoperative Phase I (Weeks 1 to 4)

GOALS
- Promote healing: reduce pain, inflammation, and swelling
- Begin to restore ROM to 30 to 90 degrees
- Independent home exercise program

PRECAUTIONS
- Brace should be worn at all times
- No PROM of the elbow

TREATMENT STRATEGIES
- Brace set at 30 to 90 degrees of flexion
- Elbow AROM in brace

- Wrist AROM
- Scapular isometrics
- Gripping exercises
- Cryotherapy
- Home exercise program

CRITERIA FOR ADVANCEMENT
- Elbow ROM: 30 to 90 degrees
- Minimal pain or swelling

Postoperative Phase II (Weeks 4 to 6)

GOALS
- ROM: 15 to 115 degrees
- Minimal pain and swelling

PRECAUTIONS
- Continue to wear brace at all times
- Avoid PROM
- Avoid valgus stress

TREATMENT STRATEGIES
- Continue AROM in brace
- Begin pain-free isometrics in brace (deltoid, wrist flexion/extension, elbow flexion/extension)
- Manual scapular stabilization exercises with proximal resistance
- Modalities as needed
- Modify home exercise program

CRITERIA FOR ADVANCEMENT
- ROM: 15 to 115 degrees
- Minimal pain and swelling

Postoperative Phase III (Weeks 6 to 12)

GOALS
- Restore full ROM
- All upper extremity strength 5/5
- Begin to restore upper extremity endurance

Continued

Postoperative Phase III (Weeks 6 to 12)—Cont'd

PRECAUTIONS
- Minimize valgus stress
- Avoid PROM by the clinician
- Avoid pain with therapeutic exercise

TREATMENT STRATEGIES
- Continue AROM
- Low intensity, long duration stretch for extension
- Isotonics for scapula, shoulder, elbow, forearm, wrist
- Begin internal/external rotation strengthening at 8 weeks
- Begin forearm pronation/supination strengthening at 8 weeks
- Upper body ergometer (if adequate ROM)
- Neuromuscular drills
- PNF patterns when strength is adequate
- Incorporate eccentric training when strength is adequate
- Modalities as needed
- Modify home exercise program

CRITERIA FOR ADVANCEMENT
- Pain-free
- Full elbow ROM
- All upper extremity strength 5/5

Postoperative Phase IV (Weeks 12 to 16)

GOALS
- Restore full strength and flexibility
- Restore normal neuromuscular function
- Prepare for return to activity

PRECAUTIONS
- Pain-free plyometrics

TREATMENT STRATEGIES
- Advance internal/external rotation to 90/90 position
- Full upper extremity flexibility program
- Neuromuscular drills
- Plyometrics program
- Continue endurance training

- Address trunk and lower extremities
- Modify home exercise program

CRITERIA FOR ADVANCEMENT
- Complete plyometrics program without symptoms
- Normal upper extremity flexibility

Postoperative Phase V (Months 4 to 9)

GOALS
- Return to activity
- Prevent reinjury

PRECAUTIONS
- Significant pain with throwing or hitting
- Avoid loss of strength or flexibility

TREATMENT STRATEGIES
- Begin interval throwing program at 4 months
- Begin hitting program at 5 months
- Continue flexibility exercises
- Continue strengthening program (incorporate training principles)

CRITERIA FOR DISCHARGE
- Pain-free
- Independent home exercise program
- Independent throwing/hitting program

Bibliography

Altchek, D.W., Hyman, J., Williams, R., Levinson, M., Paletta, G.A., Dines, D.M., Botts, J.D. Management of MCL Injuries of the Elbow in Throwers. *Tech Shoulder Elbow Surg* 2000;1:73-81.

Jobe, F.W., Elattrache, N.S. Diagnosis and Treatment of Ulnar Collateral Ligament Injuries in Athletes. In Morrey, B.F. (Ed). The Elbow and its Disorders. WB Saunders, Philidelphia, 1993, pp. 566-572.

Kal-Nan, A., Morrey, B.F. Biomechanics of the Elbow. In Morrey, B.F. (Ed). The Elbow and its Disorders. WB Saunders, Philadelphia, 1993, pp. 53-72.

Timmer, L.A., Andrews, J.R. Histology and Arthroscopic Anatomy of the Ulna Collateral Ligament of the Elbow. *J Sports Med* 1994; 22:667-673.

Index

MP joints. *See* Metacarpophalangeal
 joints
Musculocutaneous neurectomy,
 141-142

N
National Osteoporosis
 Foundation, 264
Nerve. *See* Ulnar nerve

O
OA. *See* Osteoarthritis
Osteoarthritis (OA)
 hands as affected by, 162
 of knee, 9
 nonoperative treatment
  measures for, 162
 PIP joint affected by, 178
 surgical overview for hand
  affected by, 162-163
 TKA treating, 9
Osteoporosis. *See also* Vertebral
 kyphoplasty
 anatomy overview of, 261-262
 assessment areas for, 265*b*,
  264-266
 balance treatment for, 269-270
 bone densitometry and,
  263-264
 developing, 262
 diagnosis of, 263-264
 flexibility and, 264-270
 fractures related to, 261, 262
 as new diagnosis, 261
 posture/body mechanics and,
  264-270
 primary, 262-263
 rehabilitation overview for,
  264-270
 risk factors associated with, 264*b*
 secondary, 263
 strengthening for, 267-268
 weight-bearing treatment for,
  268-269

P
Patellar tendonitis, progressive,
 304
Patellofemoral pain. *See also*
 Distal realignment; Proximal
 realignment
 as common knee
  complaint, 313
 distal realignment for, 314-315
 proximal realignment for,
  313-314
 rehabilitation after surgery for,
  315-327
 surgery for, 313
 surgical overview for, 313-315
 therapeutic interventions
  for, 313
Patient-controlled analgesia
 (PCA) pump, 3, 11
PCL. *See* Posterior cruciate
 ligament
Percutaneous vertebroplasty, 270
Peroneus brevis tendon, 375
Phalangeal fractures
 as common, 86
 management of, 86
 postoperative phase I
  following, 88-89
 postoperative phase II
  following, 90
 postoperative phase III
  following, 90-91
 rehabilitation following, 88-91
 surgical overview for, 86-87
 of thumb, 87-88
PIP joint. *See* Proximal
 interphangeal joint
Posterior cruciate ligament
 (PCL), 10
 composition of, 339
 double-bundled reconstruction
  of, 339-340
 functions of, 338